Infections, Chronic Disease, and the Epidemiological Transition

Rochester Studies in Medical History

Senior Editor: Theodore M. Brown
Professor of History and Preventive Medicine
University of Rochester

Additional Titles of Interest

The Birth Control Clinic in a Marketplace World
Rose Holz

Bacteriology in British India: Laboratory Medicine and the Tropics
Pratik Chakrabarti

Barefoot Doctors and Western Medicine in China
Xiaoping Fang

Beriberi in Modern Japan: The Making of a National Disease
Alexander R. Bay

The Lobotomy Letters
Mical Raz

Plague and Public Health in Early Modern Seville
Kristy Wilson Bowers

Medicine and the Workhouse
Edited by Jonathan Reinarz and Leonard Schwarz

Stress, Shock, and Adaptation in the Twentieth Century
Edited by David Cantor and Edmund Ramsden

Female Circumcision and Clitoridectomy in the United States: A History of a Medical Treatment
Sarah B. Rodriguez

The Spanish Influenza Pandemic of 1918–1919: Perspectives from the Iberian Peninsula and the Americas
Edited by María-Isabel Porras-Gallo and Ryan A. Davis

A complete list of titles in the Rochester Studies in Medical History series may be found on our website, www.urpress.com.

Infections, Chronic Disease, and the Epidemiological Transition

A New Perspective

Alexander Mercer

University of Rochester Press

First published 2014

University of Rochester Press
668 Mt. Hope Avenue, Rochester, NY 14620, USA
www.urpress.com
and Boydell & Brewer Limited
PO Box 9, Woodbridge, Suffolk IP12 3DF, UK
www.boydellandbrewer.com

ISBN-13: 978-1-58046-508-3
ISSN: 1526-2715

Library of Congress Cataloging-in-Publication Data

Mercer, Alex, author.
Infections, chronic disease, and the epidemiological transition : a new perspective / Alexander Mercer.
p. ; cm. — (Rochester studies in medical history, ISSN 1526-2715 ; vol. 31)
Includes bibliographical references and index.
ISBN 978-1-58046-508-3 (hardcover : alk. paper)
I. Title. II. Series: Rochester studies in medical history. 1526-2715
[DNLM: 1. Communicable Diseases—epidemiology. 2. Disease Transmission, Infectious. 3. Mortality—trends. WA 110]
RA643
616.9—dc23

2014027696

A catalogue record for this title is available from the British Library.

This publication is printed on acid-free paper.
Printed in the United States of America.

For my parents

Contents

Preface

Much has been written since the 1970s about the causes of the decline in mortality from infectious diseases, but far less about the emergence of chronic diseases. When Abdel Omran first referred to the change in predominant causes of death as an "epidemiologic transition," academic studies tended to focus more on issues raised by Thomas McKeown in his influential book *The Modern Rise of Population.* McKeown's emphasis on improvements in the "standard of living" and nutrition as key determinants of increased life expectancy aroused considerable controversy, while Omran's "theory" of transition remained a basically descriptive framework for analysis of changes in disease and mortality. The epidemiological transition is ongoing globally, and constitutes a fundamental change in the human condition; as such, the phenomenon has both contemporary relevance and historical importance.

One objective of this book is to review evidence from local, national, and international studies indicating that preventive measures and changes in behavior played a far greater role in mortality decline in England and globally than McKeown or Omran suggested. However, the aim is to go beyond the controversy over the relative importance of "human intervention" and "standard of living" as determinants of increased life expectancy. Assessment of changes in disease and mortality in England since the 18th century and their possible causes is fundamental to an understanding of how contemporary patterns of disease emerged. A very long-term perspective is particularly important as it encompasses the development of a preventive approach to disease in response to devastating epidemics of plague, smallpox, and typhus that laid the foundation for later health interventions. Records of cause-specific mortality available for England, with supporting data from other Western countries, form the basis of this review of the epidemiological transition and illustrate its main features—acute infectious diseases being superseded by chronic diseases as the predominant causes of death, a shift in age at death from childhood to older adult ages, increased life expectancy, and a larger, "aging" population.

A central theme of the book is the interrelated nature of diseases, particularly the role of microbial infection in chronic diseases, which indicates there is another dimension to epidemiological transition. The original concept oversimplified the process, viewing it as the replacement of one group of distinct diseases (infectious) by another ("degenerative" or "noncommunicable"). This fails to take into account the many interrelationships between infectious diseases, between infections and chronic diseases, and between the disorders underlying chronic diseases. For a more complete understanding of how chronic diseases came to predominate, it is essential to consider these relationships and the consequences of microbial infections that people encounter over the course of their lives. The need for a new conceptualization of epidemiological transition is indicated by statistical evidence of association between diseases and the findings of many clinical, observational, and epidemiological studies linking specific infections with chronic diseases. Common microorganisms, acute and chronic infections, related immune responses, and inflammatory processes are increasingly being recognized as contributing to the multifactorial etiology of chronic disease. The evidence considered here relates to various cancers, heart disease, stroke, peptic ulcer, diabetes, diseases of the liver and kidneys, and many other common chronic disorders with suspected infectious etiology.

The epidemiological-demographic perspective of this study complements an evolutionary-ecological perspective on contemporary disease patterns developed by microbiologists. Humans did not evolve for "modern lifestyles," but were affected by exposure to new microorganisms and infectious diseases as their way of life changed in earlier times. It is important to view the emergence of chronic diseases in the historical context of dramatic changes in the infectious disease environment. With urbanization and industrialization in the modern era, increasing exposure to environmental and lifestyle-related risk factors has exacerbated the biophysiological effects of infection, contributing to the development of chronic disorders. A consideration of some of the evidence of microbial involvement in chronic diseases in relation to historical trends in cause-specific mortality can contribute to an understanding of how contemporary patterns of disease and mortality have come about.

In the last two decades, there has been a growing awareness among epidemiologists that a multidisciplinary approach is required for a more complete understanding of variation and change in disease and mortality patterns. In the past, historical research tended to be fragmented, with studies by demographers, historians, geographers, economists, and medical specialists focusing on different aspects and phases of change, particular diseases, and issues of interest within disciplinary boundaries. For instance, my earlier monograph, *Disease, Mortality and Population in Transition,* focused on infectious disease mortality decline in England in the 18th and 19th centuries; selections from that monograph have been modified for inclusion here. Studies of mortality decline have generally not compared trends for infectious diseases and chronic diseases, while the epidemiological transition has not been comprehensively reviewed using data from one particular country. This book aims to address these issues and highlight a new perspective on the epidemiological transition reflecting the interrelated nature of diseases, particularly links between infection and chronic disease. Infectious etiology has now been established for a sufficient number of chronic diseases, accounting for a significant proportion of all morbidity and mortality, to indicate the need for a new conceptualization of epidemiological transition. This view would focus more on etiology and pathogenesis than previous adaptations of the theory, which have focused on phases of transition, and would reflect the increasingly blurred distinction between infectious diseases and chronic diseases. The new perspective is consistent with the view of epidemiologists who suggest that future research should be guided by a new disease paradigm encompassing pathogenesis as well as risk factors for disease linked with lifestyle and socioeconomic circumstances. As the global phenomenon of epidemiological transition continues, and the growing burden of chronic disease presents major challenges for public health and health care services worldwide, the topic has much contemporary relevance to the "health transition" in both low-income and high-income countries. The final chapter highlights possible implications for public health policy, particularly the importance of prioritizing disease prevention, which arguably made the greatest contribution in the past to improvements in longevity, health, and the quality of life.

Acknowledgments

I am grateful to friends who have listened to and queried ideas that I hope are now more clearly articulated here. I would especially like to thank Theodore Brown and the University of Rochester Press for the opportunity to contribute to this series, and anonymous publisher's reviewers whose comments and suggestions were both helpful and challenging. I also greatly appreciate the unstinting support of the editorial team that has made publication possible, and the many suggestions for improvement of the manuscript during copyediting.

Introduction

The decline in mortality from infectious diseases has been one of the most significant changes in human history leading to unprecedented increases in life expectancy. There is an expectation in industrialized countries that almost all children will grow up to adulthood and that most people will live at least eighty years despite the high incidence of chronic diseases. Heart disease, stroke, cancers, diabetes mellitus, ulcers, diseases of the kidneys and liver, and other chronic diseases cause much debility, long-term sickness, and "premature" death, which to some extent detracts from the sense of progress in health that has come with the control of infectious diseases. The epidemic diseases that caused high mortality in the 18th and 19th centuries generally resulted in acute short-term sickness, which was often fatal, particularly in the early years of life, while the major chronic infectious disease, tuberculosis, caused high mortality among adults. Infectious diseases restricted average life expectancy to 30–40 years in England and other European countries. A change in the predominant causes of morbidity and mortality from acute infectious diseases and tuberculosis to other chronic diseases among adults, concomitant with increasing life expectancy and a higher proportion of older people in the population, characterizes the epidemiological transition. This term distinguishes the process from Abdel Omran's original concept, "epidemiologic transition," which included phases and models of change.[1] Inadequate definition of disease categories, lack of consideration of disease etiology, and other aspects of Omran's theory have been criticized, and many refinements have been made. Nevertheless, the basic concept of epidemiological transition is widely accepted as a framework for analysis of long-term changes in disease and mortality.

A major objective of this study is to review the emergence of chronic diseases, the now predominant causes of death in industrialized countries, in the context of dramatic changes in the infectious disease environment. The study focuses on the epidemiological transition that occurred in England from the 18th century onward. This is distinct from an earlier change in the predominant infectious diseases when humans first began to live in settled communities during the "Neolithic Revolution," and a further phase of the global transition in which new infectious diseases have emerged and old ones have reemerged as a threat in recent decades, mostly as a result of human action.[2] The new perspective in Omran's "epidemiologic transition" was his focus on a shift from one group of causes of death, infectious diseases, to another group of causes considered to be distinctly different, "degenerative and man-made diseases." Omran later clarified that he included mental illness, drug dependency, radiation injury, occupational hazards, and traffic accidents.[3] Subsequently, the term "noncommunicable" has been widely used for chronic diseases and external causes of death (accidents, suicide, and violence). Greater knowledge about etiology made the term "degenerative disease" inappropriate for many chronic diseases, and use of the label "noncommunicable" is in many cases based on an assumption about noninfectious etiology.

This study takes into account interrelationships between infections and chronic diseases, and between the underlying disorders and biophysiological processes, which indicate that a concept of epidemiological transition based on a simple dichotomy of disease categories is too simplistic. A growing body of evidence indicates that microorganisms are associated with many chronic disorders previously regarded as having no infectious etiology and being noncommunicable, and a causal role has been confirmed in some cases. Given that some chronic diseases are known to have infectious etiology, and at least some microbial involvement is suspected in many others, the concept of a shift in the predominant causes of morbidity and mortality should take into account the increasingly blurred distinction between infectious and chronic disease. The possibility of infectious etiology being confirmed for more chronic diseases in the future suggests that the epidemiological transition might come to be viewed in terms of the balance between microbial and other causes of disease. Categories of disease that allow for what is known and not known about disease etiology are outlined in chapter 2, which provides a theoretical framework for this study of changes over time in disease and mortality.

Future research into the relationship between infectious disease and chronic disorders will contribute to a greater understanding of the ongoing global process of epidemiological transition. Increasing research interest in this field does not signify a tendency toward microbiological reductionism, as evidence that microorganisms, infection, and immune responses have a causal role in the pathogenesis of some chronic diseases complements evidence implicating various risk factors. Multifactorial causation of chronic diseases is now an accepted concept, encompassing biophysiological, lifestyle, behavioral, social, cultural, economic, and environmental factors. The mechanisms and pathways of causation for different diseases are often interconnected, and interrelationships and synergies between the underlying disorders can contribute to an increased risk of dying "prematurely." Interrelationships and synergies also existed between the infectious diseases that were major killers in the past, and these exacerbated the severity of sickness and increased the risk of dying. Sociodemographic factors also affect the severity of acute infectious diseases that contributed to high child mortality, and beneficial changes occurred toward the end of the 19th century. Early in the 20th century, it was recognized that more children were surviving to reach adulthood, although lifetime effects of childhood infections were suspected when age-specific adult death rates were found to vary in relation to year of birth.[4] Subsequently, many studies have found more direct evidence linking particular chronic diseases with acute infectious diseases in childhood, chronic infections, and infections contracted in adult life.

A life course perspective on the development of chronic diseases complements a historical perspective on trends over time.[5] In addition, an evolutionary-ecological perspective, using the concept of epidemiological transition as a framework, also contributes to a more comprehensive understanding of the changing relationship between disease patterns, the environment, and the consequences of human action.[6] Long before many of the well-established risk factors for chronic disease became prevalent, humans were exposed to infections and developed immune responses that can affect health throughout life. Even though many of the associations between microorganisms and chronic diseases are still under investigation and criteria for establishing causality can be difficult to apply, it is conceivable that rapid expansion of this area of research and advances in technologies for identifying pathogens could lead to a radical change in the conceptualization of disease. It has even been suggested that as more causal links between infections and chronic disease are confirmed, a "new germ theory" of disease could emerge.[7] A new epidemiological paradigm for research might encompass pathogenesis and the many levels of causation, including genetic, immunological, biophysiological, sociocultural, and economic, as well as risk factors linked with lifestyle, behavior, and the environment.[8] These aspects of disease etiology need to be taken into account when considering the emergence of the chronic diseases that have replaced acute infectious diseases and tuberculosis as the predominant causes of morbidity and mortality.

The change in predominant diseases, the shift from child to adult mortality, and the increase in life expectancy in the epidemiological transition are integral to the process of demographic transition, which encompasses changes in mortality, fertility, and population. Although different versions of demographic transition theory have been proposed since the 1940s, the basic concept is widely accepted. Mortality decline has usually preceded fertility decline, leading to more rapid population growth.[9] Societies that have undergone a process of "modernization" since the 18th century have experienced a transition from high fertility and high mortality to low fertility and low mortality. It has been questioned whether the concept of demographic transition constitutes a theory, a historical or predictive model, a generalization, a mere description, or just a useful framework for analysis of data.[10] Similar issues surround the concept of epidemiological transition, although it has focused attention on important global changes in disease and mortality. The relationship between declining mortality and fertility is complex, with improved child survival potentially having a negative impact on fertility because conception is less likely during breastfeeding, while prevention of debilitating infectious disease among young adults reduces a constraint on fertility. Of more concern here is the consequence of longer survival and lower fertility in terms of "population aging," an increasing proportion of older people that has implications for morbidity and the provision of health and social services. In this respect, a greater understanding of disease etiology and epidemiological transition is integral to the broader process of health transition. The term was originally used to distinguish cultural, social, and behavioral determinants of health from the effects of medical interventions and changes in people's economic standard of living. Health transition theory developed in the 1990s, encompassing health, morbidity, and the organized health-care response, as well as changes in mortality.[11]

Most studies of historical change in disease patterns have focused on mortality because of the availability of quantitative data, which are generally lacking for morbidity. The studies by Riley of sickness data for workingmen in England from the 19th century and studies by Fogel and Costa of records for Union Army veterans in the United States are notable exceptions. Fogel reported that a high proportion (13–22%) of males aged 16–39 years were rejected by the army in 1861 as they were found to have chronic health conditions.[12] Among those recruited, chronic diseases were more likely to develop later in life following infectious disease while in the army: acute respiratory infections followed by chronic respiratory problems and arrhythmias; measles by chronic respiratory problems and valvular heart disease; typhoid fever by valvular heart disease; rheumatic fever by heart disease, arrhythmias, congestive heart failure, and joint and back problems; diarrheal disease by arteriosclerosis; and malaria followed by joint problems.[13] Fogel and Costa analyzed data on height, body mass index, and morbidity, which indicated that Union Army veterans aged 65 years and over in 1910 were much more likely to have heart, musculoskeletal, respiratory, and digestive diseases than veterans aged 65 and over in a national survey in 1985–88. They attributed the difference to early life experience as well as health interventions and changes in lifestyle, as severity of infectious disease, undernourishment, and other types of stress in utero and in childhood may adversely affect the development of vital organs.[14] Fogel found that the onset of chronic disease had been delayed over the course of the 20th century. Compared with white males in 1895–1910, white males in 1983–92 were much more likely to be free of chronic diseases at ages 60–64 years, while arthritis, heart diseases, respiratory diseases, and cancer started 8–11 years later among men aged 65 years and over in 1983–92. He concluded that improvements in health in the second half of the 20th century were partly due to improved physiology among later cohorts who had benefited from improved technologies for food production, public health, personal hygiene, and medical interventions introduced earlier in the century.[15]

Riley found that when case fatality and mortality declined in England at the end of the 19th century, the average length of episodes of sickness among a sample of workingmen increased. This could be due to episodes of sickness being relatively short in the past because they either were not severe or quickly resulted in death, and to survival of more people predisposed to chronic sickness later in life by infectious diseases in childhood.[16] The aggregate sickness time has now become critical for health-care provision, and the challenge for health policy and programs is to promote lifestyles and working conditions conducive to longer lives spent in good health.[17] Riley also found that the profile of sickness among workingmen was substantially different from the cause-of-death profile, with only respiratory disease and accidents featuring significantly in both. Major chronic diseases causing deaths in England at the end of the 19th century such as heart disease, cancer, and nephritis were not among the causes of sickness recorded at that time.[18] Despite the limitations of mortality data, they provide a more complete record of the emergence and growing predominance of chronic diseases. This study is based on the wealth of local and national historical mortality data available for England and Wales, with data from other Western countries used for comparison on particular aspects of disease and mortality change.

It is now widely accepted that the long-term decline in mortality in England began in the mid-18th century, with subsequent downturns at the beginning of the 19th century and in the 1870s, as in much of Europe.[19] Within this overall mortality transition, there was a resurgence in the national death rate between the 1830s and 1870s when the population of industrial towns was increasing rapidly. Many people who migrated to the towns to escape rural poverty and seek new livelihoods experienced squalid living conditions, poverty, and disease in densely populated "slum" areas. Death rates were extremely high, particularly among children, with up to half of them dying before the age of 5 years. With so many very short lives, average life expectancy was only about 30 years in major industrial cities such as Manchester and Liverpool.[20] From the 1870s, the decline in the national death rate resumed and became more rapid and continuous from the beginning of the 20th century. A major study of aggregated data from several hundred parishes in England by Wrigley and Schofield provided stronger evidence of the earlier phase of mortality decline that occurred before national registration. This confirmed the major contribution to more rapid population growth made by mortality decline, and suggested that the level of fertility made a greater contribution than previously thought.[21] The estimates for England as a whole indicated a decline in the death rate from the 1740s, and an increase in the birthrate throughout the 18th century, contrary to earlier indications from small-scale studies.[22] The new national estimates led to a revision of the theory of demographic transition regarding the relative contribution of changes in mortality and fertility to population growth.

Demographic transition and epidemiological transition are closely related processes in an ongoing global phenomenon. The lag between mortality decline and fertility decline has generated unprecedented population growth. Although demographic balance has been restored in industrialized countries, high fertility rates persist in many African and Middle Eastern countries, despite considerable improvements in child survival. Population growth rates still exceed the peak rates experienced in England in the 19th century, and economic opportunities are grossly inadequate to meet the needs of a growing number of young adults. Cultural, social, economic, and political factors inhibit the process of fertility transition, and rapid population growth is projected to continue for many years. In contrast, remarkable reductions in fertility have been achieved in many low-income countries in Africa and Asia as a result of reproductive health and family planning programs, enrollment of girls in school, postponement of marriage, employment opportunities for women, and their empowerment to make decisions about childbearing and contraception. Migration from rural areas into the towns has exposed people to new ideas and values, including limitation of family size. At the same time, migration into the towns has led to rapid growth in urban population size and density, with adverse consequences for living conditions and health. As in Europe in the past, people in the poorer areas of expanding towns and cities in developing countries are exposed to infectious diseases that can transmit more rapidly in crowded conditions. The infectious diseases include many of those that caused high mortality in England in the past, such as diarrheal diseases, respiratory diseases, tuberculosis, and childhood epidemic diseases, as well as warm-climate diseases and previously unknown infectious diseases that have emerged recently.

The main focus in this study is the transition in cause of death in England from acute infectious diseases and tuberculosis to other chronic diseases, the decline in child mortality, increased survival to older ages at which chronic diseases are more likely to occur, longer lives, and a shift toward predominantly adult deaths. A primary objective is to reassess the major changes in disease and mortality since the 17th century and possible explanations. Much of the decline in mortality between the mid-18th and mid-19th century involved acute infectious diseases, although a major component after this was the declining death rate from tuberculosis. While there are acute forms,[23] it is typically regarded as a chronic infectious disease as most clinical cases are due to reactivation of a latent infection or reinfection among those already tuberculin sensitive from an earlier infection. Other chronic diseases among adults became increasingly predominant as mortality from acute infectious diseases and tuberculosis declined.

The historical change in disease and mortality patterns experienced in England during rapid urbanization has parallels in developing countries today. Many of the infectious diseases that caused high mortality in England in the past still contribute to unacceptably high child mortality in low-income countries. In addition, diseases prevalent in warm climates, particularly malaria, continue to cause much sickness and high mortality in both urban and rural areas. Infectious diseases continue to be a major cause of death, accounting directly for about one-quarter of deaths globally, and contributing to chronic conditions and complications that account for many more deaths.[24] The pandemic of HIV/AIDS has led to reductions in average life expectancy in some parts of Africa, although the disease has caused relatively few deaths in England.[25] Elsewhere, child death rates and life expectancy have generally improved, but death rates from chronic diseases have reached levels found in industrialized countries. Although the composition of the disease burden in developing countries is different from that in England in the past, and new infectious diseases are emerging and old ones reemerging, a reassessment of this transition for which there is particularly well-documented evidence can contribute to a better understanding of the ongoing process of global epidemiological transition.

Historical changes in disease and mortality in England can be seen as broadly typical of the European experience of epidemiological transition, and the main diseases recorded in the 18th century that contributed to mortality decline were similar throughout the Continent. There is wide consensus that long-term mortality decline began first in England and northwestern Europe, with an early phase characterized by diminished spikes in mortality caused by epidemic diseases.[26] Although there were different levels of mortality and different turning points in disease-specific trends, there were many common features, such as the disappearance of plague by the early 18th century, the decline of typhus, and the control of smallpox by the end of the 19th century. As tuberculosis mortality among adults declined, the other chronic diseases that came to predominate as causes of death in England were the same as those in other European countries, although the relative contribution of particular diseases to overall mortality varies. Before considering the concept of epidemiological transition further and outlining the theoretical framework for this study, it is useful to review some of the issues addressed in studies of infectious disease mortality decline in England and the more recent mortality transition in developing countries.

Chapter One

Background

The decline in mortality from the mid-18th century in England and other European countries and the more rapid growth in population that occurred up to the mid-20th century have been the subject of investigation and debate among historians, geographers, economists, demographers, and medical specialists. Attention has focused on the relative importance of different factors, such as treatment, care of the sick, measures to control and prevent infectious diseases, living conditions, "standard of living," nutrition, and changes in the nature of some diseases. Historians and economists have considered the decline in mortality in the context of agricultural and industrial revolutions leading to improvements in food supplies and expansion of economic activity. Studies of the relationship between food supply and death rates in the period leading up to the mortality transition have indicated that many epidemic diseases caused spikes in mortality that were independent of the effects of famine and poor harvests.[1] In earlier premodern times, changes in the infectious disease environment were linked with great transformations in the way of life of humans, particularly the development of agriculture and adaptation to living in settled communities.[2] Eventually urbanization and large-scale migrations led to new ways of living in very different environments, while trade and changes in population size and density brought exposure to new pathogens, different infectious diseases, and changes in the immunological status of individuals and populations.

Industrial development and economic growth in Western countries eventually brought many improvements in living conditions, but the concept of "standard of living" is too general to provide a satisfactory explanation for the decline in mortality and increased life expectancy. It reflects the values of particular sections of society, cultures, and historical periods and masks factors specific to the decline in mortality from particular diseases. It is clearly important to distinguish the specific changes in people's lives that contributed to improved survival chances. In the limited sense of people's own economic circumstances and access to food, shelter, and other basic needs, the concept of "standard of living" can generate hypotheses that are testable with reference to specific indicators. However, generalizations have often been formulated that persisted as explanations of mortality decline despite the lack of supporting evidence. McKeown in particular was an influential exponent of the view that improvements in the "standard of living" and nutrition were the main cause of mortality decline in

England in the second half of the 19th century. In his early work, he and his colleagues concluded that about half of the decline in the overall death rate was the result of improvements in the "standard of living," particularly the effect of a putative improvement in nutrition on tuberculosis mortality.[3] He attributed a further quarter of the decline to sanitary reforms and hygiene measures affecting waterborne diseases and the remainder of the decline to a suggested change in the "character" of scarlet fever. A similar explanation was given by Omran in a study of historical data from New York, in which he referred to mortality decline and the change in the predominant causes of death as an "epidemiologic transition." He concluded that mortality decline was due to improvements in nutrition, "living standards," housing, personal hygiene, and a change in the "character" of scarlet fever.[4] More recently, Fogel analyzed anthropometric data and found that much of the decline in mortality in England between 1751 and 1975 was associated with changes in physiology. He interpreted these as an indication that levels of malnutrition had been reduced, although he recognized that malnutrition was also a consequence of high infectious disease rates.[5]

McKeown emphasized the role of nutrition in the decline of mortality from airborne infectious diseases, concluding that "the most acceptable explanation of the large reductions of mortality and growth of population which preceded advances in hygiene is an improvement in nutrition due to greater food supplies."[6] This view has been widely criticized, partly because of a lack of direct evidence of an improvement in diet, or in the economic standard of living of most people between the mid-18th and mid-19th century. Szreter pointed out that McKeown's thesis came to be accepted by many professionals concerned with public health, despite being largely speculation for which no supporting evidence was provided.[7] In fact, McKeown acknowledged reaching his conclusion that nutrition must have played a part because nutritional deprivation is known to contribute to the risk of dying from infectious diseases in developing countries, and he could offer no other explanation for the decline in airborne infectious disease death rates in England.[8]

Many studies have investigated the role of nutrition in resistance to disease and its effect on the efficiency of immune responses to viral infections.[9] Inadequate nutrition is clearly an important contributing factor in many child deaths from infectious disease in developing countries, and undernourishment undoubtedly contributed to high mortality in Europe in the past. However, there is a complex interrelationship between nutrition, infectious disease, and mortality risk, with severe infectious diseases causing malnutrition, interfering with the body's ability to convert food into energy and growth, and stunting physiological and intellectual development.[10] Evidence of improvements in physiology does not necessarily indicate improved intake of nutrients (diet), and nutritional status is a measure of net nutrition after the nutrient requirements of the body have been met.[11] While agricultural development and imports improved the supply of food between the mid-18th and mid-19th century, supplies may only have kept pace with population growth, while widespread poverty greatly restricted access to food. Studies of food consumption per capita and real incomes in England in the 18th century have not indicated a consistent association with mortality decline, and the economic standard of living of many people may have deteriorated in the first quarter of the 19th century when mortality was lower and population growth more rapid. There is unlikely to have been much improvement in the "standard of living" of the new urban labor force in the period of rapid industrialization between the 1830s and 1870s, although the economic circumstances of many occupational groups probably improved in the last three decades of the century.[12]

As cities grew during the industrial revolution, health hazards increased with industrial pollution, particles from wood and coal fires in the air, poor disposal of animal and human waste, and streets contaminated with standing water, rubbish, and excrement. Many risk factors for chronic diseases became more prevalent and employment in hazardous occupations increased, contributing to longer episodes of sickness due to accidents and respiratory disease.[13] Exposure to pollution and hazardous substances in the air and food would have contributed cumulatively to chronic sickness, while severe infectious diseases in childhood contributed to chronic disease later in life (see chapters 9–12). Szreter emphasized the severe negative consequences for health of conditions in industrial towns that constituted a threat to the whole population and presented major public health challenges.[14] Material living standards were critically important for health, as they are in developing countries undergoing rapid urbanization today. Szreter suggested that the rapid industrial and economic growth in Britain between the 1830s and 1870s had socially divisive effects, including high rents for in-migrants from rural areas, residential segregation in the growing towns, and increasing economic inequality. He argued that addressing the problems in the increasingly crowded, poorer areas of industrial towns in England in the 19th century required political commitment, organization, and the application of resources;[15] and economic growth was only converted into improvements in health through political, social, and cultural influence. Municipal authorities in industrial towns eventually implemented appropriate measures in response to the public health problems and high mortality, although not without opposition from those who were expected to contribute financially; meanwhile, the wealthiest were able to move to more salubrious areas.

Although McKeown recognized the contribution made by improvements in sanitation, he made no reference to the political commitment and organization required to achieve reforms. Szreter suggested that his unsubstantiated speculation that an improvement in people's "standard of living" and nutrition was the main reason for the decline in infectious disease mortality was widely accepted by health professionals as if it were evidence based. Furthermore, it unwittingly lent support to advocates of noninterventionism and reduced public investment in health, education, and human development in the 1980s and 1990s.[16] Easterlin argued that an assumption that economic growth based on a free market can solve problems of health and development is belied by the historical experience of increasing life expectancy linked with the control of infectious diseases and public-sector intervention.[17] Fogel, in developing a theory of technological, physiological, and economic change, emphasized that human beings have gained an unprecedented degree of control over their environment in the last 300 years, which has led to a dramatic increase of 50% in average body size and over 100% in average life expectancy.[18] He recognized that this "technophysio evolution" was not necessarily stable, and that both height and life expectancy had declined in some periods of economic growth in the past.[19] Like McKeown, he emphasized the association between chronic malnutrition and mortality in the 18th and 19th centuries. Much of his research focused on agricultural development, food consumption, and human physiology. He found a strong statistical association between mortality and changes in human height and body mass index, concluding that the decline in mortality could in large part be explained in terms of a reduction in chronic malnutrition.[20] Fogel emphasized that these anthropometric measures are indicators of net nutrition, the balance between nutrient intake (diet) and the body's nutrient requirements.[21] He recognized that infectious diseases have adverse effects on nutritional status, physiological development, and the risk of chronic disease later in life;[22] however, his explanation of long-term mortality decline did not take into account the control that human beings gained over infectious diseases.

The examination here of trends in death rates from infectious diseases and efforts to control them suggests that some studies have greatly underestimated the role in mortality decline of preventive measures, public health interventions, social organization, and sociodemographic changes. Smallpox in particular would not have been eliminated without widespread use of vaccination later supported by other preventive measures. The recession of major epidemic diseases such as typhus, typhoid, and cholera in the 19th century is unlikely to have occurred without preventive measures and public health interventions. Rational responses to the threat of feared epidemic diseases had developed over centuries, along with systems for monitoring the spread of disease based on the collection of mortality statistics. This provided a foundation for further improvements when the germ theory was accepted and knowledge of transmission developed at the end of the 19th century. The evidence reviewed here indicates continuity in the key role of preventive and public health measures in bringing changes in disease and mortality globally. Studies in both industrialized and developing countries in the 20th century have contributed enormously to an empirically based understanding of the global process of mortality decline and epidemiological transition.

Evidence began to emerge in the 1940s and 1950s that mortality was declining in developing countries as well as industrialized countries.[23] The importation of public health techniques from the West into many low-income countries resulted in death rates that were lower than in industrialized countries at a similar stage of economic development.[24] A study in South India, for example, found improvements in mortality were achieved using relatively simple health technologies when basic health services were provided and used by people who responded to advice with changes in health-related behavior.[25] In Sri Lanka the death rate declined from the early 1920s, apart from spikes in mortality during outbreaks of malaria in 1935 and 1943–46. Infant mortality declined as numbers of health centers and visits to mother-and-child health clinics increased. When attendance doubled in 1937 and again in 1939, maternal mortality began to decline consistently.[26] Rapid increases in average life expectancy were also recorded in Venezuela between 1920 and 1960. A comparative analysis of mortality change in Latin American countries found slower mortality decline in the less developed countries before 1930, but similar rates of decline to those in more developed countries after this. Mortality decline had become more dependent on imported preventive and public health measures, which had a significant impact on death rates that was independent of economic development.[27] In Guyana the death rate declined between 1911 and 1940 despite economic stagnation, and again after World War II (1939–45) despite adverse economic circumstances.[28] In Chile the crude death rate declined from 31 to 8 per 1,000 between the early 1920s and 1970s, and a similar decline from 25 to 9 per 1,000 was recorded in Mexico.[29] Differential decline in infectious disease mortality between the regions of Mexico was attributed to differences in the application of public health measures.[30] Data from Cuba provided evidence of epidemiological transition, with a rapid decline in infectious disease mortality over the period 1901–53, and an increase in the proportion of deaths attributed to cardiovascular disease from 27% to 38%.[31]

In the second half of the 20th century rapid improvements in life expectancy were achieved in some developing countries in the absence of significant national wealth creation, as the governments prioritized basic health and social programs in Costa Rica, Sri Lanka, Kerala (India), Cuba, and China, in particular. Implementation was driven by ideology in China, by social and political will in the other countries,[32] and generally by a commitment to equity. Mass education and effective political participation fostered a more equitable distribution of resources and access to schools and health services in Kerala State.[33] Besides Kerala, Caldwell identified 11 countries that had health achievements well beyond those predicted by per capita incomes. He found that educational levels of women of maternal age, family planning, and male education were the factors most strongly associated with health improvement.[34] Several studies identified the particular importance of female education as a key determinant of improvement in child survival, an effect that was independent of people's income and other indicators of material well-being.[35] Even so, favorable social conditions, including greater independence for women and more egalitarian, radical, and democratic traditions, only began to foster improvements in health when appropriate technologies from the West became available. Average life expectancy in 1930 was just 30 years in Kerala and 38 years in Sri Lanka, but by the early 1980s it had increased dramatically to 66 years and 69 years, respectively, despite the lack of improvement in the average annual income of less than US$400 per capita.[36] This experience of mortality decline without much improvement in people's economic standard of living clearly does not imply that economic factors are unimportant as determinants of health. On the contrary, evidence indicates that poverty is a major contributor to high mortality in developing countries, and wide differentials in health measures exist in relation to indicators of people's economic standard of living, such as per capita income or the amount required to purchase a nutritionally adequate diet.[37]

Deaths in childhood and during childbirth are considerably more common among the poor in developing countries, and both child and maternal mortality are more poverty-sensitive health indicators than average life expectancy. Data for 1990 indicate that 35% of deaths at ages under 5 years in developing countries occurred among the poorest 20% of the population, based on a ranking of countries by per capita income.[38] The effect of poverty is much greater at younger ages, and the death rate for children aged 0–14 years was nine times higher among the poorest 20% than among the richest 20%, while at ages 45 and over it was about twice as high.[39] This reflected a poor-rich ratio for mortality that was much greater for communicable diseases than for those assumed to be noncommunicable.[40] World Health Organization data from 46 developing countries allowed more accurate identification of the poorest in terms of the income required to purchase a nutritionally adequate diet. On average, child (0–4 years) mortality around 1990 was four to five times higher for girls and boys below this poverty line compared with those above it, while among adults aged 15–59 years it was about four times higher for men below the poverty line and twice as high for women.[41] Indicators of poverty based on nonfinancial resources also identify mortality differentials, particularly mother's educational level and father's occupation.[42]

The association of higher mortality in developing countries with poverty and lack of education clearly does not imply that higher life expectancy in industrialized countries was achieved through improvements in the economic standard of living and education,[43] and much evidence to the contrary is presented in later chapters. Differences in child survival by educational level of mothers in developing countries in the second half of the 20th century were greater than they were in Western countries in the 19th century. In some cultures, adoption of Western health technologies was inhibited by traditional belief systems and attitudes, although these influences could be overcome through parental education or when people moved to the towns.[44] Caldwell found that the influence of women's education on child survival in Nigeria was independent of economic circumstances and distance to health facilities.[45] Mother's education and literacy probably explain much of the differential in child survival in developing countries because relevant behaviors, such as seeking maternal and child health services, having children vaccinated, and maintaining hygiene in the home, were more likely to be practiced by women who had attended school.[46] Caldwell concluded that evidence-based national policies for developing countries would support investment in education, particularly schooling for girls, preventive health services, and basic curative care.[47]

Clearly, growth in national income can provide more resources for health and education services;[48] however, where the political will and social organization existed, countries have implemented basic health programs in adverse economic circumstances. In the 1950s and 1960s, governments in many low-income countries provided health services based on simple health technologies and knowledge that had been successfully applied earlier in Western countries, and average life expectancy increased from 35 to 45 years. In a study of international mortality data, Preston found that the decline in death rates in developing countries was due mainly to preventive health interventions introduced from industrialized countries, together with some basic treatment measures developed since the 1940s.[49] Although gross domestic product per capita, a proxy for average income, was an important determinant of life expectancy particularly in poorer countries, he found that improvements in life expectancy in the 1950s and 1960s were not due to improvements in people's economic standard of living. Preventive interventions such as immunization, environmental sanitation, insect control, health education, and basic mother and child health services were largely responsible in developing countries, while immunization, sulfonamides, and antibiotics were the main causes of mortality decline in industrialized countries in that period.[50]

In the first three decades of the 20th century, average life expectancy increased regardless of the level of average per capita income, and it increased even more rapidly in the next three decades. Factors other than changes in the national income of countries accounted for 75–90% of the global increase in life expectancy over the whole period.[51] For almost all countries, preventive and public health interventions, simple technologies, and basic health services contributed more to the reduction in mortality than any rise in per capita incomes.[52] Preston suggested that the decline in mortality in the United States in the first few decades of the 20th century was based on application of the germ theory and knowledge about how germs spread that had indicated ways of reducing the risk of infection.[53] Caldwell emphasized the importance of people believing that the new knowledge was correct and accepting responsibility to act on it as far as they could, and also use health services that became available. He suggested that the development of education and secular rational traditions contributed to a growing belief that people could have some control over events affecting health.[54] Socioeconomic and cultural differences led to differences in the timing and course of the mortality transition between subgroups of the population, exacerbating already wide socioeconomic differentials in mortality. At the beginning of the 20th century, children of unskilled workers in England were about half as likely to survive to five years of age as children of parents with professional occupations.[55] Differentials in child mortality were not as great in the United States, but they increased as the professional classes became more aware of the dangers of infection and more rapidly adopted preventive measures such as hand-washing and food hygiene measures.[56]

Although the existence of microorganisms was not known before the bacteriological findings at the end of the 19th century, this did not preclude the development of effective preventive measures and public health interventions in England. The advances in life expectancy in the 20th century should be viewed in the context of a preventive approach to disease that had been developing over many centuries. As early as the plague pandemics of the 14th century, it was recognized that the disease was associated with certain environments and movement of people from one area to another. Ideas developed about the relationship between disease and environmental conditions, and in the second half of the 17th century demographic and statistical methods were developed by John Graunt and William Petty for monitoring historical trends in mortality and identifying meaningful associations with living conditions.[57] Various preventive measures were adopted in Europe and Asia to protect populations from devastating outbreaks of plague, and in England the disease did not recur in the 18th century. The long-term perspective of this study encompasses the development of preventive approaches to disease in response to devastating epidemics of plague, smallpox, typhus, and cholera that laid the foundation for the later rapid improvements in health and life expectancy in the 20th century.

It was well known in the 18th century that diseases were linked with environmental conditions, and a new public spiritedness infused attempts to intervene and protect people.[58] Hygiene measures were adopted in army camps and hospitals, which were amenable to the disciplines required.[59] Measures to improve cleanliness and ventilation were introduced that were appropriate for reducing the risk of patients transmitting infection to each other, and typhus recovery rates improved in British naval hospitals after the 1740s.[60] Hygiene measures for preventing the spread of infection were more widely promoted among the civilian population through dispensaries and the "lying-in" movement. Although the impact of such measures on overall mortality in the 18th century may not have been great, they were nevertheless important in the development of a preventive approach. Dispensaries and voluntary hospitals in England provided care for casualties and patients with various diseases including respiratory conditions;[61] however, death rates in some major towns had begun to decline before hospitals opened in the 1770s.[62]

The need to care for the sick was more widely recognized by the end of the 19th century, and further efforts were made to organize health care.[63] Until that time, those suffering from infectious diseases were not hospitalized on a large scale and there was still no effective treatment for major killers such as smallpox, typhus, typhoid, and tuberculosis, which caused high mortality regardless of socioeconomic circumstances. Medicines and treatment could not have made any significant contribution to the decline in infectious disease mortality before the 1940s, as McKeown emphasized.[64] Antitoxin introduced for the treatment of diphtheria in the 1890s may have been the only effective treatment for a major infectious disease before sulfonamides and antibiotics. Salvarsan was used to treat syphilis from World War I (1914–18) until the 1940s when more effective treatment with penicillin became available, although records do not suggest the disease was a major cause of death in England.[65] Sulfapyridine for the treatment of respiratory disease and sulfonamides for whooping cough and puerperal fever were not available until the late 1930s, there were no effective drugs for treatment of tuberculosis until 1947 when streptomycin became available, and chloramphenicol for the treatment of typhoid was not available until 1950. In addition to antibiotics for infectious diseases, medical interventions for chronic diseases are likely to have contributed significantly to the increase in life expectancy at adult ages in the second half of the 20th century. However, preventive measures had a major impact on chronic disease death rates, through benefits in adult life and as a result of improvements in health and physiological development in childhood, as discussed in chapters 9–12. Evidence presented in chapters 4–8 also indicates major reductions in mortality from acute infectious diseases and tuberculosis were achieved through preventive and public health measures long before effective treatments became available.

Smallpox was controlled in England over the course of the 19th century through vaccination and other preventive measures.[66] This success laid the foundation for global eradication and inspired immunization programs against other diseases, which reduced child mortality worldwide in the second half of the 20th century. McKeown greatly underestimated the contribution of smallpox vaccination and control measures against plague and typhus as a result of focusing on the second half of the 19th century.[67] By that time, plague had long since been prevented from entering the country again and typhus and smallpox mortality had been greatly reduced.[68] The decline in incidence of these three major infectious diseases had a fundamental effect on people's lives regardless of their economic circumstances or nutritional status. Even so, despite demonstration of effective preventive intervention, destructive diseases were still viewed by many as the work of God, and there was opposition to smallpox vaccination as an interference in "God's works."[69] In spite of this objection, vaccination was widely and effectively used long before the theory of germs, identification of microbial agents, or any concept of immune response provided a scientific explanation. Similarly, when cholera arrived in Britain in 1831 during a Europe-wide pandemic, it was greatly feared for the rapid wasting and horrifying death it caused, and there was little knowledge of how the disease spread or how to treat the sick. Nevertheless, control measures such as quarantine were implemented and routes of entry into the country were monitored in a preventive approach reminiscent of the response to the threat of plague in earlier times. The arrival of cholera also led to a public health movement aimed at preventing the disease, and evidence of association with sources of drinking water and suspected contamination eventually led to a theory of transmission and a scientific rationale for improving water and sewage systems, decades before the existence of germs became known and widely accepted.

The germ theory of disease causation became the subject of bitter and lasting controversy at the end of the 19th century, reminiscent of the controversy over the theory of evolution.[70] Many found these new scientific ideas incompatible with religious doctrine and the notion of an "all-wise God." The findings of bacteriological investigations based on growing pure cultures and demonstrating association with specific infectious diseases contributed to acceptance of the germ theory as a more scientific explanation for epidemics and patterns of disease.[71] This dispelled much of the mystery and irrationality that had surrounded infectious diseases, and specific microorganisms were established as the causal agents of diseases that had been major killers known for centuries. The bacteriological discoveries lent support to the idea of isolating severe cases to prevent transmission, although for some infectious diseases there was a decline in case fatality rather than incidence.[72] To explain the decline of the major infectious diseases, it is important to consider turning points in death rates in relation to changes that could affect resistance such as diet, nutritional status, coinfections, sociodemographic changes that affect severity of infection, and preventive measures that affect exposure or the immune response to infection.

The new sciences of bacteriology, virology, and immunology contributed to the development of further preventive measures, and the national registration system introduced in England in 1837 provided mortality statistics with which to monitor the impact. Records of cause-specific mortality from England, with supporting data from other Western countries, form the basis of this study of the epidemiological transition and illustrate its main characteristics—acute infectious diseases and tuberculosis being superseded by other chronic diseases as the predominant causes of death, increased average life expectancy, an increasing proportion of older people, a shift in age at death from childhood to older adult ages, and an increase in population. With the lower death rates from infectious diseases in the first half of the 20th century, concern grew about chronic diseases such as heart disease, stroke, and cancers that were seen to be increasingly common causes of death among adults in middle and older age groups. New methods and techniques were developed to determine the geographic distribution of deaths from chronic diseases,[73] and from the 1950s epidemiology focused more on identifying and quantifying risk factors.

In the second half of the 20th century, epidemiological studies investigated differentials in mortality in relation to behavior, lifestyle, socioeconomic circumstances, environment, and geographic location. Before the global HIV/AIDS pandemic from the 1980s and the growing problem of resistance to antibiotics, there had generally been a shift in scientific attention away from infectious diseases toward the chronic diseases. Nevertheless, research continued into the transmission and population dynamics of infectious diseases, partly because developing countries were at an earlier stage of epidemiological transition. Transmission theory developed and research findings greatly increased knowledge about factors affecting severity, leading to more appropriate measures for controlling acute infectious disease worldwide.[74] However, a unified approach such as that developing with the germ theory when mortality from acute infectious diseases and tuberculosis was high in Europe, became less sustainable as a mixed burden of infectious diseases and chronic diseases with very different etiologies emerged globally.[75]

In recent years, there has been a growing awareness among epidemiologists that a multidisciplinary approach is required for a more complete understanding of variation and change in disease and mortality patterns. In the past, historical research tended to be fragmented, with studies by historians, geographers, economists, demographers, and medical specialists focusing on different aspects and phases of change in mortality, particular diseases, or issues of of special interest within their discipline. Hitherto, a comprehensive overview of the epidemiological transition has not been presented using data from one country, and the emergence of chronic diseases has not been assessed in the context of changes in the infectious disease environment. Through a synthesis of findings from research in different disciplines and analysis of trends in death rates from specific diseases, this study aims to provide a more complete account of the epidemiological transition, and a new perspective that reflects the interrelated nature of diseases, particularly links between infections and chronic diseases. The limitations of the original concept of "epidemiologic transition" and theoretical framework for this study are considered in the next chapter, together with issues relating to the data available, classification of causes of death, and disease categories.

Chapter Two

Theoretical Framework, Data, and Study Outline

The Concept of Epidemiological Transition

The original concept of "epidemiologic transition" outlined by Omran in 1971 focused attention on extremely important changes in cause of death.[1] The infectious diseases that had caused very high mortality among children and adults in the past had been replaced as the main causes of death in industrialized countries by chronic diseases among adults assumed to be noninfectious in origin. There was much criticism of his concept as a "theory," and it does appear simplistic in the light of subsequent findings about the etiology of chronic diseases. Patterns of disease, mortality, and life expectancy are more complex than a simple shift to predominantly chronic diseases as infectious disease mortality declined.[2] Nevertheless, despite criticisms and revisions of the phases of "epidemiologic transition," it has provided a framework for comparison of secular trends and profiles of disease in different populations. An objective of this study is to develop a perspective on historical changes in disease and mortality that goes beyond descriptive accounts of different phases of transition, takes into account disease etiology and the interrelationships between diseases, and contributes to an understanding of how contemporary patterns of disease have come about.

Omran's first formulation of his theory consisted of five propositions, which can be summarized as follows:

1. "Mortality is a fundamental factor in population dynamics."
2. "A long-term shift occurs in mortality and disease patterns whereby pandemics of infection are gradually displaced by degenerative and man-made diseases as the chief form of morbidity and primary cause of death."
3. "The most profound changes in health and disease patterns obtain among children and young women."

4. "The shifts in health and disease patterns that characterise the epidemiologic transition are closely associated with the demographic and socioeconomic transitions that constitute the modernisation complex."
5. There are three basic models of the "epidemiologic transition" corresponding to the experience of most Western countries, countries such as Japan where the transition was more rapid, and developing countries where the decline in mortality commenced more recently.[3]

The identification of a shift in disease patterns distinguished the theory from demographic transition theory, although there was more interest among demographers than epidemiologists until the 1990s. Omran's main concern may have been fertility and the dynamics of population change rather than chronic diseases, and he later added a fourth model in which rapid mortality decline was followed by fertility decline.[4] Some aspects of Omran's concept of epidemiological-demographic change are well accepted, such as increasing life expectancy, a shift in the age distribution of populations from younger to older ages, more rapid population growth, and changes in the cause-of-death structure concomitant with increasing average life expectancy. The key role of mortality decline in the demographic transition is also generally accepted, and with some exceptions mortality decline preceded fertility decline and may have precipitated it. The decline of child mortality made limitation of family size a less risky strategy, and its particularly important contribution to the increase in average life expectancy is considered in chapter 8. The change in the predominant causes of death from acute infectious diseases and tuberculosis to other chronic diseases is uncontroversial as the main feature of epidemiological transition, although exceptions to the different phases of transition, together with etiological considerations, indicate the need for a more empirically based and scientific theory of epidemiological-demographic change.

Omran identified three categories of determinants of "epidemiologic transition": (1) ecobiologic determinants, involving the "complex balance between disease agents, the level of hostility in the environment and the resistance of the host"; (2) socioeconomic, political, and cultural determinants, including "standards of living, health habits and hygiene and nutrition"; and (3) medical and public health determinants, including "public sanitation, immunization and the development of decisive therapies." In general terms, he attributed the decline in mortality and the change in disease patterns to factors linked with "modernisation" and socioeconomic change (proposition 4). He suggested that socioeconomic changes and improvements in "standards of living" were the important changes underlying the "epidemiologic transition" in Western populations, while public health and medical technologies were more important in the later transition being experienced in developing countries. As mentioned, the current study suggests more historical continuity with respect to the role of public health and preventive measures as the main cause of increased life expectancy before and after antibiotics were introduced. Omran's generalizations about the effect on mortality of socioeconomic change and improvement in "standards of living" in Western countries were not based on any specific indicators or even more general evidence. Like McKeown, he provided no evidence of changes in the "standard of living" or nutrition in periods of mortality decline. It will also be shown that many differences in the trends and turning points in death rates for particular diseases belie such a generalization about the decline in airborne infectious disease mortality.

Omran's theory has been criticized as insufficiently epidemiological, and it lacked consideration of disease etiology and causality.[5] Reference to the chronic diseases that have replaced acute infectious diseases and tuberculosis as the main causes of death as "degenerative and man-made" has been criticized for the vaguely moralistic undertones and an assumption that pathogenesis was an age-related process of "degeneration."[6] The term "degenerative" may not be appropriate given underlying processes now known to be involved in heart disease, cerebrovascular disease, and cancer, for example. The concept of "man-made" disease, while reflecting the health consequences of human action and behavior, underestimates socioeconomic, cultural, and other determinants of health that can be difficult for individuals to control. While better-off people have the means to adopt new products and habits later discovered to be detrimental to health, they are likely to respond more quickly to advice, while the poor are more restricted by their social and economic circumstances.[7] Other characterizations of chronic disease such as "diseases of affluence" and "diseases of civilization" have no clear scientific basis,[8] and the relationship between economic standard of living and chronic disease mortality is complex. The more affluent countries have high death rates from these diseases, although even higher age-specific death rates are found in some low-income countries that have undergone little industrial development. This belies any simplistic notion of "diseases of the industrial way of life," while higher than average death rates from chronic disease among the lower socioeconomic groups within high-income countries indicate that the term "diseases of affluence" is not appropriate.[9]

There has also been criticism and considerable modification of Omran's phases of transition in disease patterns: "age of pestilence and famine," "age of receding pandemics," and "age of degenerative and man-made diseases." Reference to an "age of receding pandemics" is inappropriate as smallpox, tuberculosis, dysentery, and pneumonia were endemic in 19th-century England.[10] The global pandemic of influenza in 1918 was also a significant anomaly, as it probably caused more deaths than any pandemic in history during Omran's era of "degenerative and man-made diseases." The HIV/AIDS pandemic had yet to emerge at the time he was writing, but this clearly constitutes a major exception. The emphasis on a decline of infectious disease has been called into question as new diseases including HIV/AIDS and reemerging diseases such as tuberculosis have challenged the implicit assumption of inevitable progress with the control of infectious diseases leading to improved quality of life.[11] Historically, epidemic diseases have had their own dynamics,[12] and a resurgence of some acute infectious diseases of childhood, including whooping cough, measles, and streptococcus-A infection in the United States, for example, has raised further doubts about the sustainability of infectious disease control.[13]

In recent years there has been renewed interest in defining significant phases in the global epidemiological transition and comparing changes in different countries. Three main components that distinguish stages of epidemiological change have been identified: Omran's shift in recorded cause of death, the age and sex groups affected by mortality decline, and the effects of changes in cause of death on survival.[14] His first stage of "pestilence and famine" was characterized by a stagnation of death rates at very high levels for thousands of years. During the second stage, in which acute infectious disease mortality declined, age at death shifted from the young to older age groups; while in the third phase, chronic diseases other than tuberculosis came to predominate and cause death nearer to the supposed end of the "natural" life span. However, death rates from major chronic diseases such as cardiovascular disease declined in the second half of the 20th century in many industrialized countries. In view of this, a distinct fourth phase of transition has been identified: "the age of delayed degenerative diseases," in which the risk of dying shifted to older adult ages.[15] A fifth phase, "the age of obesity and inactivity," has been suggested, marked by a rapid increase in obesity and being overweight, and mental disorders associated with living to much older ages.[16] The growth of the human population and related consumption patterns also have consequences for global environmental systems that may affect human health in hitherto undetected ways.[17]

Since the 1990s, models of epidemiological transition have been applied in comparative studies of national disease profiles and secular trends over time, facilitating understanding of the process and the public health interventions required.[18] Although countries in different phases of transition have different health-care priorities, an understanding of the global process can help to anticipate future needs. The recent phases of transition have important implications for health and social care as the number of older people increases together with the burden of disability and ill health associated with old age. The emerging and reemerging infectious diseases indicate the need for preventive measures that are sustainable and appropriate for specific diseases and sociocultural contexts. Kunitz warned against a historicist assumption that the stages of development would be the same everywhere, and sociocultural context has become an important consideration for health policy and programs in different countries.[19] Omran only briefly referred to differences in the experience of epidemiological transition between socioeconomic and ethnic groups, and attention has also been drawn to regional variation within countries.[20] A revised concept of epidemiological transition highlighting the shift from acute infectious disease to chronic diseases can provide the basis for a more complete understanding of the diversity of changing disease profiles in populations, which together with a greater understanding of etiology can contribute to the development of appropriate health and social interventions.

Health care and the organized social response to the epidemiological transition in disease and disability were included in the broader concept of "health transition" in the 1990s. There had been seeds of a broader theory encompassing social and behavioral determinants of health, disease, and mortality even in the early 1970s when Omran first coined the term "epidemiologic transition."[21] Caldwell and others began to focus on the dynamic process whereby health and disease patterns respond to demographic, socioeconomic, technological, political, cultural, and biological changes. Based on a conceptual framework for determinants of child mortality,[22] a comprehensive framework was developed that integrated multiple determinants of health.[23] This theoretical framework consisted of systemic determinants of health such as the population genome, the environment, and social organization; social structure, including wealth and redistributive mechanisms, social stratification, and occupational structure; and intermediate determinants including working conditions, living conditions (particularly housing and food), lifestyle, and the health-care system.[24] Family structure and living conditions influence the way that lifestyle factors affect health, and these in turn are affected by culture, ideology, laws, regulations, taxes, subsidies, and commercial pressures. Working conditions, living conditions, and lifestyle factors converge to affect proximate determinants of health, biophysiological processes, and the functioning of the body. Health status can be seen as the outcome of exposure to disease agents and the susceptibility of individuals resulting from a complex network of risks, which have social as well as biological determinants.

Research into social, economic, cultural, lifestyle, and behavioral determinants has contributed enormously to an understanding of health and disease. However, in the past this was often distinct from research into pathogenesis and the processes underlying chronic diseases. The aim here is to develop a historical perspective on the epidemiological transition that is consistent with the health transition theoretical framework, while also encompassing pathogenesis. A particular focus is empirical evidence linking the biophysiological processes underlying chronic diseases with microorganisms, infection, and immune responses. Omran recognized the importance of identifying the characteristics and determinants of changes in disease patterns;[25] however, developments in the "theory of epidemiologic transition" have tended to focus on identifying phases in the changing pattern of morbidity and cause of death. Further development of a more scientific theory of epidemiological change could focus on pathogenesis and the multifactorial causality of chronic diseases that includes infectious etiology. A more scientific theory would take into account evidence that common microorganisms, infections, related immune responses, and inflammatory processes are associated with chronic diseases, including the major causes of morbidity and mortality such as heart disease, stroke, cancers, peptic ulcer, diabetes, and diseases of the liver and kidneys. For some chronic diseases, infection is now known to be necessary for their development; for others, onset can occur without infection but it increases the risk; and in some diseases it is an immune response after acute infection that produces a chronic disorder.[26] Three categories of causal relationship have been distinguished: (1) an infectious agent or immune response after the infectious agent is cleared, or during persistent infection, produces chronic disease or disability through progressive tissue pathology or organ decomposition; (2) the initial stages of acute infection cause permanent deficit or disability (e.g., poliomyelitis); and

(3) infection indirectly predisposes to chronic sequelae (e.g., maternal infection during pregnancy leading to premature birth and an increased risk of neurologic and pulmonary deficits).[27]

It would be premature to attempt to estimate the proportion of chronic disease that involves microorganisms, infection, and immune responses, as many studies of associations are ongoing and new research findings relevant to the assessment of causality are continually emerging. Various observations can lead researchers to suspect a possible microbial cause of a chronic disease, including pathogens being present in diseased tissues, an increased risk of the disease among the immune-suppressed, or a favorable response of the condition to antimicrobial therapy. In 2005 the American Academy of Microbiology reported on microbial causes of chronic disease and identified problems for investigation of suspected microbial links.[28] These include the difficulty of establishing the relationship between a specific infection and a specific chronic disease if the infectious disease agent is ubiquitous. The criteria for establishing whether a specific microorganism has a causal role in a disease date back to the work of Koch on infectious diseases at the end of the 19th century. Koch proposed criteria for experimental proof of pathogenicity in 1883 in his postulates, which can be summarized as follows: (a) the suspected causal organism must be constantly associated with the disease; (b) the suspected causal organisms must be isolated from an infected host and grown in pure culture; (c) when a healthy susceptible host is inoculated with the pathogen from pure culture, symptoms of the original disease must develop; and (d) the same pathogen must be reisolated from hosts who have been infected under these experimental conditions.[29]

In the current epidemiological context, these rules are not entirely appropriate because of problems specific to chronic diseases. Many of the microorganisms suspected of being involved cannot be cultivated, some microorganisms may locate in tissues that are difficult to access, and in some cases the length of time between infection and onset of chronic disease is too long to assess the effect of reintroducing a cultured organism into a healthy host. Although powerful assay techniques have been developed in recent years for detection of pathogens in human tissues, research is subject to the limitations of current techniques. Failure to detect pathogen proteins or nucleic acids does not constitute proof that the pathogen is not involved in a particular chronic disease. Other epidemiological criteria can be applied when assessing evidence that might allow a conclusion to be reached about whether a particular microorganism has a causal role in a particular chronic disease. Hill proposed criteria for establishing causality at a time when epidemiological and other evidence suggested that smoking might be a cause of lung cancer.[30] These criteria can be adapted and applied when suspected links between specific microorganisms and chronic diseases are being assessed. The criteria include consistency, strength and specificity of association, existence of a dose-response relationship, exposure to infection preceding disease, and the plausibility of a suggested causal link.

A revised concept of epidemiological transition encompassing evidence of the role of microorganisms in chronic disease would take into account these theoretical, empirical, and practical issues. The question of whether the involvement of microorganisms in chronic disease already indicated by a growing body of evidence can be accommodated within a new "eco-epidemiology paradigm" proposed by some epidemiologists, or even a "new germ theory" of disease as suggested by Ewald, will be considered briefly in the final chapter.[31] Regardless of any conclusions that might be drawn about the relative importance of microorganisms in the etiology of chronic disease, the historical perspective on changes in disease and mortality developed here can contribute to a better understanding of how contemporary patterns of disease have emerged and clearly indicates the need for a new conceptualization of epidemiological transition.

Mortality Data, Disease Categories, and Study Outline

One of the objectives of the present study is to document the major changes in disease and mortality in England since the 18th century and reassess the causes of the decline in infectious disease death rates. However, the study aims to go beyond the issue of the relative importance of "standard of living" and "human intervention" as determinants of increased life expectancy, and consider the emergence of chronic diseases in the context of urbanization, industrialization, and a changing infectious disease environment. Evidence of changes in established risk factors and association with common infectious diseases can contribute to an understanding of contemporary patterns of chronic disease. Their predominance as causes of death in England reflects widely prevalent disorders and an increasing burden of long-term sickness that constitutes a major challenge for health-care provision as many more people live longer.

In the absence of historical morbidity data, much can be learned about the emergence of chronic diseases from recorded death rates. In the 18th century, infectious diseases predominated and relatively few deaths were recorded as due to heart disease or cancer, although there is little reason to doubt that some adults died from these and other chronic diseases.[32] National registration data from the second half of the 19th century provide the basis for documenting the emergence of chronic diseases as the predominant causes of death, allowing for the effect of increasing recognition. In some respects the trends in this period are a proxy for morbidity trends as many of the same risk factors contribute to both morbidity and mortality, and there was little effective treatment. In outlining changes in disease and mortality based on preregistration data and national registration statistics, data from local areas and other Western countries are used for comparison and assessment of the universality of changes and possible explanations for them.

Mortality Data and Disease Categories

Despite the many limitations of early historical records such as the London Bills of Mortality, which include many ill-defined categories of cause,[33] these sources indicate major turning points in mortality. Medical writers such as Black and Heberden used the data to monitor disease and mortality patterns.[34] Black recognized that the records were incomplete as burials outside the parochial churchyard and deaths in "mad houses" and among certain religious sects were not included, and "causes" of death were recorded by women "searchers" with no medical training. Nevertheless, the data support the view of contemporary historians that infectious diseases accounted for most deaths in England in the 18th century. There was also continuity between the infectious diseases recorded in the London Bills in the 1830s and in the early years of national registration when "fevers," tuberculosis, respiratory diseases, and the epidemic diseases of childhood were prominent in the records for London.[35]

Under civil registration introduced in 1837, efforts were made to ensure complete recording of deaths, which was to be done within five days. Edwin Chadwick and Joseph Lister requested medical practitioners to provide a written statement on the cause of all deaths in their practice.[36] William Farr also encouraged medical practitioners to cooperate, and he influenced the development of techniques and procedures for collecting and analyzing mortality statistics. There was widespread support for the new system, which was designed to improve on recording of deaths by the unqualified "searchers." Later, printed forms were supplied for certification of a death and its cause. By 1870, 92% of all deaths in England and 98% in London were medically certified.[37] Clearly, much caution is required when interpreting trends in mortality in view of doubts about the veracity of some certificates and other deficiencies.[38] This particularly applies to disease-specific death rates before the causal pathogens were identified at the end of the 19th century. Even so, medical practitioners would have been experienced in all types of infectious disease, and the specific disease is likely to have been identified on the basis of valid clinical symptoms.[39] Although little can be done to correct for misclassification, taking cause-specific data at face value allows relative trends and turning points to be considered despite doubts about the actual level of mortality from specific diseases. This is particularly important when considering long-term trends, because of possible transfers due to new knowledge, improved diagnosis, or changes in classification preference. Bearing this in mind, the registration data and earlier records provide a useful statistical framework for assessing changes in the profile of diseases that were the main causes of death. However, attempts to quantify the arithmetic contribution of different diseases to mortality decline can be misleading, partly because of misclassification, but also because the risk of dying is affected by coinfections, interrelated diseases, multiple chronic disorders, and the cumulative and long-term effects of infections.

Historians assessing the contribution of infectious diseases to mortality decline have considered changes that may have affected identification.[40] Knowledge about diseases developed over the period of mortality decline from the mid-18th century, and this could affect the recording of infectious diseases, particularly after the bacteriological discoveries at the end of the 19th century. Identification of microorganisms as causal agents led to a paradigm shift in the concept of disease, and the germ theory and new scientific methods affected clinical identification. With this in mind, some basic definitions, terminology, and disease categories can be considered. Infection is the process by which microorganisms are transferred to a new host from another person or source, and *an* infection refers to the presence of pathogenic microorganisms (pathogens) that can multiply in the body. An infectious disease is a clinical manifestation of symptoms and biophysiological changes caused by microorganisms such as bacteria, bacilli, viruses, fungi, or parasites. Many infectious diseases are considered to be communicable, in the sense that the causal microorganisms are transmissible from one infected person to another by contact (contagious), through discharges from an infected person, through an animal vector, or through a medium such as the air, water, or food. Infectious diseases may be acute and short term (e.g., measles and smallpox), chronic (i.e., long term or persistent, such as tuberculosis and HIV/AIDS), or recurrent (e.g., malaria). This distinction is not clear-cut, as the duration of disease, the period during which microorganisms can be transmitted to another person or detected in the body, and the length of time from infection to onset of sickness are not fixed. The distinction between infectious and chronic diseases has become even more problematic with the confirmation of infectious etiology for more chronic diseases previously considered as not infectious in origin and noncommunicable (e.g., peptic ulcer).

Industrial societies have now reached a stage of epidemiological transition in which chronic diseases rather than acute infectious diseases account for most deaths. Many of the chronic diseases have been labeled as "noncommunicable" because the underlying manifestations cannot be transmitted from one person to another as can microorganisms causing infectious diseases. In a rather different sense of cultural "communicability," risk behaviors can be transferred when people adopt practices that appear socially acceptable and desirable, while socioeconomic circumstances can inhibit healthy lifestyle choices.[41] More problematic for the assumption of noncommunicability is the growing body of evidence that microorganisms are associated with many chronic diseases previously considered to be "noncommunicable," with infectious etiology already established in some cases. The simple dichotomy of disease categories used to characterize the epidemiological transition in terms of a shift from infectious diseases to "degenerative diseases" or "noncommunicable diseases" is no longer tenable. Although some disorders and chronic diseases are definitely not infectious in origin or communicable, the possibility that microorganisms, infections, or immune responses might have at least some role in other chronic diseases undermines the general validity of the "noncommunicable disease" label. It also makes the distinction between infectious diseases and chronic diseases less clear-cut, and a more unified epidemiological approach to these diseases may be required.[42] Although the epidemiological transition is referred to succinctly here as a shift from acute infectious diseases to chronic diseases, the profile of diseases is more complex. Chronic diseases include chronic infectious diseases with known and necessary infectious causal agents (e.g., tuberculosis and HIV/

AIDS), diseases for which infectious etiology has now been established (e.g., peptic ulcer and cervical cancer), other chronic diseases for which at least some role for microorganisms or immune responses has not been ruled out, and disorders that definitely do not have any infectious causal agent (e.g., radiation sickness and some genetic disorders).

A specific microorganism may act as a causal agent in more than one chronic disease, and diverse pathogens may contribute to some underlying disorders.[43] Infectious etiology makes some chronic diseases communicable but only slightly, or not conspicuously (e.g., peptic ulcer), while for some other diseases an assumption of noncommunicability could turn out to be false. Diseases differ in terms of cause (infectious agent—known, possible, or none) and effect (manifestation—acute or chronic), and communicability, which could vary and change over time.[44] When considering changes in the profile of disease in a population over time, it is useful to bear in mind categories based on the different possible combinations of these characteristics. The following disease categories provide a framework for this study of historical disease trends in England: acute infectious diseases (e.g., measles and smallpox) and chronic infectious diseases (e.g., tuberculosis) caused by a microorganism(s) that is necessary for the disease to occur and communicable; chronic diseases with confirmed infectious etiology (microorganism[s] communicable at some stage may contribute to this or a different chronic disease in some recipients); chronic diseases in which microbial agents might act in conjunction with known causal agents or have some other role in the development process (suspected microorganism[s] may or may not have a causal role, and may or may not be communicable); and chronic diseases that definitely do not have infectious etiology and are not communicable (e.g., some genetically inherited conditions). Some clearly noncommunicable conditions with external causes (mainly accidents, violence, and suicide attempts) are of less concern here as the focus is on changes in disease and mortality. Other categories of disease are relevant to the ongoing global epidemiological transition: acute and communicable infectious diseases resistant to control because of variation (e.g., influenza) or antibiotic resistance (e.g., methicillin-resistant *Staphylococcus aureus*—MRSA); and zoonotic infectious diseases that are generally not communicable, or only slightly communicable (e.g., severe acute respiratory syndrome—SARS). The whole set of disease categories is relevant to the rather different disease profiles of warm-climate countries including infectious diseases of zoonotic origin and many emerging infectious diseases.

When considering the changing profile of disease in the epidemiological transition in England, other groupings of disease can be used to overcome some of the limitations of the data due to changes in diagnostic preference and accuracy of certification. Chronic diseases such as different cancers, and cardiovascular diseases including heart disease and stroke, can be grouped together on the basis of common underlying disorders and disease processes, although the manifestations are very different in terms of symptoms and site in the body. This aggregation of data can be particularly useful for comparability over time, as changes in classification affect subcategories more than larger groups of disease. Subcategories have become much more narrowly defined under successive revisions of the International Classification of Diseases (ICD) system (appendix A), and very specific diagnosis is clearly important for clinicians concerned with treatment and monitoring outcomes. Even so, analysis of trends for larger categories can be useful because of possible transfers of recording. Smaller subcategories are likely to be more subject to diagnostic error and changes in clinical preference for certification of the primary cause of death. Classification errors tend to cancel each other out for large groups of diseases, such as all malignant neoplasms and all cardiovascular diseases.[45] The broad groups can also be more than a means to ensure greater consistency over time. For example, monitoring trends in the death rate for all cardiovascular diseases combined allows for the possibility that the underlying biophysiological disorders might have resulted in a different cardiovascular outcome with a different primary cause of death being recorded.

Risk factors for subcategories of chronic disease can be different, although many are common to very different manifestations of disease. Pathways link the underlying cellular, immunological, and biophysiological processes with exogenous risk factors for morbidity and mortality, including lifestyle, behavior, sociocultural, economic, and environmental factors. A multidisciplinary approach is required for a more comprehensive understanding of the causes of disease, variation in morbidity and mortality between populations and trends over time. A synthesis of the findings of many disciplines, including microbiology, evolutionary ecology, virology, bacteriology, immunology, epidemiology, demography, and other social sciences can contribute to a more comprehensive understanding of the epidemiological transition. Possible explanations of changes in disease and mortality will be considered here in relation to socioeconomic change, while the growing predominance of chronic diseases is considered in the context of a changing infectious disease environment. The existence of intercurrent infections and debilitating sequelae meant that particular diseases did not always have an independent impact on morbidity and mortality as often assumed in earlier studies. A more complete understanding of epidemiological transition needs to take into account interrelationships between diseases, including the effects of intercurrent infections, debilitating and long-term effects of infections, links between infections and chronic diseases, and the combined effect of underlying chronic disorders.

Outline of Chapters

As background to the major changes in disease and mortality in England since the 18th century, chapter 3 provides a brief overview of changes in the infectious disease environment in earlier phases of human history. Major changes in ways of living are considered, such as the shift from hunting and gathering to a more settled existence based on agriculture, living in larger urban communities, and the upheavals during the industrial revolution. These changes had ecological consequences including exposure to different microorganisms and susceptibility to new infectious diseases. Migration, population movements, and trade fostered transmission of infections, and new diseases were introduced into Europe from Asia, including plague, smallpox, and cholera. Devastating epidemics of plague from the 14th century through the 17th century led to efforts to prevent the disease. The absence of plague from England in the 18th century is contrasted with continuingly high mortality from typhus, a disease associated with war, deprivation, crowded living conditions, and poor personal hygiene. The rapid growth of towns brought adverse changes in the infectious disease environment, while the decline in mortality from the mid-18th century onward contributed to natural population growth. The relationship between the decline in mortality, continuing high fertility, population growth, economic circumstances, and food supply is a central theme of chapter 4.

In chapter 5 the relationship between the main categories of disease and total mortality is considered with reference to different sets of records, particularly the association between smallpox epidemics and spikes in mortality. Evidence of the impact of vaccination will be considered in some detail as the contribution of immunization has been underestimated in earlier studies. The disease was ubiquitous in England in the 18th century, and surveys throughout the country found an average case fatality of 17%. Evidence suggests that inoculation prevented smallpox deaths in some parts of England, while data from many locations and different Western countries indicate that vaccination dramatically reduced smallpox deaths and total mortality after 1800. A resurgence of the disease after a few decades was followed by a pandemic in 1870–71, which led to more concerted efforts to vaccinate, revaccinate, and isolate cases. The final decline and virtual elimination of smallpox from England before the end of the 19th century was remarkable. Evidence from England and other parts of Europe indicates that vaccination, later supported by other preventive measures, had a dramatic epidemiological-demographic impact.

Chapter 6 documents the importance of other infectious diseases as major killers in the 18th century, including different "fevers." Epidemics of typhus fever were reported throughout Europe, particularly in times of war and food shortages. The observed association with jails, ships, and military camps provided a focus for preventive efforts in England, while hygiene measures were introduced that reduced mortality from other diseases and "fevers" generally. The possible impact of specific preventive measures on typhus and typhoid is considered, while much of the chapter focuses on the response to cholera, which arrived from Asia in the 1830s. The public health movement and the timing of improvements in water supplies, sewerage, domestic sanitation, and hygiene are considered in relation to trends in mortality from cholera and other diseases that could have been affected. A hypothesis that improved water supplies contributed to prevention of typhoid as well as cholera is supported by evidence from other countries in the 20th century.

In chapters 7 and 8 the persistently high infant mortality from diarrheal diseases in the second half of the 19th century is contrasted with the decline among older children linked with improvements in water and sewage systems. The vulnerability of infants to poor domestic, personal, and food hygiene, as well as dangerous weaning practices, is considered in chapter 7. The plateau in infant mortality is viewed as a setback following an earlier decline, followed by a more rapid decline after 1900. The findings of studies in developing countries and local area studies in England indicate the likely causes of the national decline in infant and child mortality. The decline in the child (1–4 years) death rate from the 1860s is considered in chapter 8, including the major contribution of the decline in scarlet fever mortality. The correspondence of the trends for scarlet fever and for typhoid combined with other fevers, in conjunction with recent evidence that enteric fevers and dysentery impede absorption of micronutrients, suggests that typhoid may have lowered resistance to streptococcal infections, increasing the severity of scarlet fever attacks. The decline in child (1–4 years) death rates from some infectious diseases from the 1860s is contrasted with a much later decline in measles and respiratory disease death rates. Evidence from developing countries indicates that sociodemographic factors affect the severity of airborne epidemic diseases, suggesting that historical changes in these factors may explain the downturn in some disease-specific death rates in England. The final section of chapter 8 compares the contribution of changes in infant, child (1–4 years), adolescent, and adult mortality to overall mortality decline and increasing life expectancy, emphasizing the shift from high child mortality to deaths predominantly among older adults.

In chapters 9 and 10 the decline in respiratory tuberculosis death rates among infants, children, and other age groups is contrasted with the lack of decline in respiratory disease death rates before the 1890s. Age-specific death rates presented by year of birth indicate that respiratory tuberculosis mortality declined over successive birth cohorts throughout the 19th century. Explanations of the long-term decline in tuberculosis mortality in other studies, in terms of natural selection, improved resistance to infection, a diminution in virulence, and putative improvements in nutrition, have not been supported by convincing evidence. Contact with the causal bacillus was universal, and case fatality remained high. It is suggested that the risk of tuberculosis developing was reduced by avoiding smallpox, and evidence of a statistical association between smallpox and tuberculosis mortality trends is consistent with this. Vaccination protected children from smallpox, a disease that is likely to have increased the risk of clinical tuberculosis developing from a latent tubercular infection or a new infection. The downturn in respiratory disease and measles death rates may be explained by a reduction in the severity of infections as a result of smaller families and other sociodemographic changes, in view of findings in population biology and studies in developing countries. The lifetime repercussions of severe infectious diseases in childhood are considered, along with exposure to risk factors for respiratory disease during adult life, such as cigarette smoking and air pollution.

In chapter 11 the fairly continuous decline in respiratory disease death rates is compared with four phases of a unique long-term trend in the death rate from cardiovascular disease—an increase in the second half of the 19th century, a decline between 1891 and 1910, an increase between 1920 and 1940, and a more continuous decline after 1951. The trends for cardiovascular disease and respiratory disease death rates were similar between 1875 and 1916 with regard to a major turning point around 1891 and correspondence of short-term fluctuations. Evidence of association between common respiratory infections and atherosclerosis, heart disease, and stroke is considered, which suggests they may have a role in the underlying disorders as well as in acute cardiovascular attacks. Other lifestyle-related risk factors are discussed in relation to differentials in cardiovascular mortality, trends over time, and changes in health-related behavior. In particular, the influence of cigarette smoking on the risk for cardiovascular disease and cancer is considered in relation to mortality trends and differentials.

Data on deaths by site of cancer available from the period 1911–15 onward are presented in chapter 12, which indicate that lung cancer was not a significant cause of death until the 1920s, and cancers of the digestive system are likely to have contributed most to increasing cancer mortality in the second half of the 19th century. Risk factors identified in cross-sectional studies are considered along with trends in death rates by site and for all sites combined. Age-specific cancer death rates presented by year of birth reveal a turning point in cohort mortality among females after the mid-19th century, which could reflect the reduced impact of childhood infectious disease. Evidence of a statistical association between tuberculosis and cancer mortality is discussed, together with epidemiological evidence of an increased risk of lung cancer following pulmonary tuberculosis, and evidence that neonatal vaccination with BCG (Bacillus Calmette-Guérin) can offer some protection against childhood cancers. Other examples of association between microorganisms and different types of cancer are considered, including the confirmed causal link between bacterial infection with *Helicobacter pylori* and gastric cancer.

The theme that the infectious disease environment continues to be highly significant for morbidity and mortality from chronic diseases is developed further in chapter 13. The focus is on trends in death rates from ulcers, nephritis, cirrhosis of the liver, and diabetes mellitus, diseases for which there is evidence of microbial involvement. The confirmed role of *Helicobacter pylori* as the main cause of peptic ulcer is considered in relation to long-term trends in period and cohort death rates. Changes in the domestic environment and experience of infections in childhood are considered with regard to the development of chronic disease in later life. The suspected involvement of enterovirus infection in type-1 diabetes, particularly Coxsackie B virus, and the role of hepatitis C virus in type-2 diabetes and cirrhosis of the liver are considered in relation to changes in death rates across birth cohorts. The relationship between streptococcal infection and chronic nephritis is considered in relation to long-term trends in cohort mortality. The final section of the chapter summarizes many other chronic diseases that exhibit signs of possible microbial involvement. The issue of what criteria should be applied to establish causality is briefly considered in the final chapter.

Chapter 14 summarizes the decline in infectious disease mortality since the 18th century, the most likely contributing factors, the rise to prominence of chronic diseases, and evidence that microorganisms and immune responses are among the main causes. It is suggested that the virtual elimination of the major epidemic killers of the 18th century before the 20th century was due to preventive measures and public health interventions. The most likely causes of the more rapid decline in overall mortality in the first half of the 20th century are summarized, including improved hygiene, isolation of infectious cases, better care of the sick, smaller families, other sociodemographic changes reducing the severity of infections, better nutritional status, and immunization. Despite dramatic changes in the infectious disease environment, many of the microorganisms remain widely prevalent, some still cause many deaths in developing countries, and other common pathogens are associated with chronic diseases. The implications of causal links for the concept of epidemiological transition are considered, along with the idea of a new "eco-epidemiology paradigm" for research suggested by some epidemiologists, which requires interdisciplinary collaboration. This would encompass pathogenesis as well as lifestyle-related factors and the wider social and economic determinants of morbidity and mortality. Further research into the role of microorganisms and immune responses will enhance understanding of the pathogenic processes underlying chronic disease. The implications of the global epidemiological transition for public health and prevention of disease, including the growing burden of chronic disease and the continuing threat from infectious diseases, are considered with regard to the needs of both low-income and relatively high-income countries.

Chapter Three

A New Infectious Disease Environment

Human history has been marked by significant migrations and adaptation to new methods of survival, with consequences for the infectious disease environment, health, longevity, and population. This chapter briefly outlines evolutionary changes in the human condition that led to agriculture, the growth of towns, and exposure to new infections, and considers the infectious disease environment in England when the long-term decline in mortality began. The infectious diseases that contributed to high mortality in the 18th century and the relationship of mortality decline to population growth and food supply are a particular focus. Population increased despite adverse changes in the infectious disease environment, and survival was dependent on immune defenses as well as food supplies. The importance of immunity may be less obvious now that infectious diseases in Western countries are relatively mild and appear to cause few deaths, although immune responses to invasive microorganisms occur continuously throughout life, whether or not there is any discernible acute sickness. In some cases the immune response can become less efficient with age, while other microorganisms, or the immune response to them, can have adverse biophysiological consequences resulting in chronic disease.

Although microorganisms causing some of the infectious diseases that were major killers in the 17th and 18th century are no longer prevalent in England, other common microorganisms continue to cause childhood epidemic diseases, respiratory infections, and gastrointestinal disorders. Some of these microorganisms are associated with chronic diseases that are now major causes of death. Although environmental, socioeconomic, lifestyle, and behavior-related risk factors contribute to the development of these diseases, common microorganisms have been confirmed as causal agents in some chronic diseases, while the involvement of infection in the underlying biophysiological processes in other chronic diseases is strongly suspected. Some chronic disorders have been linked with long-term effects of childhood infections or exposure to microorganisms during adult life, which will be considered in chapters 10–13 along with the issue of the criteria that can be applied to assess causality. At this stage, the possibility of infections being involved in chronic diseases can be borne in mind in considering evolutionary changes that have affected humans, their infectious disease environment, and their immune responses. Changes in the way of life of our human ancestors as they sought to address basic needs for food affected their exposure to microorganisms, and eventually with the development of agriculture, trade, and the division of labor, human interactions affected the transmission of infectious diseases and the immune status of individuals and populations.

Human beings, other vertebrates, and invertebrates require an effective means of protection against infection, although invertebrates produce no antibodies. Vertebrates evolved an additional immune mechanism beyond that required to fight bacterial infection, possibly as a means of responding to cellular anomalies. In humans, this may have enabled more effective defenses against invading microorganisms to evolve with the two systems developing in an interrelated way in response to a changing infectious disease environment.[1] Writers on the evolution of infectious diseases such as Burnet, Cockburn, and McNeill emphasized ecological aspects of competition among microorganisms seeking human hosts in which to replicate.[2] For example, Cockburn linked the decline of leprosy, which was common in Europe in the Middle Ages, with the rise of tuberculosis, suggesting that leprosy may have been replaced as tuberculosis conveyed some cross-immunity and spread more rapidly when the rural population began to have more regular contact with people in towns.[3] This hypothesis is supported by evidence from many studies that BCG vaccine for protection against tuberculosis also protects against leprosy, although effectiveness varies.[4] An evolutionary perspective on changing infectious disease patterns highlights the importance of changes in the immune status of individuals—and of populations, as encapsulated in the phrase "the ever varying state of the immunological constitution of the herd."[5] McNeill pointed out that the immune status of populations affected the interval between epidemic "mortality crises," while increased human contacts and migration led to global transmission of many infectious diseases before the 18th century.

Evolution, Settlement, Migration, and the Infectious Disease Environment

Our human ancestors living in the rain forest were probably exposed to infections among wild animals, such as yellow fever among monkeys and rabies among bats, together with a variety of parasites that thrived in the humid conditions, such as worms and trypanosomes (single-celled protozoa). With small groups moving into grassy woodland or onto the savanna in search of food, the change of habitat would have brought contact with new microorganisms and possibly reduced exposure to some parasites. Humans would still have been troubled by a great variety of parasites, although many would not necessarily produce symptoms that would be recognized as illness. Some parasites that spread from host to host directly, such as spirochetes and those causing yaws infection, may have survived among small migratory communities.[6] A variety of foods would have been required to sustain nomadic groups in different seasons, and new infections were probably contracted by following herds of wild animals. So long as the biological evolution of early humans kept pace with the evolution of their parasites, predators, and prey, no great change in the ecological balance would have occurred. Numbers probably increased steadily with some of the young moving away to form new nomadic groups. Humans learned to live in particular microenvironments, adapting to different climatic conditions in different parts of the world. Their success in temperate zones may have been enhanced by a relative lack of predators and natural parasites. Although migration to such areas is likely to have been disruptive ecologically, life would have been sustained through an ability to adapt behaviors as difficulties were encountered or created. The colder the climate, the more survival would have depended on the ability to find suitable large-bodied plants and animals for food. One advantage for humans living this way of life would have been less diversity of infections compared with the tropics, and a balance with parasitic organisms may have been less important than in a warmer climate.

Following the retreat of the ice cap in Europe from 19,000 to 11,000 years ago, humans developed methods of fishing and cultivation of plants for food over a long period of the "Neolithic Revolution." The ability to generate a regular supply of food through agriculture and to store it became the basis for a settled way of life and increasingly large communities. Nomadic tribes from the steppes and mountains of eastern Europe and central Asia began to live in settlements from about 10,000 years ago. Eventually towns, cities, and civilizations developed in China, India, Mesopotamia, the Nile Valley, the Mediterranean area, western Europe, and the Americas. There has been considerable debate as to whether the concentration of people into relatively small areas for cultivation and animal husbandry was initially beneficial for diet and health.[7] The way of life brought contact with new microorganisms that found the human body a suitable environment in which to feed and proliferate. Some pathogens have life cycles that would not be completed in nomadic people, and schistosomiasis probably started to cause sickness when humans began to live in settled communities near slow-moving water.[8] Cockburn referred to the risk of infestation with hookworm and ascarids because of living near exposed excreta; infections carried by rats, mice, ticks, fleas, and certain mosquitoes; and cross-species infections with diseases associated with denser populations.[9] Although living in one relatively small area could have reduced the variety of parasites to which humans were exposed, and tolerance would develop to those locally prevalent, trade and travel would eventually have led to contact with other forms of parasite.[10]

People living in settled communities became exposed to new infectious diseases as a result of proximity to exposed human and animal excreta. Diarrheal diseases transmitted by fecal contamination of hands, water, and food are likely to have occurred as communities became larger and waste was more difficult to avoid than in a nomadic way of life. Cohen noted the mixed blessings of some new sources of food, such as milk from domesticated cattle. This carried the risk of infection with *Mycobacterium bovis*, the cause of bovine tuberculosis, a disease that may have originally transferred to cattle from wild animals. The ability to store food would have brought nutritional benefits, although food could become contaminated with fungi, bacteria, and rodent feces.[11] Living in close proximity to rats also made communities vulnerable to bubonic plague, which originated from foci of infection among burrowing rodents. McNeill suggested that many diseases are likely to have transferred from rats and mice, and also from domesticated animals.[12] For example, measles is related to canine distemper, smallpox is related to cowpox, and influenza is shared by humans, pigs, and birds. As populations grew and became more dense, transmission of various bacterial and viral infections would have been sustained in the population without intermediate hosts. People became dependent on immune mechanisms for survival as well relying on agriculture for food. For some infectious diseases, the immune reaction ensured that when death did not occur, and there was recovery following elimination of the invading microorganism by antibodies, the immune mechanism would prevent the disease occurring again for a period of months, years, or throughout life.

The epidemic cycle of some infectious diseases became independent of the original animal source, and measles is the classic example of an airborne infectious disease that has become dependent on human population size and density. It became an acute disease of childhood among urban populations because most people first contracted the virus early in life and immunity is conveyed on those who survive. Statistical studies of how the disease propagates in modern urban communities identified a pattern of regularly occurring epidemics linked with the proportion of "new susceptibles" in the population who had not previously been infected.[13] The disease probably requires a population of at least 7,000 individuals, while 250,000 could be a critical threshold above which the virus can remain endemic. Smaller populations have been devastated by infection brought in from outside, when both children and adults have had no previous contact with the disease, and hence have no immunity.[14] Until relatively recently, many cities in industrialized countries experienced in-migration from rural areas, which contributed to higher population density. In the crowded living conditions conducive to transmission of infectious diseases, there was often an annual excess of deaths over births. Even so, populations continued to grow through in-migration, and some cities became large enough to sustain airborne infectious diseases. For example, smallpox became endemic in London before the 18th century. In addition to airborne infectious diseases and waterborne infections, insect-borne diseases such as typhus, and malaria in warmer climates, may have made urban life for many people less healthy than the life of hunter-gatherers in earlier times.

The effects of large-scale migration on infectious disease patterns are illustrated by European settlement in North America and migration through ports of entry such as New York and New Orleans, which had very transient populations.[15] More rapid population growth in these cities than elsewhere contributed to higher mortality because of inadequate quarantine measures for ships, the pressure on existing facilities, improper disposal of untreated sewage, and explosive growth of poor housing. Airborne, density-dependent infectious diseases such as smallpox and measles caused regular spikes in mortality. Respiratory tuberculosis became endemic and the biggest killer in the

19th century as in England and other European countries, while some other diseases were already endemic. Kunitz found that dysentery and malaria were the most significant of these between the first settlement and the end of the 18th century, while yellow fever eventually became endemic in urban populations.[16] This acute infection, caused by a flavivirus, is transmitted to humans and other primates by mosquitoes in Africa and Latin America, and an urban cycle developed in North America with the mosquito *Aedes aegypti* transmitting infection from person to person. Cholera also became a major killer during the 19th century, partly because the disease does not convey lasting immunity and people were vulnerable in successive epidemics.

Cholera and smallpox were involved in most of the regular mortality spikes in North America in the 19th century, together with some significant outbreaks of yellow fever and typhus. Yellow fever and typhoid became endemic and caused significant spikes in mortality in New York.[17] Together with cholera, these diseases were even greater contributors to overall mortality in New Orleans.[18] The endemic diseases became more demographically significant when airborne, density-dependent infectious diseases became predominantly diseases of childhood because survivors gained immunity. Smallpox was known as a severe epidemic disease affecting the Mid-Atlantic colonies most, followed by the South and New England.[19] The large spikes in mortality caused by this airborne, density-dependent infectious disease became less significant at the beginning of the 19th century despite more rapid population growth. In New York smallpox continued to produce mortality spikes until vaccination was widely used in the first few decades of the 19th century (the role of vaccination in controlling smallpox in England and other European countries is discussed in chapter 5).

Within Europe migration from areas of high incidence of infectious disease is likely to have increased mortality rates, along with migration to the expanding towns and cities where people sought to escape rural poverty and find new livelihoods. Many studies have considered other broad influences and economic, political, and military factors affecting the infectious disease environment. Flinn identified several general factors that could have reduced mortality in Europe in the 17th and 18th centuries.[20] A reduction in military activity and reorganization of armies that limited the sources of epidemics, greater military discipline and restraint in dealing with civilian populations, changes in naval warfare and efforts to improve hygiene on board ships could all have prevented deaths. Improvements in agriculture, including the settlement of new land, the use of crop rotation, and introduction of new crops from the Americas, probably contributed to increased food production in response to the needs of a growing population.

McNeill suggested that some of the agricultural changes in the period 1650–1750, such as the "new husbandry," had important consequences for the infectious disease environment. New crops provided feed for cattle on a scale not previously possible, leading to an expansion of meat and dairy production. This may have had ecological consequences such as the transfer of mosquitoes to feed on the larger population of cattle.[21] Malaria is likely to have been a major cause of death in preindustrial times, both directly and indirectly, being a chronic disease that increased susceptibility to other infectious diseases. Malaria does not feature separately in all the mortality records from Europe in the 18th century, although it was still an important cause of death in Sweden, for example. Major outbreaks were reported in parts of England, with cause of death being recorded as "ague." Drainage measures and agricultural changes probably contributed to declining mortality from the disease even before the downturn in overall mortality in the mid-18th century.[22] The decline of malaria in northern Europe contrasted with its continuing prevalence in warmer Mediterranean countries. In France with its mixed climate, the disease was still endemic in the 18th century. Administrative records from France for 1775 indicate a whole series of other infectious diseases, including influenza ("grippe"), dysentery, pneumonia, and a fever known as "military sweats." Records from Brittany in northwestern France from the 18th century also reveal regular epidemics of dysentery, fevers (most likely typhus and typhoid), and smallpox. These diseases continued to cause epidemics among the French peasantry in the late 18th century, while the chronic infectious disease tuberculosis was endemic.[23]

Most records from the 18th century showing cause of death are from northwestern Europe, with smallpox, tuberculosis, "fevers," epidemic childhood diseases, and gastrointestinal disorders being the main causes recorded. Kunitz noted the differential in overall death rates between countries in the northwest and those in the south and east of Europe in the 18th century, as well as differences in life expectancy between commoners and aristocrats.[24] Living conditions varied, and there was higher infant mortality in Germany and Spain in the second half of the 18th century compared with England, France, and Sweden in the northwest. There is evidence of higher mortality in areas of Europe that had large estates worked by an impoverished peasantry, and high mortality was associated with the deleterious consequences of exploitation of women for agricultural labor.[25] Mothers were required to work long hours; and being unable to breastfeed properly, they often used unhygienic "pacifiers," which probably contributed to gastrointestinal disorders among infants. Large estates were common in the south and east of Europe, while other areas where mortality declined in the 18th century were characterized by mixed arable and dairy farming on medium-sized landholdings. Epidemics caused by enteric pathogens (typhoid and paratyphoid), bacterial diseases, and viral infections may have been less frequent in parts of northwestern Europe due to the isolation of farms. Even so, dysentery could be devastating, as in Akershus in Norway, where about half the deaths between 1801 and 1815 were attributed to the disease. Together with smallpox, dysentery was the main disease recorded in years when the number of deaths exceeded the number of births. Records for 1785–1807 from one small port town, Larvik in Norway, indicate that 15% of deaths were attributed to dysentery.[26] Records indicate that plague, which had been devastating in the 17th century, did not reappear in many parts of Europe in the 18th century, although some port towns had major outbreaks.

Plague and Its Absence after the 17th Century

Different phases in the changing pattern of cause of death can be identified, although there is often considerable overlap in terms of the diseases that characterize different periods. The recession of the epidemics of plague that had terrorized Europe for three hundred years from the 14th through the 17th century, and its disappearance from England after the epidemic of the 1660s, prepared the way for a new era of epidemiological-demographic change. The reason for the recession of plague epidemics in Europe has been the subject of much research and debate, and it is important to consider explanations here in view of their possible relevance to the mortality transition that began in Europe in the 18th century.

The pandemic of 1347–49 known as the "Black Death" caused a dramatic reduction in the population of Europe that lasted for more than a century. Although the disease flourished in the overcrowded living conditions prevailing at that time, it is unlikely that the pandemic was mainly a consequence of population growth. Hatcher found that changes in the population of England in the preindustrial period between the 13th and the 17th century were largely due to changes in mortality. The major killers were epidemic diseases, and there was little association between changes in mortality and the economic standard of living.[27] The plague pandemic may have begun as a result of changes in trade patterns affecting contacts between the East and the West, and it is widely accepted that it had its origins in Russia. The plague bacillus, *Yersinia pestis,* is likely to have transferred from burrowing rodents to rats that found their way onto ships bound for European ports. The black rat, *Rattus rattus,* has been identified as the main carrier of fleas that can transmit the plague bacillus. Originally a native of India, it appears to have reached Europe in the 14th century where it rapidly replaced indigenous rats and flourished around human habitations.[28] In overcrowded and unhygienic living conditions, rat fleas separated from their usual host had the opportunity to transfer to humans to feed.

Fleas carried by rodents can become infected with *Y. pestis,* and these vectors would have caused the spread of the disease into Europe from Asia. Many different types of rodent have played a part in maintaining reservoirs of infection, such as marmots, susliks, and tarbagans in Siberia and Mongolia.[29] During the winter, bacteria probably survive in the tissues of rodents that only have mild infections, and irrespective of the type of host, bacilli would spread to other rodents via fleas. Burnet suggested it was reasonably certain that when the epidemic of 1348–49 was developing in England, transmission of the bacillus from rats to humans via fleas was superseded by human to human transmission, either via fleas or by airborne transmission of bacilli in the pneumonic form of plague. Pneumonic plague can develop when bacilli reach the lungs in severe cases of infection and produce pneumonia.[30] In certain circumstances the bacteria can then be transmitted to other people via airborne droplets, resulting in pneumonia, which in turn can be transmitted to others. Transmission becomes much more rapid, making pneumonic plague one of the most lethal forms of infectious disease.

The plague epidemic of 1348–49 in England eventually ran its course, but not before over a quarter of the population had died.[31] The population of Europe probably did not recover until the 15th century, but increased steadily during the 16th century. The period 1565–85 in England was noticeably free of epidemic spikes in mortality. Although population growth was quite rapid, most of the growth was only recovery from the effects of the Black Death. Between that pandemic and the major plague epidemics in the 17th century, outbreaks continued to occur in some parts of Europe and the Mediterranean. It is possible that infection remained prevalent among the rat population, causing epidemics when living conditions deteriorated and allowed rat fleas to transfer to humans to feed. However, in the 17th century there were particularly cold winters in Europe that could have killed off rat fleas carrying *Y. pestis*, and infection may have been reintroduced from outside. People living in overcrowded rat-infested conditions near ports or along trade routes from Asia were particularly vulnerable. In the early stages of the pandemic it was recognized that the disease had spread rapidly from outside Europe, across the Continent, from town to town and from house to house. As early as 1347, city authorities in Italy tried to prevent travelers coming from areas where the disease had been reported.[32] Despite a widely held religious view and fatalism that plague was a manifestation of "God's anger at man's sinfulness," people began to organize practical protective measures.[33] Over the next few centuries a more rational response developed with prevention and control measures based on systematic surveillance and authorities being given powers to enforce segregation and isolation of the infected.[34]

Information coming from other areas provided early warning of possible epidemics, and knowledge increased about how the disease spread from Asia to Europe. This eventually led to the implementation of a cordon sanitaire along the border between the Hapsburg Empire and the Ottoman Empire in the 18th century. Civil reports on plague incidence in Asia provided a basis for deploying soldiers to at-risk areas to conduct routine border patrols, procedures that took many years to develop. Other measures introduced for the protection of town populations included stationing a watch at the gates to screen travelers coming from plague-affected areas. The draconian measure of enforced isolation of households where cases had occurred aroused both hostility and support.[35] Although it was attempted in England in the major epidemic in the 1660s, it is unlikely to have been effective as rats could move from house to house in search of food. The London Bills of Mortality recorded 97,306 deaths in 1665, and about two-thirds (68,596) were directly attributed to plague. Many more deaths are likely to have been assigned to other ill-defined categories.[36] An estimated 7–20% of the population of London died in the epidemic, which was the last major outbreak of plague in England.

Understandably there was considerable concern in Britain as a whole that plague could be reintroduced from abroad. Once plague reached northwestern Europe, it was likely to reach England because of the frequent trade and shipping contacts.[37] Port sanitary authorities were given powers to remove infected people to a "hospital." Information networks provided early warning of outbreaks in Baltic and Mediterranean ports, and orders were issued against ships coming to Britain from several infected areas after the 1660s. Elsewhere in Europe, quarantine and other preventive measures were not always effective, and a disastrous outbreak of plague occurred in Marseilles in 1720, in which an estimated 50,000 people died.[38] Quarantine retained its particular importance for Britain after the recession of plague in Europe in the 18th century, because of its trade with many countries outside Europe that had not adopted the measure.[39] Plague remained a major threat, with a disastrous epidemic occurring in Canton and Hong Kong as late as 1894 when an estimated 90,000 people died.[40] Port authorities in Britain became increasingly active in the control of communicable diseases in the last three decades of the 19th century following the cholera epidemic in the 1860s.[41] However, thousands of ships arrived each year at many different ports. Standards of monitoring are likely to have varied, and some steamships on their way to England from Asia were able to bypass European ports that had quarantine controls. A small outbreak of plague occurred in Essex in 1909, after an absence of the disease from the country for over two centuries.[42]

Many studies have considered other possible explanations for the recession of plague in Europe, such as changes in the rodent population that carried fleas infected with *Y. pestis.* The black rat has been identified as the main carrier of fleas that can transmit the plague bacillus when they transfer to humans to feed. However, the displacement of the black rat by the brown rat has been discounted as an explanation for the recession of plague, as the brown rat appears to have been predominant in London in the 18th century.[43] The brown rat, *Rattus norvegicus,* which was less inclined to nest close to humans, probably did not arrive in England until the 1720s.[44] Although the susceptible rat population could have been reduced by plague, wild rodents in remote areas continued to act as a reservoir of infection in parts of Asia where the disease still persists today. Eventually, improvements in hygiene and housing conditions in Europe would have reduced exposure to rodents and fleas, but significant changes came much too late to account for the absence of plague in England in the 18th century. There is unlikely to have been any significant improvement in housing conditions with regard to rat infestation and overcrowding that might account for the absence of plague, and typhus with a similar mode of transmission was still a major killer in the poorer areas of English towns as late as the mid-19th century (see chapter 6).

The fact that plague epidemics continued to cause massive mortality in some European cities in the 18th century indicates that the virulence of *Y. pestis* had not diminished. Although mild infection might allow survival of people with some immunity, there appears to be no convincing evidence that this resulted in a level of herd immunity that could account for the recession of epidemics. The possibility of a buildup of immunity in human populations through centuries of contact seems inconsistent with the occurrence of outbreaks of plague in parts of Asia that have always been a major focus of the disease. However, other ecoimmunological changes relating to the prevalence of different forms of bacillus might have played a part in the recession of plague. Three main varieties of *Y. pestis* have been found to cause plague in Asia, and these have antigens in common with a closely related bacillus, *Yersinia pseudotuberculosis.* This microorganism is relatively innocuous to humans, producing a mild disease with fever and abdominal pain, especially in children. It is possible that infection with *Y. pseudotuberculosis* conveys cross-immunity to *Y. pestis,* giving both humans and rats immunity to plague. This particular bacillus only recently became widespread, as did a further related bacillus, *Yersinia enterocolitica,* although this suggests that transformations could have occurred in the past. It is possible that a milder form of bacillus with an ecological advantage over *Y. pestis* became predominant, conveying cross-immunity to plague and contributing to its recession.[45]

The hypothesis of cross-immunity would be difficult to test historically, while there is much documented evidence indicating that human intervention is a plausible and sufficient explanation for the recession of plague in Europe.[46] Although human intervention and cross-immunity are not mutually exclusive as explanations, preventive intervention based on monitoring epidemics, restricting people's movements, isolating the infected, and enforcing quarantine of ships could by itself explain the absence of plague in England after the 1660s, and the recession in Europe in the 18th century. Preventive measures were developed over many centuries, and it seems plausible that they gradually became effective enough to control the disease. The rationale for public health intervention, developed through attempts to prevent the spread of plague epidemics,[47] arguably lent support to the development of preventive interventions that eliminated smallpox and cholera from England by the end of the 19th century (see chapters 5 and 6).

Infectious Diseases in England in the 18th Century

Apart from the absence of plague in the 18th century, the main cause-groups to which deaths were attributed in England and other European countries were similar to those recorded in the 17th century, with smallpox being particularly prominent. McNeill suggested that smallpox had spread to Europe by the 16th century with the expansion of sea trade and the development of commerce, which led to regular contact between all the principal centers of population worldwide.[48] Smallpox epidemics occurred regularly throughout Europe, and the disease directly caused at least 1 in 10 and possibly 1 in 5 deaths in the 18th century.[49] Records from Geneva for the periods 1730–39 and 1775–86 indicate that smallpox was endemic, with up to 10% of deaths regularly attributed to the disease.[50] In national records from Sweden for 1779–82, specific causes were identified for about half of all deaths, with 10% of deaths attributed to smallpox and 10–11% to tuberculosis.[51] Data from southern Sweden confirm the importance of these diseases over a longer period, 1749–1801.[52] National records for Finland indicate that over 40% of deaths were attributed to specified infectious diseases in the 18th century.[53] For the years 1751–60, the six main specified diseases were smallpox/measles (12.8%), whooping cough (6.9%), pulmonary tuberculosis (8.4%), typhus (9.5%), dysentery (2.8%), and malaria (2.1%).

The London Bills of Mortality indicate that plague had periodically caused massive mortality, although smallpox epidemics were a much more regular check on population growth (fig. 3.1). In the period 1701–1800, 40% of all deaths recorded in the London Bills were attributed to smallpox, "consumption," and "fevers," with the proportion in each decade ranging from 34–47%. The proportion of deaths involving "convulsions" increased from 5% to 30% between the 1650s and the 1730s, and Creighton suggested that many of these deaths would previously have been recorded in the category "infancy" (deaths at ages under two years). After the 1730s, the decline in the convulsions death rate made a major contribution to overall mortality decline (see fig. 3.1 and chapter 5). Dysentery and other diarrheal diseases are also likely to have been significant causes of death, as in other parts of Europe, and Creighton suggested that deaths classified as "griping of the guts," "bloody flux," and "surfeit" probably involved gastrointestinal infections.[54] These categories accounted for 5.5% of all deaths recorded in the London Bills in the 1650s, and this portion rose to 17.0% and 13.8%, respectively, in the 1670s and 1680s, the two decades after the last plague epidemic. The decline to 1.4% of total deaths by the 1730s may be due in part to a transfer of recording to other categories.

The main categories to which deaths were consistently assigned in the London Bills of Mortality were smallpox, consumption (mostly respiratory tuberculosis), "fevers,"and infant deaths often attributed to "convulsions" (table 3.1). These are comparable to the main categories in the bills for Northampton and Carlisle (table 3.2). The Northampton data indicate that smallpox epidemics were the main cause of spikes in the annual number of deaths in the 18th century (see fig. 5.3). The bills available for Carlisle for eight years between 1779 and 1787 were compiled by Heysham at his medical practice in the town.[55] Over 50% of deaths were attributed to specified infectious diseases typical of other records from northwestern Europe, including smallpox, consumption, measles, whooping cough, thrush, and jaundice. The broad category of "fevers" was subdivided into inflammatory, nervous, putrid, worm, and jail fever (typhus). The proportion of deaths attributed to consumption in Carlisle (13.3%) was within the range for London in the 18th century (10–25%), although lower than for London and Northampton in the period 1779–87. The higher proportion of deaths attributed to smallpox in Carlisle (14.7%) could reflect epidemic variation or Heysham's greater awareness of different manifestations of the disease. The detailed breakdown of deaths by cause and age indicates that most smallpox deaths were among children under age five (appendix B). These bills, together with some parish records showing deaths attributed to smallpox (see chapter 5) and aggregated data for several hundred parishes, provide valuable evidence of changing patterns of mortality spikes, the onset of mortality decline in the mid-18th century, and natural population growth (baptisms minus burials), which are considered further in the next chapter.

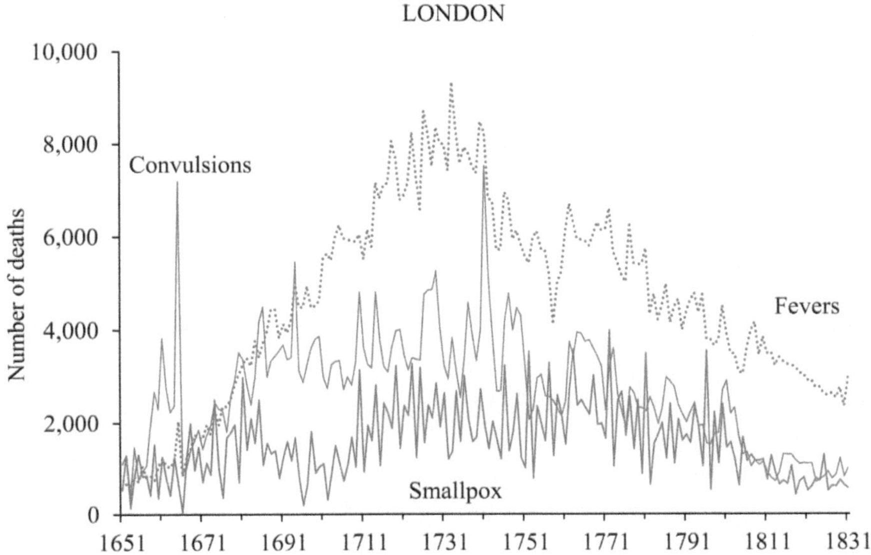

Figure 3.1. Annual deaths in the area of the London Bills of Mortality recorded as due to smallpox, fevers, and convulsions, 1651–1831. *Source:* Marshall, *Mortality in the Metropolis.*

Table 3.1. Percentage of deaths in different cause groups in the London Bills of Mortality, 1650–1829

	Percentage of all deaths in 50-year period			
Cause of death recorded	1650–99	1700–1749	1750–99	1800–1829
Measles	0.5	0.7	1.1	3.2
Whooping cough	—	—	1.5	3.2
Smallpox	5.9	7.6	9.7	5.0
Consumption[a]	16.0	14.2	21.8	23.4
Asthma/tissik	—	1.9	1.9	3.6
Fevers	11.4	11.5	12.8	6.4
Dropsy	3.9	3.2	4.3	4.3
Rickets	1.8	0.6	0.0	0.0
Convulsions/teething	17.6	33.0	28.3	19.0
Apoplexy/sudden death	0.5	0.7	1.1	1.9
Old age	5.5	8.1	6.7	8.7
Abortion/stillborn	2.8	2.8	3.2	3.3
Griping of the guts[b]	8.5	2.1	—	—
Plague[c]	6.9	—	—	—
All above causes	81.3	86.4	92.4	82.0
Average annual deaths	20,414	24,467	20,874	19,544

Source: Marshall, *Mortality in the Metropolis.*

[a] Consumption probably includes some other respiratory and wasting diseases as well as tuberculosis.

[b] Recording of deaths in this category gradually declined until 1739.

[c] Of the 70,882 deaths attributed to plague between 1650 and 1699, 68,596 occurred in 1665 and 1,998 in 1666.

Table 3.2. Cause-specific deaths as a percentage of all deaths for Carlisle, London, and Northampton, 1779–87

	Percentage of all recorded deaths		
Cause recorded	Carlisle	London	Northampton
Infant deaths	13.2	24.9	17.9*
Fevers	11.2	12.5	10.3
Dropsy	3.0	4.6	7.6
Measles	1.9	1.1	3.3
Whooping cough	1.2	1.4	0.8
Scarlet fever	2.4	†	†
Thrush	4.0	†	0.4
Smallpox	14.7	9.4	8.2
Consumption (TB)	13.3	24.0	19.8
Asthma	1.7	1.5	1.1
Apoplexy	2.0	1.2	1.0
Palsy	0.9	0.3	1.0
Old age	14.0	6.5	9.8
Accidents	1.8	0.6	1.0
Other and unknown	14.7	12.0	17.8
Total deaths	1,615	175,143	828

Sources: Lonsdale, *Life of John Heysham MD*; Marshall, *Mortality in the Metropolis*; Northampton Bills of Mortality (1779–87).

Note: Data are missing for 1780 in Carlisle and 1787 in Northampton.

* "Fits" included in Northampton Bills.

† Cause not specified until later bills.

Chapter Four

Mortality Decline, Food, and Population Growth

"Standard of Living" and Nutrition

Despite many limitations of the records showing cause of death and some degree of inaccuracy in the level of cause-specific mortality, the historical data indicate that infectious diseases predominated in the mid-18th century when overall mortality began to decline in England and other parts of Europe. Wrigley and Schofield's analysis of aggregated data from several hundred parishes in England confirmed the findings of earlier studies that mortality in England declined from the mid-18th century. All of the 11 severe mortality crises (30% above trend) occurred before 1750, and the last secondary crisis (20–30% above trend) was in 1762–63. After 1802–3 there were only two years in which mortality was more than 10% above the trend level, in 1846–47 and 1848–49.[1] Figure 4.1 shows the dramatic change in the pattern of annual fluctuations in the crude death rate from the 1740s, and the greatly diminished spikes in annual mortality compared with earlier years. The death rate had generally been lower than the birthrate between 1540 and 1640, and population may have approached the limit that could be fed given the land available and the state of agricultural technology. Although there does not appear to have been an increase in subsistence crises, the increase in demand would have led to increased food prices, exacerbating poverty.[2] From the 1740s, the more rapid population growth put further pressure on food supplies, which had to be increased just to maintain existing levels of average consumption per capita.

Wrigley and Schofield found that short-term variations in mortality were determined by factors other than food supply and there was little correlation between food supply and mortality over the long run.[3] Using their aggregate data, Fogel found that less than 10% of "crisis mortality" (50–100% above normal) in England between 1541 and 1871 was due to famines, and that the decline in mortality was not due primarily to a reduction in "crisis mortality," whether caused by famines or not.[4] About three-quarters of the decline between 1726–50 and 1851–71 was due to a reduction in underlying mortality, excluding

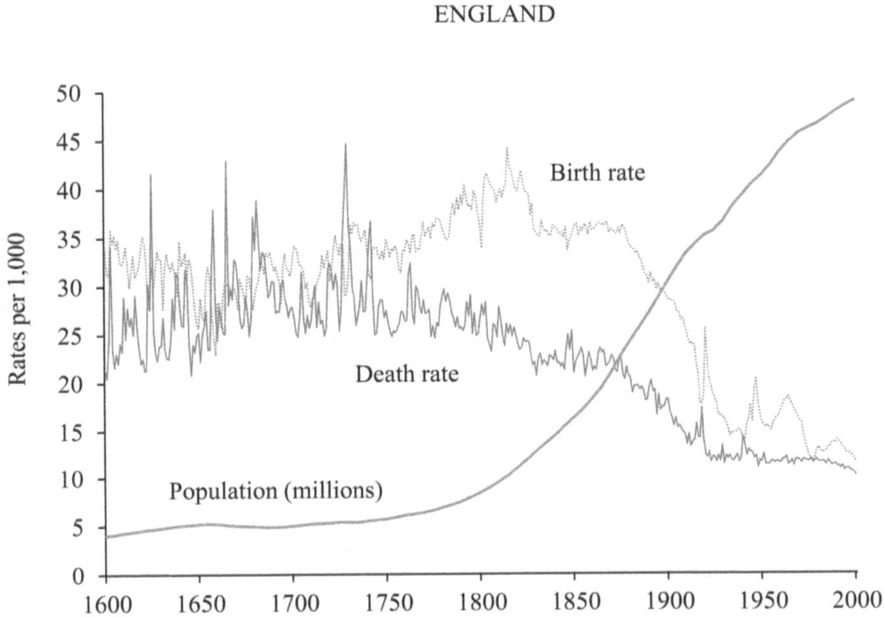

Figure 4.1. Annual crude death rates and birth rates in England, 1600–2000. *Source:* Wrigley and Schofield, *Population History of England,* 531–35.

excess in "mortality crises." His statistical analysis suggested that over 80% of the decline in mortality between 1775–99 and 1850–74, and half of the decline between 1875–99 and 1950–74, was associated with changes in height and body mass index, indicating improved nutritional status.[5] However, he emphasized that these anthropometric measures reflect net nutrition, the balance between nutrient intake (diet) and the body's nutrient requirements for vital systems to function at rest, to combat disease, and for activity including work. He recognized that the high prevalence of infectious diseases would have caused malnutrition even if diets had been high in calories, proteins, and other critical nutrients, which was certainly not the case for lower socioeconomic groups.[6] A hypothesis that physiological changes reflect a reduction in the level of chronic malnutrition, which contributed significantly to mortality decline,[7] has to take into account the effect on nutritional status of changes in the infectious disease environment.

McKeown had concluded that the decline in mortality and more rapid population growth in England were due largely to improvements in the "standard of living" and nutrition, although he recognized the importance of purer water supplies and sanitation. Although he could not find direct evidence that diet had improved, he speculated that increased food supplies led to better nutrition and improved resistance to infectious diseases, causing a sustained decline in the death rate and population growth.[8] His thesis has been summarized as follows: "Population growth was not influenced by improved sanitation before about 1870 or by specific medical measures before the introduction of sulfonamides in 1935. . . . The rise of population in the eighteenth and early nineteenth centuries [was due] to a decline of mortality which resulted from improvement of diet . . . [through] a large increase in food production."[9] McKeown's analysis of mortality decline relied on national registration data, with little reference to evidence of important changes in disease, mortality, and economic circumstances between the mid-18th and mid-19th century. Other studies had found no consistent association between changes in economic indicators and phases of rapid population growth.[10] The specific issues for his explanation would be whether changes in mortality before the long-term decline were associated with changes in food supply and access to food, whether any significant increase in food consumption per capita corresponded with the main turning points in the overall death rate, and whether any improvement in diet would have reduced case fatality from major epidemic diseases. Shortages of food and malnutrition would have contributed to the risk of children dying from acute infectious diseases that are still prevalent, such as measles, as in developing countries today.[11] However, even members of the well-fed aristocracy and royalty were at high risk in epidemics of smallpox and typhus. These two diseases were major contributors to spikes in the annual death rate in excess of 35 per 1,000 in the first half of the 18th century. In London the annual number of deaths from smallpox leveled off from the 1740s, and deaths attributed to "fevers," including typhus, declined, thus contributing to the decline in overall mortality (see fig. 3.1).

The movement of people to the towns and increasing contacts between rural populations and town dwellers favored more widespread transmission of infectious diseases such as smallpox, typhus, and tuberculosis. In the hundred years before the downturn in mortality, the increase is likely to have been due to changes in the infectious disease environment rather than adverse changes in food supplies. Studies in Scandinavia indicated that smallpox epidemics occurred independently of fluctuations in harvest yields, and there was little correlation between bread prices and the number of smallpox deaths.[12] There was no consistent association between higher food prices and spikes in overall mortality in England in the first half of the 18th century, and the country was not significantly affected by harvest failure. Even before this, overall burial rates in England were not consistently associated with changes in food output.[13] There may have been more association between spikes in mortality, harvest failure, and food shortages in other parts of Europe,[14] and short-term effects of harvest failure on mortality and fertility continued to act as a check on population growth in the poorer regions of Europe in the 18th century.[15] In the more developed areas, reduced incidence of harvest failure and food shortage is likely to have reduced mortality spikes linked with typhus, while smallpox with its more independent cycle of epidemics and other infectious diseases continued to be a major cause of mortality spikes, as in England.[16]

When mortality decline began in the mid-18th century, the increase in population would have put further pressure on food supplies in many parts of Europe. Subdivision of small holdings is unlikely to have increased supplies without an increase in yield per acre, and use of less fertile land appears to have been less common in the west compared with the east of Europe.[17] Data from Scandinavia suggest that per capita food consumption did not increase before the mid-19th century,[18] and the decline in mortality before this occurred in regions that differed socioeconomically and geographically, as it did in France.[19] In England enclosure of lands caused much social disruption and poverty among people evicted from land on which they depended for food. The introduction of new crops such as the potato, corn, and buckwheat may have reduced famine crises because crops were less susceptible to weather damage.[20] However, an increase in potato growing in the first four decades of the 19th century when population was growing more rapidly may only have provided a substitute for other foods, and per capita consumption of wheat flour declined between the 1770s and 1830s.[21] Imports contributed to food supplies,[22] which probably became more regular from the early 18th century onward. Even so, supplies may only have kept pace with the demands of a growing population, and there is little evidence of improvement in the diet of most people in England between 1750 and 1850 in terms of quality or daily calories per capita.[23]

Fogel suggested that contrary to Malthusian predictions, population and food supply had been maintained in equilibrium in England through a reduction in body size as well as higher mortality.[24] Estimates of average daily calorie consumption indicated that mature adults in England must have been very small in the 18th century to have had sufficient energy for economic production, and up to 20% of the population may have been unable to contribute significantly because of their extremely poor diet.[25] Fogel suggested that the annual aggregate food supply in England had actually been sufficient to prevent subsistence crises since the 16th century. However, with an unregulated market for grain, as well as gross inequalities in income and in sources of wealth, particularly land, the price of food frequently became prohibitive for people in lower socioeconomic groups during subsistence crises. There were government efforts to gain control of surplus grain and sell it at a reduced price in times of shortage, but these were inadequate even when measures were implemented more widely in the 1630s.[26] Food relief initiatives were abandoned after this, and although food shortages may have become more localized after a national crisis in the 1690s,[27] there were periodic famines and food riots in the 18th century.

Local food shortages exacerbated epidemics of infectious diseases, with large numbers of vagrants, homeless, and unemployed people fostering the spread of disease from these foci.[28] The risk of contracting the louse-borne disease typhus increased during food shortages and famines because of social disruption, deteriorating living conditions, and neglect of personal hygiene. The body louse transmitting infection would have transferred from rats to humans when people were scavenging for food in times of shortage and high prices. An analysis of data from London indicated an association between high bread prices and deaths from typhus ("spotted fever").[29] From the mid-18th century, national and local governments once again moved toward intervention in the grain market, and the system of poor relief was expanded. A more regular food supply and better distribution would have alleviated some of the conditions that fostered typhus epidemics. Improvements in transportation infrastructure such as canals, harbors, navigation aids, roads, and bridges enabled food distribution and alleviation of local shortages through development of "famine relief" interventions.[30] By the mid-19th century, greater government control over food stocks and prices had eliminated famines in England.[31]

Evidence of changes in nutritional status in relation to mortality decline comes from studies of average height based on records for subsets of the population of England and other European countries.[32] Again, it is important to emphasize that many exogenous and environmental factors determine physical growth as well as food intake, including climate, clothing, shelter, work, sanitation, and the experience of infectious diseases. The nutritional and health status of the mother also affects her child's birthweight, physical growth, mental development, and future health. Maternity care and health during pregnancy are known to affect the birth weight of a child and its chances of survival.[33] The efficiency of the body in utilizing nutrients is a further influence on physical development, and the ability to ingest and convert food into nutrients, energy, and growth can be adversely affected by gastrointestinal and other infections. Stature is a function of proximate determinants such as diet and "catch-up" growth after a period of deprivation, but it also depends on work and disease episodes, both of which make competing demands on nutrients required for physical growth.[34]

Interpretation of trends in average height in the 18th and 19th centuries has been controversial, although it is recognized that an increase does not necessarily reflect an improvement in diet and nutrition.[35] Different methods of analysis of pooled data for marine recruits from poor backgrounds between 1770 and 1870, and military recruits between 1740 and 1914, raised doubts about any increase in average height in the second half of the 18th century.[36] There is more certainty that average height was higher for those born between 1790 and 1820, and a few centimeters lower for those born between 1820 and 1850.[37] Evidence from studies of other subsets of the population in Britain supports the view that average height was lower for those born in the second quarter of the 19th century.[38] After this setback, average height of military recruits increased slowly over successive birth cohorts born in the second half of the 19th century, while the increase among conscripts in some other European countries was more rapid.[39] In the first half of the 20th century, average height for five-year-old boys increased in different towns in England and Wales, and data from Leeds indicate similar trends for boys and girls.[40]

The lower average height found among boys and young men born in London and other towns in the second quarter of the 19th century probably reflects the effects of rapid urbanization and adverse changes in the infectious disease environment. Floud and colleagues found that much of the decline in average height was due mainly to a decline in urban areas. As men born in towns were shorter on average than those born in rural areas, it might be expected that an increase in the proportion of the national population being born in towns would have reduced national average height.[41] The increasingly crowded living conditions and higher density of population in the poorer areas of towns were conducive to rapid transmission of infectious diseases. However, the introduction of vaccination dramatically reduced smallpox mortality in the first quarter of the 19th century (see chapter 5). Average height was higher between 1790 and 1820 when population growth in England was at its peak. There was a resurgence of smallpox in the second quarter, and a reduction in average height compared with the previous quarter may reflect increased incidence of this severe infectious disease. Records indicate that children who had experienced an attack of smallpox grew to be shorter on average than those who had not had the disease. For each of the ages between 14 and 17, there was a difference of a few centimeters in the most frequently recorded height (mode) between the two groups, despite a similar composition in terms of the proportion of children from "disadvantaged" backgrounds.[42]

The studies of average height of boys and men in England found large differences between those from different social backgrounds.[43] The shorter height of those from poorer backgrounds is consistent with evidence of much higher mortality rates. Contemporary reports indicated large differences in child survival between socioeconomic groups in the 1840s. An estimated 90% of children of the gentry survived to their first birthday, compared with 80% among tradespeople, and 68% among factory operatives. Rates of survival to 5 years of age were 82%, 62%, and 45%, respectively. An estimated 63% of the gentry would have lived for 40 years, compared with only about 20% of the children of factory operatives.[44] Survival chances in families not supported by regular work and for those in workhouses are likely to have been even worse. Although workers in some occupations may have benefited from rising real wages in the second half of the 19th century, the living conditions of the poor in Manchester in the 1840s led Engels to accuse the ruling classes of "social murder" for not taking action.[45] The majority of people in industrial towns still lived in appalling conditions, and many had no regular work. Reduction in the population of vagrants, homeless, and unemployed people as a result of confining them in workhouses is unlikely to have reduced death rates because of the high risk of infectious disease, particularly tuberculosis (see chapter 9).

Long-term trends in real wages and other indicators of people's economic standard of living do not indicate consistent improvements that might have allowed better diet and nutrition and hence improved resistance to infectious diseases. Although real wages of many manual workers may have increased in the first half of the 18th century, studies indicate stagnation or decline for these and other workers in the second half of the century when mortality was declining.[46] Food prices may actually have increased in this period of more rapid population growth.[47] In the first half of the 19th century, there is evidence that real wages increased for many occupational groups, although some of this might be due to deflation following the Napoleonic Wars.[48] There is also evidence that real wages of farm laborers did not increase very much, with only a 25% increase over the 30-year period 1820–50.[49] Many people in rural areas still suffered "crushing poverty," even in the so-called golden age of agricultural prosperity from 1850 to 1873, a period of rising real wages for many of the working poor in the towns.[50] In the period 1872–96, families of many workingmen may have been better off despite higher rents, as wages increased and food prices fell.[51] Even so, there was still no consistent association between economic standard of living and mortality, and the death rate continued to decline when real wages were falling at the beginning of the 20th century.

The disclosures of Booth and Rowntree at the beginning of the 20th century appear to have had little influence on the government's "laissez-faire" attitude toward poverty.[52] Investigations just prior to World War I revealed continuingly low standards of nutrition among women, children, and much of the working class, which were only alleviated as a result of food rationing and virtually full employment during the war.[53] In contrast, higher socioeconomic groups and the wealthy are likely to have been well-fed throughout the 18th and 19th centuries, and improved nutrition is unlikely to explain the increase in their life expectancy. A plausible explanation for national mortality decline must take into account improvements among the peerage, which are unlikely to have been due to changes in their economic circumstances, food availability, or nutrition. Estimates for the British peerage indicate that average life expectancy at birth (e0) among females remained around 33 years from the 14th to the 17th century, then increased from 36.7 years in 1725–49 to 45.7 in 1750–74, 51.7 in 1800–24, and 58.4 years in 1825–49.[54] For the population of England as a whole, Wrigley and Schofield estimated that life expectancy at birth was around 30 years in the 17th century and increased to 35–40 in the second half of the 18th century.[55] After 1800 there was a more sustained increase in average life expectancy throughout the 19th century (fig. 4.2). There is little evidence of any consistent improvement in the economic standard of living or diet of the majority of people in England that might have contributed significantly to the decline in mortality between the mid-18th and mid-19th century.

Mortality Decline, Fertility, and Population Growth

From the mid-18th century the declining death rate diverged from the birthrate (see fig. 4.3) in the demographic transition that lasted until the mid-20th century. Rates of population growth in England were higher in all decades of the 19th century than in any earlier period. The highest growth rates were in the first three decades when annual spikes in mortality were greatly diminished and the birthrate remained high. In other European countries for which data are available, such as Norway and Sweden, there was a continuous gap between the birthrate and the death rate from the 1810s when smallpox vaccination was widely adopted (see chapter 5 and fig. 5.11). Population increased by about 1.5% per

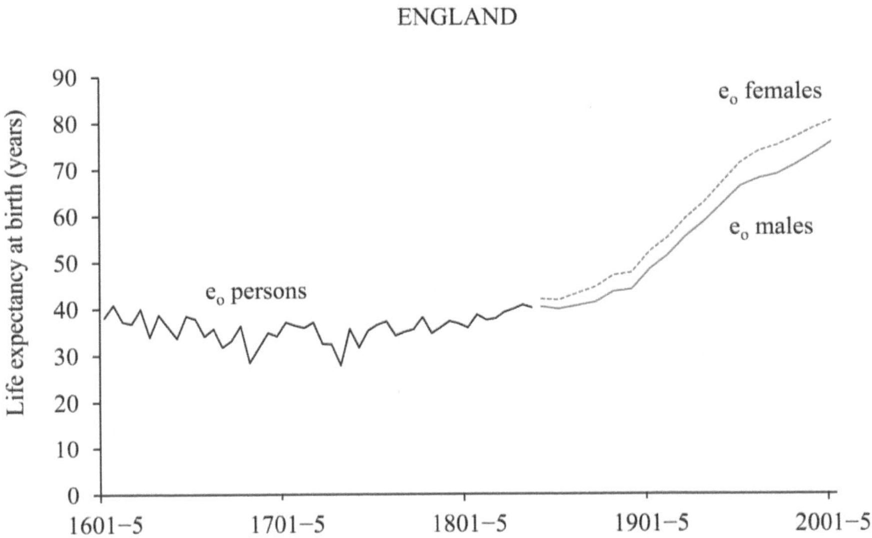

Figure 4.2. Estimates of life expectancy at birth (eo) in England for 5-year periods: 1601–5 to 2001–5. *Sources:* Wrigley and Schofield, *Population History of England,* 531–35; Preston, Keyfitz, and Schoen. *Life Tables for National Populations,* 224–66. Office for National Statistics "Report: Decennial life tables," 110.

year on average in England, and by over 1% per year in many European countries. The total population of Europe increased by an estimated 29% between 1750 and 1800, and by 47% between 1800 and 1850, and again between 1850 and 1900.[56] The growth rate in the 19th century was unprecedented, although more recent growth rates in some countries of the Middle East and Africa have been much higher due to the lack of decline in fertility rates.

The contribution of changes in mortality and fertility to more rapid population growth differed among European countries, and the relative contribution of mortality decline was greater in Sweden and France than in England, where fertility increased.[57] Wrigley and Schofield estimated that the gross reproduction rate (GRR), which takes into account the number of women of reproductive age, remained around 2.2–2.3 between 1701 and 1756, then increased continuously to reach a peak of 3.0 in 1816. They suggested that the increase was linked with changing marriage patterns,[58] and there is some evidence of a lower age at marriage.[59] Short-term variations in marriage rates and fertility were associated with variations in real wages and the economic standard of living,[60] and a later study found a lag of 15–20 years, which suggested that changes in real wages may have affected the ability to save for marriage.[61]

The increase in the birthrate in England in the second half of the 18th century was exceptional in the context of increasing food prices. However, epidemics as

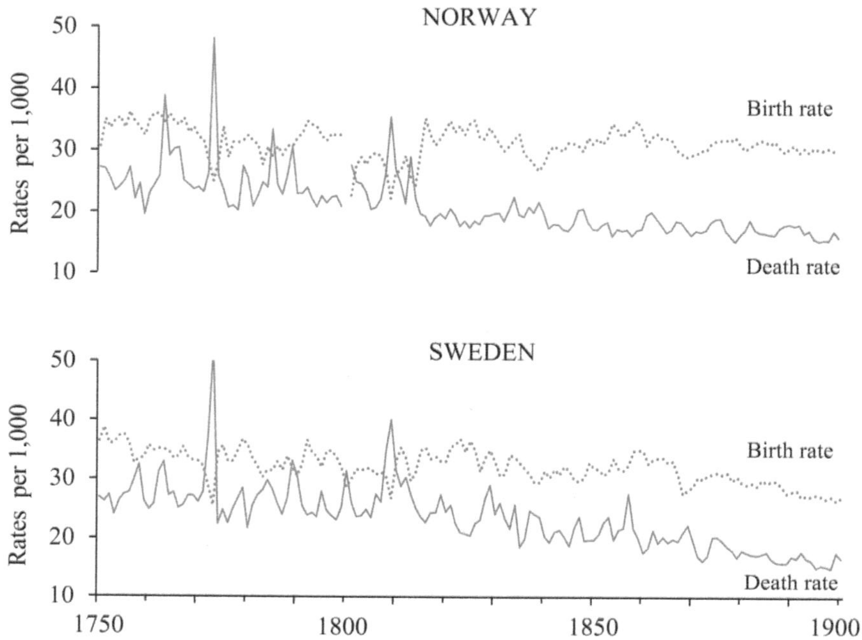

Figure 4.3. Annual crude death rates and birth rates in Norway and Sweden, 1750–1900. *Source:* National records in Mitchell, *European Historical Statistics*, 104–119.

well as food shortages affected people of reproductive age, and a decline in the number of baptisms following mortality crises is a well-known demographic feature of preindustrial Europe.[62] Short-term changes in the birthrate in England were negatively associated with fluctuations in the death rate, and sharp dips in fertility became less frequent from the mid-18th century along with the reduction in mortality spikes. Of the 15 years in which the birthrate fell more than 10% below a 25-year moving average, 13 occurred before the 1740s.[63] After 1802, the birthrate did not fall this low in any year, and the pattern of annual birthrates and death rates became much less subject to short-term fluctuation. There were regular spikes in the annual death rate in the period 1541–1741 reaching 35–40 per 1,000 in some years, while after the 1740s the death rate reached 30 per 1,000 in only 3 years, all in the 1760s. Flinn noted that the decline in death rates from the mid-18th century in European countries reflected a changing pattern of annual fluctuation, with less frequent and diminished spikes in mortality.[64] The long series of registration data for Sweden and Norway indicate that the pattern of annual fluctuations in death rates changed dramatically after 1800, with greatly diminished spikes creating a wide divergence from the birthrate (fig. 4.3). Changes in the population growth rate in Sweden between 1750 and 1850 were consistently due to falling mortality—as in France, where fertility declined consistently.[65] The greatly diminished spikes in mortality and declining death rate in England contributed to exceptionally rapid population growth (see fig. 4.1).

In the next chapter, the changing pattern of mortality spikes in the 18th and 19th centuries is considered in the context of increasing efforts to prevent smallpox. In rural areas, smallpox epidemics occurred at longer intervals of several years, and children were more likely to grow up without contracting the disease. Consequently, many adolescents and young adults were either killed or severely debilitated when an epidemic did occur. Razzell suggested that smallpox could have reduced marriage rates and increased childlessness as a result of male sterility.[66] Studies in India have indicated a much higher incidence of azoospermia (absence of viable sperm) among men who survived smallpox infection.[67] Childlessness among the British peerage increased from about 14% in the 17th century to 23% in the 1740s when smallpox was at its peak, after which it declined to around 18–19% by the end of the 18th century. The average number of children per married female declined from about 5 in 1550 to 3.5 in 1724, then increased to 5 by 1815.[68] It is very unlikely that these changes in fertility among the peerage were due to changes in their economic standard of living, and equally unlikely that increases in their average life expectancy were due to improved nutrition. These broad trends in fertility and mortality among the peerage correspond with the rise and fall of smallpox in England. Regular epidemics caused high mortality and severe debility among all strata of society, and the rise and decline of the disease had enormous repercussions for health and population. The changing pattern of smallpox epidemics, with increasing mortality up to the 1740s and a sharp decline after 1800 when vaccination was introduced, had a major epidemiological-demographic impact, as discussed in the next chapter.

Chapter Five

Smallpox

The mortality decline in England between the mid-18th and the mid-19th century does not appear to have coincided with any consistent improvement in the economic standard of living, and there is no convincing evidence of a significant improvement in diet and nutrition that could have increased resistance to the major infectious diseases. The pattern of cause of death in England and other parts of Europe in the 18th century was characterized by severe infectious diseases such as smallpox, typhus, typhoid, dysentery, and tuberculosis. Although plague caused a dramatic reduction in population in the 14th century, and periodically massive mortality until the 1660s, the recession of the disease did not result in more rapid population growth. By the end of the 17th century in England and other European countries, epidemics of smallpox had become a much more regular cause of high mortality checking population growth, and many towns would not have grown much without in-migration. Data from towns in the British Isles and from Sweden and Finland presented by Razzell indicate 8–20% of all deaths were directly attributed to smallpox in the first half of the 18th century (table 5.1).[1]

With the growth of towns, the number and concentration of people who had not previously been infected with smallpox ("new susceptibles") reached levels that allowed the virus to maintain a presence in England. Smallpox predominated in a competitive environment in which microorganisms required human hosts in which to replicate. There are likely to have been different strains of the smallpox virus, which differed in virulence, although those who survived infection with any of these strains would usually have gained lifelong immunity to the disease. *Variola major* would have been highly destructive of life even without intercurrent infections or under-nutrition. Different infectious diseases had different epidemic cycles, and the cycle of smallpox epidemics would have been linked with sociodemographic factors such population size and the number of "new susceptibles" who had no immunity.[2]

The immunity gained by those who survived infection resulted in smallpox becoming predominantly a disease of childhood in the towns of England in the 18th century. The smallpox censuses in the 1720s compiled by Jurin were based on reports of epidemics by medical practitioners in thirty-two areas, and these indicate a case fatality of 17% overall and 24% in six rural areas.[3] Razzell found that the age pattern of smallpox mortality was consistent with universal contact with the disease;[4] however, some rural parish records from the 18th century

Table 5.1. Percentage of smallpox deaths in parts of the United Kingdom and Europe in the eighteenth century

Area	Period	Smallpox Deaths	All Deaths	Smallpox as % of all deaths
Britain				
London[a]	1710–39	63,579	772,751	8.2
Boston, Lincs[b]	1749–57	106	691	15.3
Maidstone	1752–61	252	1,462	17.2
Whitehaven[c] *	1752–80	570	2,969	19.2
Northampton[d] *	1740–74	377	3,536	10.7
Edinburgh[b] *	1744–63	2,441	24,322	10.0
Kilmarnock	1728–62	621	4,514	13.8
Other Europe				
Dublin	1661–90	14,160†	67,080†	21.1
Dublin	1715–46	13,759	74,585	18.4
Copenhagen[e]	1750–69	6,276	71,170	8.8
Sweden[e]	1749–73	171,058††	1,382,834	12.4††
Finland rural[f]	1749–73	2,730††	18,920	14.4††
Finland urban[f]	1749–73	1,640††	12,390	13.2††

Source: The table is adapted from one presented by Razzell, *The Conquest of Smallpox,* 133.
[a] Marshall, *Mortality in the Metropolis;* [b] Creighton, *History of Epidemics in Britain,* 525–26, 540; [c] Parish registers for Holy Trinity, Whitehaven, County Records Office, Carlisle; [d] Northampton Bills of Mortality (1779–86); [e] Great Britain, Royal Commission on Vaccination, *First Report,* appendix, 107–13; [f] Turpeinen, "Fertility and mortality in Finland" (death rates were used to calculate the number of deaths, rounded).
* Data from one parish.
† Based on annual average (472 smallpox deaths and 2,236 all deaths).
†† Figures include a few measles deaths.

did not show smallpox deaths.[5] In the towns, where very young children were often the victims, smallpox deaths in the first few months of life may have been underreported because the disease was less easily recognized. The Bills of Mortality for Warrington and Chester indicate more smallpox deaths at ages 6–11 months than at ages 0–5 months.[6] Some manifestations of smallpox, particularly in young infants, would not have produced the distinctive and highly visible symptoms of smallpox seen at older ages.[7] Fulminating smallpox, *Purpura variolosa,* rapidly caused death without an eruption of lesions in very young children, although it often caused convulsions. Many smallpox deaths among infants were probably recorded as "convulsions" in the absence of other distinctive symptoms of the disease. When the death rate from smallpox leveled off in London from the 1730s, the death rate from convulsions declined considerably making a major contribution to overall mortality decline (fig. 5.1).

In large towns, and in the industrializing north of England generally, smallpox appears to have been a disease of childhood with most deaths occurring at ages under 10 years, whereas in the more rural south both adults and children were infected. Creighton cited the case of Banbury where many deaths from smallpox occurred in early adulthood. He observed that epidemics were less frequent in rural areas and suggested that many children grew up without experiencing an epidemic unless they visited a nearby town where epidemics were much more frequent.[8] For example, in the town of Northampton, deaths from smallpox were recorded in epidemics occurring once or twice every 10 years, and in larger cities such as Glasgow, Edinburgh, and London the disease was endemic.[9] However, the burial registers of the London Quakers indicate that a substantial proportion of smallpox deaths in London between 1650 and 1800 occurred at ages over 10 years, which would not be expected as smallpox was continually present and likely to be contracted early in childhood. Landers suggested that many of the older children and adults who died from smallpox in London could have been in-migrants from rural areas who arrived in London without immunity. An unusual association between smallpox deaths and bread prices might reflect inflows of "new susceptibles" from rural areas in harsh economic times when food prices were high.[10] The lack of immunity among in-migrants has been questioned,[11] although this would depend on the frequency of epidemics in their rural area and the extent to which inoculation had been practiced there.

Inoculation, Vaccination, and Smallpox Mortality Decline

The contribution that immunization against smallpox made to overall mortality decline has often been greatly underestimated. McKeown, for example, concluded that immunization made little contribution to overall mortality decline, because he focused on registration data after the mid-19th century and the decline in smallpox mortality after 1870, by which time it had already declined from the very high levels of the 18th century. Considerable evidence indicates that immunization had a major impact on smallpox and overall mortality, although it is important to distinguish between inoculation and vaccination. Inoculation involved the potentially dangerous practice of infecting people by injecting matter taken from smallpox sores, while matter from cowpox sores on humans was used for vaccination. Inoculation had been used in Tibet from at least the eleventh century,[12] and reports on the practice were made to the Royal Society in London at the beginning of the 18th century.[13] Knowledge of the method used in Turkey was brought to England by a member of the aristocracy in 1721, and after experiments on prisoners, two royal children were inoculated in 1722. Statistical surveys by Jurin in the 1720s suggested there was much less risk of dying from inoculated smallpox than from natural infection. It was widely used in England from the 1740s, and a Smallpox and Inoculation Hospital was established in London in 1746. A less invasive method (Suttonian) was practiced by a surgeon in Norfolk. Sutton and his sons performed thousands of

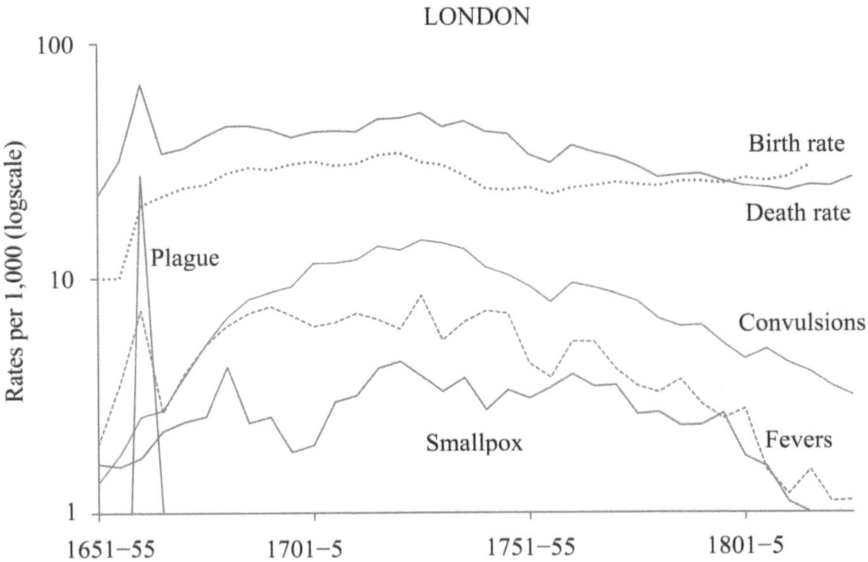

Figure 5.1. Death rates for the main causes recorded in the London Bills of Mortality, crude death rates and birth rates—annual averages for 5-year periods, 1651–55 to 1801–5. *Source:* Marshall, *Mortality in the Metropolis.*

inoculations in East Anglia, reportedly with very few deaths.[14] Inoculation became common medical practice throughout the country, particularly in the south. Although the practice may not have been extensively used in London until the 1790s,[15] by that time many in-migrants from the south of England may have been inoculated before arriving in the city.

There was much opposition to inoculation in England as in other European countries and some believed it was an interference with "God's will."[16] Inoculation was crude and dangerous by today's standards, and its effectiveness in preventing smallpox deaths in England and elsewhere has been a controversial issue. Opposition to the practice was challenged by the statistical evidence collected in pioneering studies conducted by the Royal Society and in smallpox censuses. The basis for its effectiveness is plausible, that those deliberately infected with a small dose of virus, and preferably a mild strain, would be more likely to survive exposure to a severe strain during an epidemic. There is some evidence from particular locations that case fatality was much lower among those inoculated than among the rest of the population. For example, there was a dramatic reduction in mortality from smallpox when large numbers of people were inoculated in Boston, Massachusetts, in the 18th century (table 5.2). Creighton also reported a greatly reduced number of smallpox deaths when inoculation was performed on about one in seven of the population of Blandford, a small rural market town in the south of England.[17]

Table 5.2. Smallpox deaths and numbers inoculated in epidemics in Boston, in the United States

Year	Smallpox cases (natural)	Smallpox deaths	Case fatality (%)	Number Inoculated	Smallpox deaths among the inoculated	Case Fatality (%)
1721	5,759	844	14.7	247	6	2.4
1730	3,600	488	13.6	400	12	3.0
1752	5,545	539	9.7	2,124	30	1.4
1764	669	124	18.5	4,977	46	0.9
1776	304	29	9.5	4,988	28	0.6
1778	122	42	34.4	2,121	19	0.9
1792	232	33	14.2	8,114	165	2.0

Source: Great Britain, Royal Commission on Vaccination, *Third Report*, appendix, 200.

In larger towns, epidemics were relatively frequent or the disease was endemic, so "new susceptibles" were mainly infants and young children because other people had survived infection in earlier outbreaks and gained immunity. People may have been more fatalistic about the chances of infants surviving, as they were vulnerable to a whole series of infectious diseases and mortality was extremely high. However, many victims of smallpox in rural areas were older children and young adults who had not experienced an epidemic as these occurred much less frequently. The older victims would already be well known in the community, and the disease produced highly visible and much feared symptoms. McNeill suggested that the later age-incidence of smallpox could underlie the resort to mass inoculation in rural areas, as inoculation offered some protection to older children and young adults. While deaths among infants would be expected, deaths among older children and young adults would be far more costly to families and to the community as whole.[18] Mass inoculations became a common response to the threat of epidemics in the rural south of England after the 1760s, and Razzell documented examples from other parts of the country as well.[19]

The issue of the impact of inoculation and its possible role in mortality decline in the second half of the 18th century has been controversial among demographers and historians. Razzell compiled a great deal of evidence, suggesting considerable variation in use of the practice in different parts of England, and the likelihood of a more significant impact in terms of preventing deaths in the south of England.[20] Studies of records in Scotland also suggest wide variation in the use of inoculation both geographically and socially. The practice was readily adopted by people who were well-off, while religious objections may have been more of a negative influence on its use among lower socioeconomic groups and the poor. Inoculation appears to have been deeply unpopular in some regions of Scotland, although readily adopted by at least half the population in other areas.[21] In Britain as a whole, including major towns, use of inoculation was probably at its peak in the 1790s, after which it was rapidly replaced by vaccination, which had an immediate impact on smallpox mortality.

Vaccination developed as a preventive measure in rural communities in the southwest of England in the second half of the 18th century. There is considerable evidence that when it became widely used at the beginning of the 19th century, it had a much more dramatic epidemiological-demographic impact than inoculation.[22] The practice was more readily adopted in major towns and cities than inoculation had been, despite being "rural folk medicine." It became known as vaccination because of its association with cows, since it involved injecting people with matter from cowpox sores. These often developed on the hands of farm workers and milkmaids who contracted the infection from cattle. Edward Jenner, a country doctor in Gloucestershire, heard local stories about cowhands and milkmaids being protected from the much more severe disease, smallpox.[23] Vaccination had already been in use for many years in rural England, and the case of a farmer who deliberately infected his wife and sons with matter from cowpox sores in 1774 was later documented by the Royal Commission on Vaccination.[24] The commission reviewed evidence from around the country, which indicated that the practice had spread rapidly after Jenner reported the results of his investigations in 1798 in his *Inquiry into the Causes and Effects of Variolae Vaccinae.* This publication included persuasive evidence of effectiveness long before microorganisms were known to exist, and before any scientific concept of immunity, cross-immunity, or an understanding of how cowpox infection prevented smallpox. Within a few weeks, smallpox vaccination was widely used in different parts of England, and in much of Europe and the United States within a decade. It was even made compulsory in Denmark in 1810, Norway in 1811, and Sweden in 1816.[25]

There is some suggestion that cowpox matter used for vaccination in the early years of the 19th century became adulterated with smallpox matter.[26] Even so, the method was based on the vaccination procedure that Jenner had tested on a young boy in 1796.[27] Jenner's publication of the results was influential in convincing the medical profession to support the method as he showed that the vaccinated boy did not contract smallpox when inoculated with virulent smallpox matter. Eventually the experience with vaccination in England led to its worldwide acceptance and use, and together with other preventive measures this led to eradication of the disease worldwide by 1977.[28] Remarkably, the disease was virtually eliminated from England and some other European countries before the end of the 19th century. The unprecedented burst of population growth that occurred in England and many parts of Europe in the first few decades of the 19th century may have been largely due to prevention of smallpox through vaccination.[29]

The population of London probably did not increase through "natural growth" in the 18th century, as the annual number of burials consistently exceeded the number of baptisms. However, estimates suggest that the population increased as a result of large scale in-migration.[30] The leveling off in the number of smallpox deaths recorded in the London Bills of Mortality between the 1720s and 1760s, and the subsequent decline, indicates a considerable reduction in the death rate assuming that population increased as estimates suggest. The gap between annual burials and baptisms narrowed from the 1740s; infant mortality declined; and the total death rate, based on a range of population estimates, also declined.[31] These changes correspond with a leveling off in the smallpox death rate between 1721–25 and 1761–65, and a subsequent decline, which accelerated in the early decades of the 19th century (fig. 5.1). Data from the London Bills of Mortality also indicate several other turning points in recorded smallpox deaths that coincide with changes in total mortality. Apart from the plague years in the 1660s, the main turning points in the long-term trend in annual deaths from smallpox and all causes correspond—around 1681–85, 1721–25, 1761–65, and after 1796–1800. In the period 1780–1820, the spikes in the annual number of smallpox deaths diminished considerably, and the beginning of an excess of baptisms over burials after 1800 indicates unprecedented natural population growth (figs. 3.1 and 5.1).

Records from other towns in England also indicate a dramatic change in smallpox epidemics and mortality after 1800. Data from St. John's Parish in the town of Chester in the north of England indicate correspondence between spikes in annual smallpox deaths and total deaths in the second half of the 18th century. A dramatic change occurred in the 1800s when vaccination came into use. No deaths were attributed to smallpox after 1811, and there was unprecedented natural population growth (fig. 5.2).

One of the longest series of data is the Bills of Mortality for All Saints Parish in the midland town of Northampton. These indicate many spikes in mortality associated with smallpox epidemics in the second half of the 18th century. Although data for some years are missing, the evidence suggests that spikes in smallpox deaths were greatly diminished after 1800 (fig. 5.3). The decline in smallpox deaths was not offset by an increase in other causes of death, and the total number of deaths was thus much reduced.[32] The numbers of deaths declined between 1780–99 and 1800–1819 for smallpox (210 to 66), measles (70 to 41), and whooping cough (40 to 32). As in London, the number of deaths from consumption was lower in the first two decades of the 19th century following the downturn in smallpox deaths (fig. 5.4), an association considered further in chapter 9.

Data from Glasgow indicate a dramatic reduction in the smallpox death rate after 1800 when vaccination was introduced, and this is reflected in a lower overall death rate, despite a measles epidemic in the period 1807–12 (table 5.3). The national data from Sweden also indicate that a reduction in the smallpox death rate was not offset by any increase in measles, diphtheria, and scarlet fever mortality (table 5.4).

Other Bills of Mortality and parish registers indicate that deaths recognized as due to smallpox contributed significantly to spikes in overall mortality. Smallpox was recorded in 19% of deaths in the northern town of Whitehaven in the

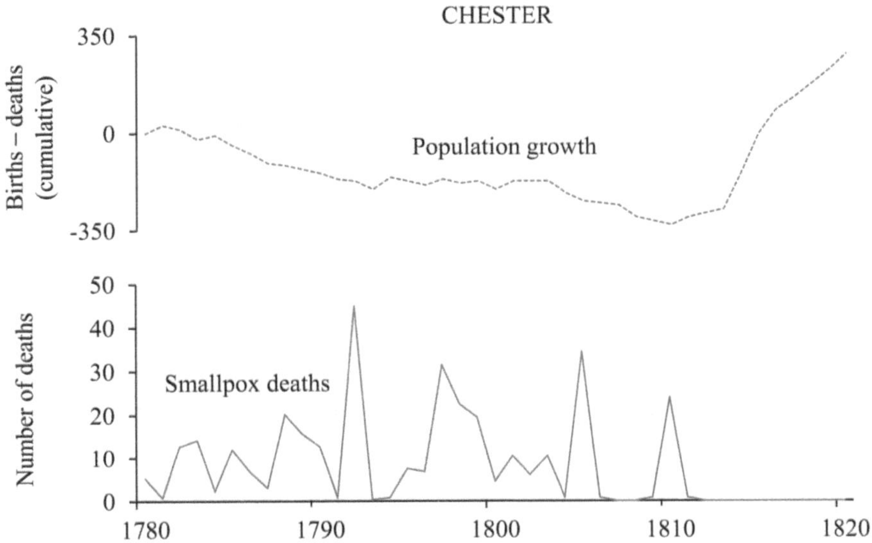

Figure 5.2. Smallpox deaths in St. John's Parish, Chester, and natural population change, 1780–1820. *Source:* Parish Register of St. John's, Chester.

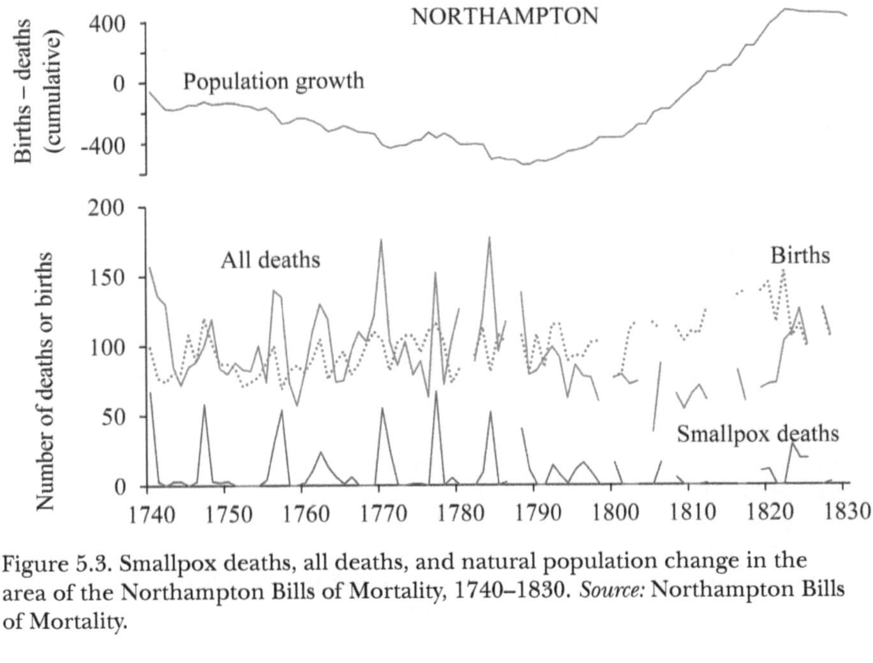

Figure 5.3. Smallpox deaths, all deaths, and natural population change in the area of the Northampton Bills of Mortality, 1740–1830. *Source:* Northampton Bills of Mortality.

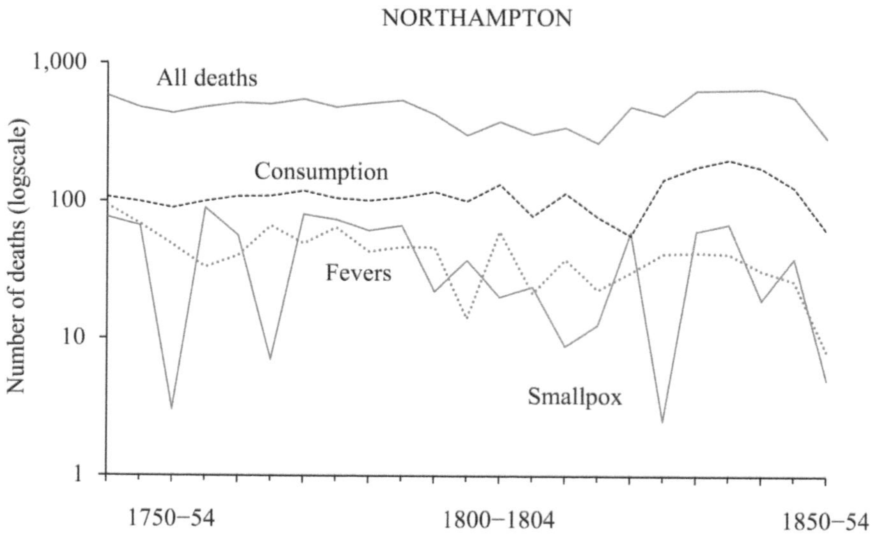

Figure 5.4. Deaths from smallpox, fevers, consumption, and all causes in the Northampton Bills of Mortality in 5-year periods: 1740–44 to 1850–54. *Source:* Northampton Bills of Mortality.

second half of the 18th century, and epidemic spikes in smallpox deaths correspond with spikes in total mortality.[33] In Manchester 14% of deaths were attributed to smallpox over the period 1754–74,[34] over 15% in the 1760s, and 13% in the 1780s.[35] The Bills of Mortality available for the nearby town of Warrington between 1791 and 1800 indicate a crude death rate of 31.4 per 1,000 population, while the bills available for 1818–29 indicate that the rate had fallen to 27.4 per 1,000.[36] Most of the decline of 4.0 per 1,000 was due to a reduction in the smallpox death rate from 4.6 to 1.3 per 1,000, and the proportion of all deaths attributed to smallpox fell from 14.6% to 4.7%. The Bills of Mortality for Carlisle for 1779–87, compiled by Heysham, also show that about 14% of deaths were attributed to smallpox. Lonsdale pointed out that after vaccination was introduced in the town in 1800, 12 years elapsed before any death from smallpox was recorded,[37] and there was unprecedented population growth between 1811 and 1831.[38]

The data from the Northampton bills indicate that after two decades of greatly diminished spikes in smallpox deaths between 1800 and 1820, there was a resurgence of deaths from the disease (fig. 5.3 and 5.4). A destructive epidemic of smallpox was also recorded in Norwich in 1819 when 39% of all deaths were attributed to the disease. Edwardes suggested that vaccination coverage lapsed after the initial success in preventing the disease, which could account for the resurgence in many towns. People may have become less concerned

Table 5.3. Crude death rates from smallpox, measles, whooping cough, and all causes in Glasgow, 1789–1812

		Death rates per 1,000			
Years	Total deaths	All causes	Smallpox	Measles	Whooping cough
1789–1794	11,103	27.8	5.1	0.3	1.4
1795–1800	9,991	21.6	4.0	0.5	1.2
1801–1806	10,304	18.3	1.6	0.7	1.1
1807–1812	13,354	20.6	0.8	2.3	1.2

Source: Creighton, *History of Epidemics in Britain*, 513, 635.
Note: Death rates are based on Creighton's population figure for 1791 (66,578) and census figure for 1801 (84,122).

Table 5.4. Average death rates from smallpox, measles, diphtheria, and scarlet fever in Sweden, 1779 to 1811

	Death rates per 1,000			
Years	Smallpox	Measles	Diphtheria	Scarlet fever
1779–1789	2.1	0.3	0.2	0.1
1790–1800	1.9	0.5	0.2	0.1
1801–1811	0.8	0.4	0.1	0.1

Source: Siljeström, *En studie i Sjukdomsstatistik.*

about the disease when there were few fatalities for several years.[39] Smallpox returned to contribute to higher overall death rates in the second quarter of the 19th century in many towns, including the major industrial cities of Manchester and Glasgow (fig. 5.5). An analysis of data from parish registers from the industrial towns of Walsall, West Bromwich, and Sedgeley in the West Midlands, and Ashton-under-Lyme and Wigan in the northwest of England, also indicate an increase in mortality in the second quarter of the 19th century, as in other towns.[40] Estimates for provincial cities with populations over 100,000 suggest that average life expectancy fell from 35 years in the 1820s to about 30 years in the 1830s and 1840s, before increasing again in the last few decades of the 19th century.[41] These trends are consistent with the evidence of lower average height in the second quarter of the 19th century discussed in chapter 4.

The Vaccination Law of 1853 made infant vaccination compulsory, and it was supported by further legislation in 1863. Compulsion understandably aroused controversy, and the policy was not fully enforced. Even so, it is estimated that about half of the infants in British towns were vaccinated between 1800 and 1870. By the time a pandemic struck in 1870–71, vaccination efforts had again diminished and local sanitary departments were more focused on tracing

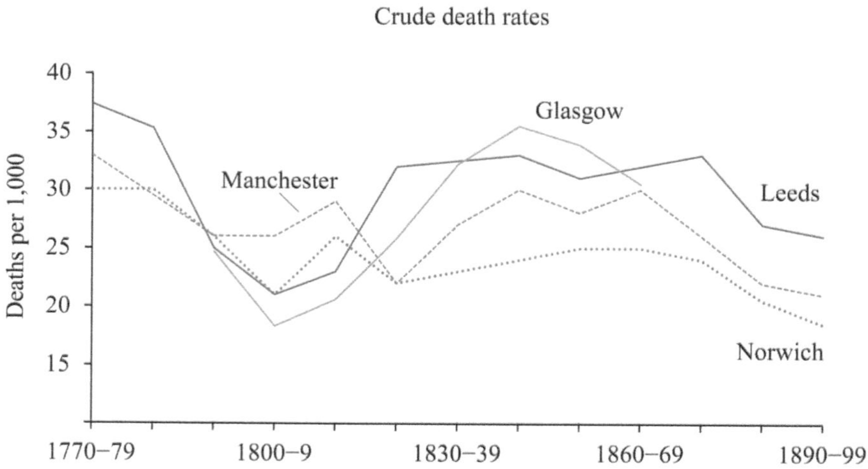

Figure 5.5. Crude death rates for selected towns in Britain—annual averages for decades 1770–79 to 1890–99. *Sources:* Cherry, "Hospitals and population growth, pt. 1," 64–65; Great Britain, Royal Commission on Vaccination, *Final Report*, appendix 4, 41; Flinn, *Scottish Population History*, 377, 383.

infected people, isolating them in their homes or in a hospital, and cleansing their houses.[42] The pandemic was so severe that measures were taken to implement compulsory vaccination, and the need for revaccination was recognized. These measures played a major part in efforts to control the disease.[43] Vaccination officers achieved greater coverage of infants, and separation of deaths among the vaccinated and nonvaccinated in the Registrar General's reports provided evidence of lapsed immunity. Renewed efforts to vaccinate and revaccinate are likely to have reduced the number of people who could transmit the disease, thereby reducing incidence. At this stage, other preventive measures may have been sufficient to eliminate the disease. In the town of Leicester in the Midlands, where there was much opposition to compulsory vaccination, the control strategy after 1877 was based on notification of cases, isolation of those infected in the Fever and Smallpox Hospital, and quarantine for contacts who were financially compensated.[44]

Isolation had been a strategy for preventing the spread of disease since the plague epidemics, and it was introduced for smallpox in the 1860s.[45] As with plague, an effective prevention strategy evolved over many years, with different interventions being tried to offer some protection against a much-feared disease. It was recognized that effective surveillance, notification of cases, and vaccination of hospital staff could contribute to smallpox prevention. Provincial councils were responsible for a relatively small population, making notification more manageable than in London. The relatively high number of smallpox deaths in the capital may have been due to a lack of coordination of control measures over the whole city. However, the idea of "stamping out" smallpox without relying on infant vaccination seems to have influenced the strategy from the 1860s. Sanitary departments focused on isolating the sick or hospitalizing them, tracing and vaccinating contacts, and cleansing and disinfecting their dwellings. Although isolation aroused much opposition, it was central to the "stamping out" approach after the 1870–71 pandemic.[46] Smallpox deaths were rare in London after 1885, and by the 1890s the smallpox death rate had been reduced to 0.2 per 100,000, compared with 200–300 per 100,000 at the beginning of the century (fig. 5.6).

In the last smallpox outbreak in London in 1901, in which 24 people died, preventive measures were effective in limiting the disease to a few areas of the city. It had been recognized in the pandemic of 1870–71 that port towns such as London were vulnerable to infection being introduced from overseas. The final phase of the control of smallpox in England in the last three decades of the 19th century reflects tighter prevention measures, including inspection of ships; monitoring of outbreaks occurring abroad as well as in the country; and tracing and isolating those infected. Over the course of the 19th century, initially vaccination, then revaccination and the other preventive measures dramatically reduced smallpox deaths, and the national death rate from smallpox was down to 1.3 per 100,000 by the 1890s.

Vaccination and Smallpox Mortality Decline in Europe

Evidence of the control of smallpox in England in the 19th century through vaccination is supported by data from other European countries. Major turning points in the smallpox death rate coincide with the introduction of vaccination at the beginning of the 19th century. Together with other preventive measures implemented later, vaccination is the most likely explanation for the recession of epidemics, as in England. The main sources indicate that smallpox epidemics had begun to predominate in the pattern of mortality fluctuations in European countries in the 18th century. The growth of towns had created "pools of new susceptibles" and populations of the size and density required to sustain an airborne disease such as smallpox. As contacts between people in rural areas and towns increased, they would be increasingly exposed to infection. The suggestion that resistance to the most virulent smallpox virus, *Variola major*, increased through long exposure of the population is not supported by any firm evidence.[47] It is also unlikely that the decline in the death rate from smallpox was due to a decline in the virulence of the disease as case fatality among the "naturally" infected remained high.[48] There was little consistent relationship between smallpox epidemics and poor harvests as in the case of typhus epidemics. Many poor harvests were not accompanied or immediately followed by smallpox epidemics, and a major pandemic in 1778–79 followed a good harvest.[49] Although under-nutrition would have contributed to higher case fatality from some infectious diseases, *Variola major* caused high mortality even in well-fed populations.

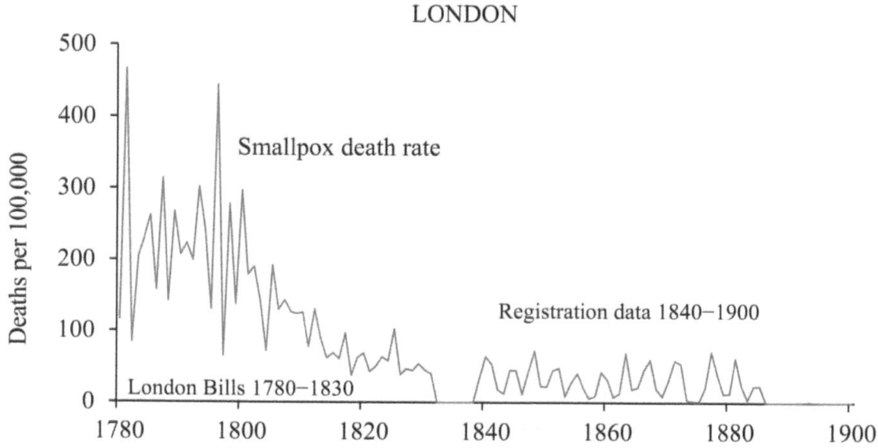

Figure 5.6. Annual death rates from smallpox in London, 1780–1900. *Source:* Marshall, *Mortality in the Metropolis.*

The use of inoculation seems to have varied considerably between different parts of Europe. In France, there was organized resistance to the practice, which continued until the death of Louis XV from smallpox in 1774.[50] Estimates indicate a more rapid decline in mortality in the 1790s and in the first few decades of the 19th century.[51] In Denmark, inoculation was introduced in the 1750s, and a special clinic was opened on the outskirts of Copenhagen in 1770.[52] The pattern of smallpox epidemics and mortality spikes changed dramatically, and even more dramatically after 1810 when vaccination was made compulsory (fig. 5.7). Before the inoculation facility opened, the overall death rate fluctuated from 40 to 80 per 1,000, and an excess of burials over baptisms indicated that without in-migration the population would have declined. However, between 1770 and 1810, the crude death rate was generally 30–50 per 1,000, and the number of recorded burials was about the same as the number of baptisms. Following the introduction of vaccination, the ratio of vaccinations to births reached 0.7 in 1808 and remained above this when vaccination became compulsory. In the period 1810–50, very few smallpox deaths were recorded, the overall death rate was down to around 30 per 1,000, and there was natural population growth despite a declining birthrate.

In contrast to Denmark, inoculation did not become popular or widespread in Sweden after it was introduced in 1756. Only an estimated 50,000 inoculations were performed in the second half of the 18th century.[53] National records for this period indicate several spikes in smallpox deaths corresponding with peaks in total deaths. The immediate impact of vaccination on overall mortality was masked by a major epidemic of typhus, which caused high mortality between 1804 and 1813 during the war with Finland. However, after vaccination became compulsory in 1816, the number of deaths attributed to smallpox

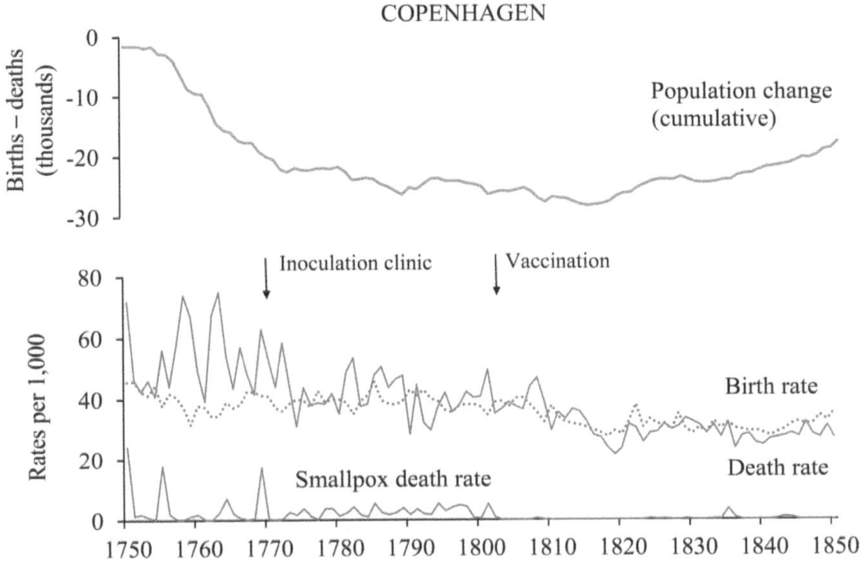

Figure 5.7. Annual smallpox death rates, crude death rates and birth rates, and natural population change in Copenhagen: 1750–1850. *Source:* Great Britain, Royal Commission on Vaccination, *First Report*, appendix 1, 107–8.

quickly became negligible.[54] In the period 1816–20 smallpox accounted for less than 1% of deaths in many districts, compared with around 10% in the second half of the 18th century.[55] The pattern of mortality fluctuations changed dramatically when vaccination was introduced, and very few smallpox deaths were recorded between 1810 and 1850 (fig. 5.8). As in England, the overall death rate was reduced, and it was consistently well below the birthrate. Census data confirm the more rapid growth in population.[56]

Studies of infant mortality also indicate the predominance of smallpox in the 18th century in Sweden, with 15 of the 20 spikes in mortality between 1752 and 1801 involving smallpox epidemics.[57] In frequent epidemics, smallpox was one of the major killers of children in the 18th century, but records from Stockholm, Gotland, and the northern provinces of Sweden indicate that the disease was largely absent after 1810.[58] Although there had been limited use of inoculation, vaccination was readily adopted and the number recorded increased rapidly in the first two decades of the 19th century. Sweden was one of the first countries to introduce compulsory vaccination, in 1816, and more than 70% of children were vaccinated between 1816 and 1820.[59] The 10 spikes in infant mortality between 1806 and 1830 were due mainly to dysentery, whooping cough, and measles; smallpox was no longer a significant cause of death. As mentioned, the decline in the death rate from smallpox was not offset by increases in mortality from other diseases (table 5.4). Although some studies suggest that whooping

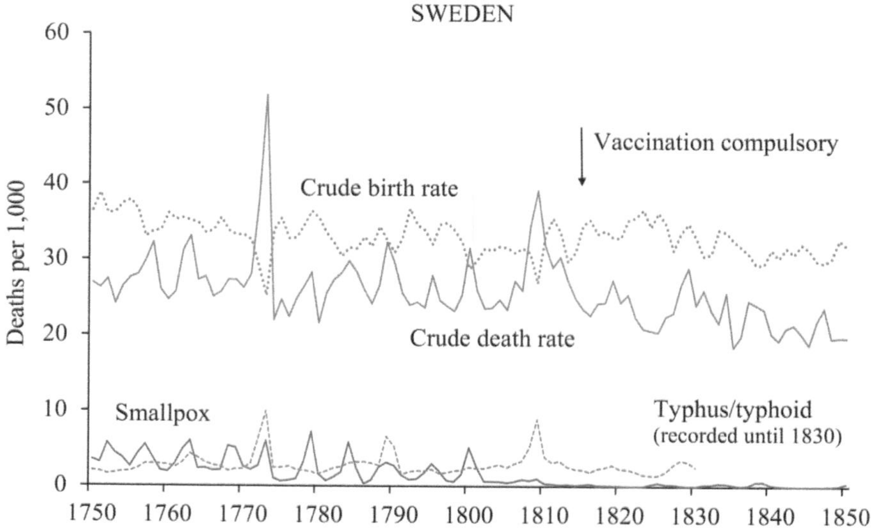

Figure 5.8. Annual death rates from smallpox and typhus/typhoid, crude death rates and birth rates in Sweden, 1750–1850. *Source:* Great Britain, Royal Commission on Vaccination, *First Report*, appendix 1, 112–13.

cough mortality increased,[60] the overall death rate declined in the first half of the 19th century, which was largely due to the control of smallpox through vaccination. Not only were the 10% of deaths that had been directly attributed to smallpox prevented, but lives were also saved by preventing severe sequelae of the disease.[61]

In Finland, which was part of Sweden until 1809, inoculation was also rarely practiced and only in certain areas. Fluctuations in the death rate in the second half of the 18th century were not associated with poor harvests, and many of the spikes in mortality corresponded with smallpox epidemics (fig. 5.9). Records indicate that in the period 1749–73, 14.4% of deaths in rural parishes and 13.2% in town parishes were attributed to smallpox or measles, and the death rate from these diseases did not decline between 1751–75 and 1776–1800. Under separate recording between 1776 and 1800, 87% of deaths from these diseases were due to smallpox, suggesting that at least 9% of all deaths in the second half of the 18th century were caused by the disease.[62] A further study of cause of death statistics found that the annual average death rate from smallpox was 237 per 100,000 for the years 1751–75 and 302 per 100,000 for 1776–1800, but declined dramatically from the 1810s when an increasing proportion of children were vaccinated. The smallpox death rate among infants fell from 17.1 per 1,000 births between 1776 and 1800 to 9.4 per 1,000 between 1801 and 1825, and the overall infant mortality rate declined.[63] Data from Finland's Åland islands suggest that vaccination programs after 1805

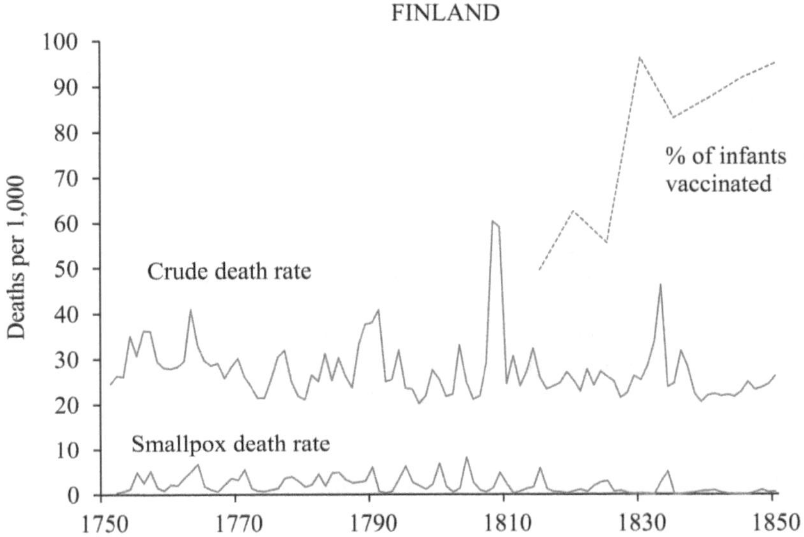

Figure 5.9. Annual death rates from smallpox, crude death rates, and estimated proportion of infants vaccinated in Finland, 1750–1850. *Sources:* Pitkänen, Mielke, and Jorde, "Smallpox and its eradication in Finland"; Turpeinen, "Fertility and mortality in Finland."

were extremely efficient with the majority of children being vaccinated. The number of smallpox deaths was dramatically reduced, and the overall death rate declined in the 19th century.[64]

Studies in Finland and Sweden indicate that the near elimination of smallpox by the end of the 19th century was due mainly to vaccination, revaccination, and isolation of cases. As in other European countries, the major smallpox pandemic in the 1870s led to a recognition among the medical profession that revaccination should be promoted. Although the number of revaccinations in Finland was relatively small, smallpox was almost completely eradicated from the country by the end of the 19th century (1896–1910).[65] The disease was also largely absent from most countries close to Finland apart from Russia, which was probably the source of smallpox cases along the border in eastern Finland. When the germ theory of infectious disease was accepted, the importance of preventing the spread of infectious diseases had a rational basis and notification of cases was made more efficient. Patients were isolated in communicable disease hospitals; homes were disinfected; and vaccination, revaccination, or isolation of contacts was enforced. Despite the effectiveness of preventive measures in virtually eliminating smallpox from Finland during the 19th century, the impact on overall mortality was less dramatic than elsewhere in northern Europe, because epidemics of "fevers" linked with wars and famine continued to cause massive mortality.

For Norway, there are few data on smallpox deaths, although trends in death rates are consistent with vaccination having a major impact. As in Sweden, there was a marked change in the birth and death rates after 1810 when vaccination was made compulsory (fig. 4.3). The overall death rate declined dramatically, the birthrate returned to the previously high level of 30–35 per 1,000, and population growth became more rapid and uninterrupted. This contrasts with the regular mortality spikes in the 18th century, which constituted a check on population growth. In Iceland, there were devastating smallpox epidemics in the 18th century, in 1707 when about 18,000 deaths were recorded in a population of 50,000, and in 1785–87 when 1,425 deaths from smallpox were recorded.[66] In the 19th century the ratio of vaccinations to births increased, indicating almost complete coverage by 1817. There was only one further major outbreak of smallpox, in 1839 when the epidemic was contained by isolation measures. Census data indicate that population growth was much more rapid in the first half of the 19th century compared with the decades prior to the introduction of vaccination.[67]

Evidence from many other parts of Europe indicates that smallpox death rates were much lower in the first half of the 19th century when vaccination was introduced (table 5.5). In the provinces of Moravia and Silesia, the smallpox death rate declined from over 5,000 per million to less than 300 per million. In many other areas, the death rate declined from over 2,000 per million to less than 500 per million, and the decline in the smallpox death rate from 14,000 per million to less than 200 per million in Trieste indicates a massive reduction in mortality through control of just one disease. Dramatic reductions in smallpox mortality when vaccination was introduced were recorded in cities and provinces of Germany (table 5.5). A very high ratio of vaccinations to births was achieved in Berlin by 1810,[68] and the annual average death rate from smallpox between 1810 and 1850 was 176 per million compared with 3,422 per million between 1781 and 1805, before vaccination was introduced. Similar reductions in the smallpox death rate of more than 90% were recorded in the provinces of Brandenburg and Westphalia. In the pandemic of 1870–75, it was recognized that some of the vaccinated caught smallpox, and revaccination was therefore introduced in Germany, as in England. The German Vaccination Law of 1874 provided support for compulsory vaccination, and data from Bavaria, Prussia, and Württemberg indicate a rapid decline in the smallpox death rate after this (table 5.6). There were no further significant epidemics of smallpox in these provinces, and the death rate from the disease was below 5 per million after 1886.

There were only two major epidemics of smallpox in Europe after the 1800s when vaccination was introduced—in the 1830s and in the early 1870s.[69] The Europe-wide pandemic of smallpox between 1870 and 1875 led to renewed efforts to vaccinate children in England and on the Continent. Compulsory vaccination was carried out despite varying degrees of opposition, and together with revaccination and other preventive measures this led to the virtual elimination of smallpox from England and other parts of Europe by the end of the 19th century. The importance of worldwide eradication of smallpox, which was

Table 5.5. Annual death rates from smallpox in selected locations in Europe, before and after introduction of smallpox vaccination

Area of Europe	Years before vaccination	Death rate/ million	Years with vaccination	Death rate/ million	% decline in death rate
Brandenberg	1776–1780	2,181	1810–1850	181	91.7
Prussia (East)	"	321	"	56	82.6
Westphalia	"	2,643	1816–1850	114	95.7
Rhenish Province	"	908	"	90	90.1
Saxony (Prussian)	"	719	"	170	76.4
Tyrol/Voralberg	1777–1803	911	1807–1850	170	81.3
Austria (Lower)	1777–1806	2,481	"	340	86.3
Austria (Upper)	"	1,421	"	501	64.7
Styria	"	1,052	"	446	57.6
Illyria	"	518	"	224	56.8
Bohemia	"	2,174	"	215	90.1
Moravia	"	5,402	"	255	95.3
Silesia (Austria)	"	5,812	"	198	96.6
Gallicia	"	1,194	"	676	43.4
Trieste	"	14,046	1838–1850	182	98.7
Posen	1780	1,911	1816–1850	743	61.1
Prussia (West)	1780	2,272	1810–1850	356	84.3
Pomerania	1780	1,774	"	130	92.7
Berlin	1781–1805	3,422	"	176	94.9
Bukowina	1787–1806	3,527	1807–1850	516	85.4
Sweden	1775–1800	2,067	1801–1850	278	86.6

Sources: Edwardes, *Concise History of Smallpox and Vaccination,* 18–19, 48–50, 180–82; Great Britain, Royal Commission on Vaccination, *First Report,* 72; *First Report,* appendix 1, 112–13.

achieved in 1977, is illustrated by the outbreak that occurred in England as late as 1962 when the disease was introduced from abroad. In a relatively well fed and housed population, 26 of the 66 confirmed cases were fatal (39%) before the outbreak was controlled through isolation measures.[70] This compares with case fatality of 17% found in the smallpox censuses in England in the 18th century, and 16–47% in several European countries in the first half of the 19th century.[71]

Records from different parts of England and Europe in the 18th century indicate that between 8% and 20% of deaths were directly attributed to smallpox, and a further unquantifiable proportion of deaths involving unrecognized

Table 5.6. Smallpox death rates in Germany before and after the Vaccination Law of 1874, and percentage decline from 1868–74 to 1875–80

	Smallpox deaths per million		
Year	Prussia	Bavaria	Württemberg
1868	620	120	133
1869	432	250	63
1870	188	190	19
1871	194	101	74
1872	175	75	293
1873	2,432	1,045	1,130
1874	2,624	611	637
1868–74	952.1	341.7	335.6
1875	356	176	30
1876	95	47	3
1877	36	17	1
1878	31	13	2
1879	3	17	0
1880	7	13	0
1875–80	88.0	47.2	6.0
Decline	90.8%	86.2%	98.2%

Source: Edwardes, *Concise History of Smallpox and Vaccination*, 181–82.

symptoms and secondary complications would have been recorded in other categories. In the first few decades of the 19th century, when vaccination became widely used, deaths from smallpox were greatly reduced, overall death rates were lower, and population growth was at its most rapid. Vaccination was all the more important because of migration into the towns at that time, which exacerbated the crowded living conditions conducive to the transmission of infectious diseases. A resurgence in the overall death rate in English towns in the second quarter of the 19th century may in part reflect a resurgence of smallpox. As in other countries of Europe, mortality declined more consistently from the 1870s when efforts were renewed to vaccinate children. The organized efforts to control smallpox through vaccination and other preventive measures that led to the virtual elimination of the disease during the course of the 19th century constitute a remarkable public health achievement. The role of other preventive and public health measures in the decline in mortality in England after the mid-19th century is considered in the next chapter.

Chapter Six

Typhus, Typhoid, Cholera, Diarrhea, and Dysentery

Although smallpox epidemics predominated in the pattern of mortality fluctuations in the 18th century in England and other European countries, many deaths among children and adults were attributed to "fevers." Hospital statistics and medical writings suggest that typhus was probably a more significant component of "fevers" mortality in England in the 18th century than typhoid.[1] Typhus and typhoid were first distinguished under national registration in 1869, by which time typhus mortality had declined and typhoid accounted for a higher proportion of deaths. Of the 18,390 "fevers" deaths in that year, 47% were attributed to typhoid, 23% to typhus, and 30% to "simple fever." "Convulsions" was often recorded as the "cause" of death in the first two years of life, although the symptoms are likely to have been due to bacterial infections linked with poor hygiene and fecal contamination of water and food, and with viral diseases such as smallpox that had not displayed the recognized symptoms. Many other deaths involving gastrointestinal disorders among children and adults were probably recorded in the London Bills of Mortality as "griping of the guts," "bloody flux," and "surfeit."[2]

The vagueness of some cause-of-death categories and increasing recognition of diseases clearly affect the assessment of their contribution to overall mortality decline. Even for the registration period, quantification based on cause-specific death rates is simplistic because of concurrent infections and interrelationships between diseases. Nevertheless, a summary of the simple components of mortality change provides some indication of the relative importance of different categories of disease and symptoms (see appendix C1). Estimates based on the London Bills of Mortality suggest that the death rate declined by 32% between 1751 and 1801. In simple arithmetic terms, the main contributions to each unit of change were "fevers" (–0.25), convulsions/teething (–0.40), consumption (–0.09), and smallpox (–0.08).[3] National registration data indicate that the death rate in England and Wales declined by 22% between 1851 and 1901, with contributions to each unit of change from typhus/typhoid fevers (–0.17), cholera, diarrhea and dysentery (–0.12), convulsions/teething (–0.14), consumption (–0.33), and smallpox (–0.05). This chapter considers the decline in mortality from typhus, typhoid, cholera, dysentery, and diarrheal diseases, and the impact of improvements in hygiene, domestic sanitation, water supplies, sewerage, and other environmental health measures.

The Decline in Mortality from Typhus and Other Fevers

The Northampton Bills of Mortality indicate a decline in the number of deaths from "fevers" between 1740–44 and 1850–54 (fig. 5.4), and the London bills also indicate a downturn from the 1740s (figs. 3.1 and 5.1). Although "spotted fever" (typhus) had been separately recorded earlier,[4] it was included in the general category of "fevers" at this time. Even so, Creighton believed that a major typhus epidemic occurred in London in 1741–42 when 1 in 5 deaths were attributed to "fevers." An epidemic of "spotted fever" was reported in Tiverton in the southwest of England where 1 in 12 deaths was recorded as due to "fevers," and he suggested that this epidemic affected London as well as the weaving towns of Devon. High mortality also occurred in towns further north, including Norwich, Newcastle, and Edinburgh, where about 16% of deaths were attributed to "fevers," 16% to smallpox, 12% to measles and whooping cough, and 22% to consumption. Creighton was not certain that typhus was the main cause of high "fevers" mortality in these northern towns but was convinced that typhus mortality declined after the 1740s epidemic.[5]

Differentiation of infectious diseases causing "fevers" deaths was difficult even when disease-specific symptoms were well known because the symptoms would not all be present in every case. Zinsser pointed out that when a rash with red spots together with fever, headache, delirium, and extreme weakness was observed, there could be little doubt that the disease was typhus. However, the red spots would not always be distinctive, particularly among children, and cases could have been mistaken for measles, or later for scarlet fever. In adults, typhus fever would sometimes have been indistinguishable from typhoid, or even malaria where it was prevalent.[6] Malaria probably accounted for some deaths in England, as well as debilitating illness, particularly in East Anglia where marshland provided a suitable habitat for mosquitoes. However, malaria is unlikely to have been a major component of mortality decline in England, and the proportion of deaths attributed to "ague" was also quite low in other European countries in the 18th century.

From descriptions of epidemics, it is clear that typhus occurred throughout Europe in the 17th and 18th centuries, although it may have been mainly an infection among rodents until the prolonged wars in Europe in the 16th century.[7] The disease was associated with war and famine, and conditions in army camps and famine areas would foster close proximity to rats. This provided opportunities for rat fleas carrying the causal agent, *Rickettsia prowazeki*, to transfer to humans and infect them. Human lice and fleas would ingest blood from infected people and pass on the disease through bites if they transferred to another person. The disease could also have been transmitted when insect feces entered the skin through lesions or got inhaled from clothes and bedding.

Transmission through clothes was suspected on board ships, although it was not known until 1910 that human lice were involved.[8]

The first unmistakable outbreaks of typhus in England were in jails, and the disease would have spread from these foci of infection into the most crowded areas of towns. When typhus was first named in the 18th century, it was correctly linked with prisons, ships, overcrowded places, filthy living conditions, and poor personal hygiene. In the absence of plague, it may have been the only major "fever" that was famine related, causing subsistence-related mortality spikes particularly in really backward areas of Europe.[9] As mentioned earlier, disruption of social and economic activities, scavenging for food, and deterioration of personal hygiene would have fostered transmission. Although nutrition per se is unlikely to have contributed to the decline in typhus mortality, a more consistent food supply and reduction of "famine crises" probably prevented some of the disruption of daily life that had contributed to epidemics.[10] However, reduction in major outbreaks of typhus resulting from interventions to prevent subsistence crises and famine between the mid-18th and mid-19th century (see chapter 4) would have been partially offset by the adverse effect of increasingly crowded and unhygienic living conditions in the rapidly growing towns of England.[11]

Medical personnel with experience of typhus epidemics in army camps probably contributed to dissemination of ideas about conditions in which diseases spread. It became widely known in the 18th century that armies, ships, and jails were foci of typhus.[12] Toward the end of the century, investigations into conditions in jails led to local initiatives to improve conditions,[13] which may have reduced transmission from some of these sources. It was also recognized that typhus could be prevented on board ships and in hospitals by applying hygiene measures, and that poor hygiene contributed to outbreaks of dysentery in army camps. Although the mechanism was not known, a link between environmental conditions and "fevers" epidemics was recognized, and this lay behind increasing efforts at the local level to prevent disease in the second half of the 18th century.[14] It was known that urban filth, slums, overcrowding, and ignorance about hygiene contributed to epidemics in the growing towns. In London, parishes appointed commissioners who were authorized by private acts of Parliament in the 1760s to collect rates (local taxes) to be used for contracting street maintenance, cleaning, and refuse removal.[15] Several companies were formed that provided piped water and sewers were constructed—initiatives that spread to other towns.[16] Many municipal authorities in England and other parts of Europe had begun some environmental improvements from around the 1740s, such as drainage schemes, sewage disposal, cleaning and paving streets, and ventilation of jails. The contribution to declining mortality in the second half of the 18th century is difficult to assess, although sanitation interventions and ventilation are likely to have had more impact in urban areas where population was more dense.[17] There were proposals for ventilation of meeting halls, hospitals, ships, and prisons, and for cleaning up stinking refuse and pools of stagnant water in towns. However, effective local powers to control many environmental hazards were not granted until the mid-19th century, and there was no central government intervention to improve conditions.[18]

People better-off could try to avoid locations thought to be unhealthy because of the stench, or they could move temporarily to avoid an epidemic. Domestic and personal hygiene measures introduced in their households may have been adopted by some of the servants.[19] Eventually, ideas about cleanliness and hygiene disseminated among the less well off, and the dispensary movement may have contributed to this from the end of the 18th century. The first dispensary opened in London in 1773, and outpatient services were provided for the sick poor. Attendance at dispensaries provided an opportunity to inform people about hygiene and caring for sick relatives and infants. Physicians learned from home visits about the dreadful sanitation and housing conditions that fostered infectious diseases among the poor,[20] long before knowledge about microbes and modes of transmission. Two major groups of disease could have been affected by appropriate advice to people concerning personal hygiene: the louse-borne diseases (typhus, relapsing fever, and trench fever) and gastrointestinal diseases (e.g., typhoid, dysentery). The enteric fevers (typhoid fever and paratyphoid fever) are caused by bacterial infection with *Salmonella typhi* and *Salmonella paratyphi*, transmitted via water, milk, and food contaminated with fecal matter. Even before these sources of infection were known, improvements in personal hygiene could have prevented pathogens in fecal matter being transmitted via the hands to food, or directly to the mouth. Improvements in personal hygiene and the washing of clothes and bedding could also have reduced the risk of typhus infection. Razzell suggested that increasing availability of washable cotton clothes might have contributed to the prevention of louse-borne infectious diseases among those who could afford them. He noted that contemporaries had reported improvements in cleanliness that could have contributed to the reductions in "fevers" deaths in London in the second half of the 18th century.[21]

Although there may have been some improvements in personal hygiene and a reduction in foci of typhus epidemics in England from the mid-18th century, the disease remained endemic in the poorest areas of major cities, particularly among people without regular wages, the destitute, and vagrants. The resurgence of the disease in the mid-19th century may have been linked with economic hardship caused by the Crimean War, although Hardy suggested that the epidemic of 1856 started shortly before the return of soldiers. Immigration from Ireland peaked in London in the 1850s, but major typhus epidemics have not been traced to that source.[22] The epidemic in London in the 1860s particularly affected unemployed men, overcrowded lodging houses, and poor areas disrupted by slum clearance, street building, and railway projects, and the disease spread from these sources to other communities.[23] Slum clearance schemes were driven by public health concern to eliminate "fever-nests," and measures to clean tenements were adopted in London following their introduction in Liverpool.[24]

Provision of regular water supplies in typhus-prone areas of London between the 1850s and 1870s may have made it easier for working people to wash their clothes and themselves. A drainage project was completed in the 1860s, and the removal of large quantities of refuse from inner London could have reduced the number of rats living around human habitations. The impact of these improvements on typhus incidence is difficult to assess, although the typhus/typhoid death rate in London was down to 5 per 100,000 by the 1870s. There were still large mortality differentials, with a death rate of 58 per 100,000 in Liverpool, which had trade and transport links with Dublin and Belfast, where the death rate was still over 90 per 100,000.[25] However, typhus had ceased to be a major killer in most towns in England, and the national death rate was below 2 per 100,000. In the last three decades of the century, improvements in the general economic circumstances may have reduced social dislocation and the need for the poor to share overcrowded dwellings, while isolation of cases in hospitals could have had some impact on the spread of the disease toward the end of the century. The decline of typhus benefited both children and adults, and the final recession of the disease from the 1870s contributed to the downturn in child mortality and total mortality.

Cholera, Public Health Reforms, and Mortality Decline

The 1870s marked a major turning point for disease and mortality in England. In the last three decades of the 19th century, typhus and smallpox, the major epidemic diseases of the 18th century, were practically eliminated, there was no major outbreak of cholera, and the typhoid death rate was down to a very low level (fig. 6.1). Cholera, which had arrived in Britain in 1831 during a Europe-wide pandemic, was greatly feared. This led to implementation of quarantine measures and cordon sanitaires of the kind imposed earlier to prevent the spread of plague. The cause of cholera, how it spread, and how to treat the sick were largely unknown, although boiling water for drinking to prevent the disease and to rehydrate victims may have been practiced on a limited scale in some parts of Europe.[26] The causal microorganism, *Vibrio cholerae*, is highly pathogenic to humans, and those infected have very visible symptoms of severe diarrhea, vomiting, and rapid wasting. It spreads rapidly where water supplies are contaminated and sanitation is poor. People are infected by consuming water, milk, or food contaminated by fecal matter, or by direct contact with infected people resulting in hand-to-mouth transmission. Case fatality in untreated epidemics can be over 50%,[27] and the first cases of the disease not surprisingly caused great consternation. The Board of Health in England accepted the "contagion theory" and imposed quarantine on ships arriving from the Baltic. However, this public health measure was suspended in 1832 following pressure from businessmen and merchants whose profits were negatively affected.[28]

In the years 1831–35, the annual numbers of deaths recorded as due to cholera in the London Bills of Mortality were 48, 3,200, 1,150, 630, and 5, respectively. In the peak year of 1832, 11% of all deaths were attributed directly to the disease, which was probably an underreporting since many more deaths than usual were recorded in the categories "old age" and "unknown causes." Fear of

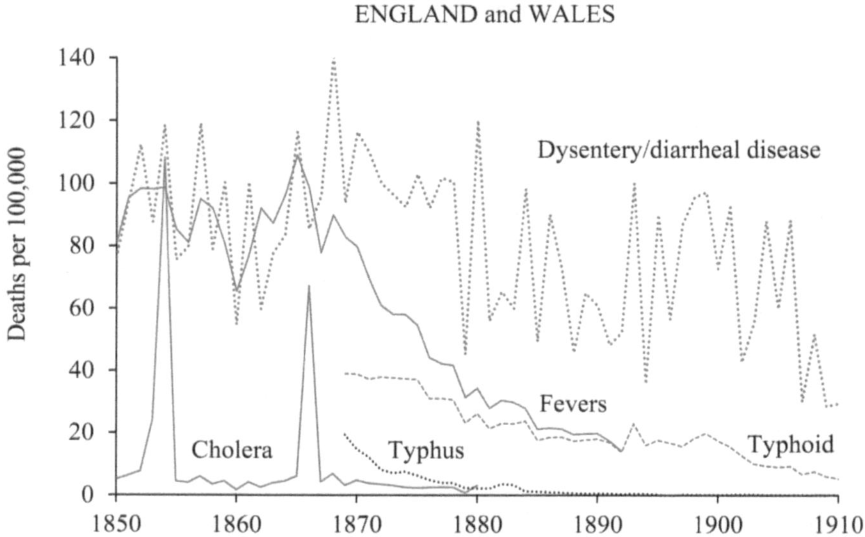

Figure 6.1. Annual death rates from typhus, typhoid and simple fever, cholera, dysentery, and diarrheal disease in England and Wales, 1850–1910. *Sources:* Registrar General, *Annual Reports*; *Annual Statistical Reviews.*

cholera encouraged authorities in many towns and rural districts to set up local boards of health. However, the epidemic also caused great concern that slum areas would become breeding grounds for social unrest as well as the disease itself. Chadwick's revelations in 1842 about living conditions in industrial towns raised awareness among the middle classes;[29] however, it is unlikely that most landowners or the government were concerned on humanitarian grounds. In fact, a Royal Commission was established to review the workings of the Poor Law with the aim of finding a cheaper system of relief rather than making improvements to benefit the poor. The local system of relief under the Poor Laws had provided some social security in England, particularly during food shortages, but at the beginning of the 19th century large numbers of the new urban poor were not covered. Many had recently moved from rural areas to seek a livelihood in the towns, and were thus not included in the parish registers on which local poor relief was based.[30] Despite this, influential advocates of laissez-faire and unregulated economic activity secured a dramatic reduction in government support for the parish-based system of relief. Under a new Poor Law in 1834, enforced labor in workhouses was instituted for those who had no work or means of support. Chadwick, who had originally supported the revision of the Poor Law, later recognized that disease was a fundamental problem that needed to be urgently addressed.

The environmentalist approach was aimed at health problems associated with standing water, animal waste, polluted wells, and inadequate sewerage and drains. The publication by Chadwick and others of the *Report of an Inquiry into the Sanitary Condition of the Labouring Population of Great Britain* in 1842, together with the Public Health Act of 1848 that he sponsored, sought to coerce major towns into implementing a radical environmental health program. This effort met with considerable opposition from property-owners who would have to pay local taxes to fund the program. Initially, the government adopted only the repressive measures from Chadwick's program, ignoring his proposals for sanitation and free education. He produced sanitary maps showing higher incidence of disease in the most overcrowded areas.[31] The new national registration system provided statistical data on crowding and disease in industrial towns and cities, which were used by supporters of public health reform to raise awareness of conditions. However, a General Board of Health was established in 1848, not because of evidence of deprivation but because of concerns in Parliament about the possibility of another cholera epidemic.[32]

Chadwick favored prevention rather than cure of disease, and most champions of public health reform were not medical professionals, with the notable exception of John Snow. Until the 1840s, sewers had been little more than elongated cesspools with an overflow at one end. Chadwick proposed that waste matter should be deposited away from human habitation through sewers constructed out of smooth ceramic pipes that could be flushed with water. Compensation payments and fear of cholera helped to overcome opposition to his scheme from owners of private property.[33] Snow's investigations during the cholera epidemics of 1848–49 and 1853 in London, and the evidence he collected implicating particular water sources, contributed to a more evidence-based theory of transmission and a scientific rationale for improving water and sewage systems. In the 1849 epidemic, he investigated deaths from cholera in the neighborhood of Broad Street in Soho, suspecting that water from a local street pump had been contaminated. By interviewing families of those who had died in the surrounding subdistricts, he found that most drank water from that pump. He suggested that the dramatic decline in the daily number of deaths in the week before the pump handle was removed was due to people fleeing the area.[34] He observed that the districts of London with the highest cholera death rates in 1849 were those supplied with water from the nearby River Thames by the Southwark and Vauxhall Company and the Lambeth Water Company, and a subsequent change in the water source of the latter provided an opportunity for further epidemiological investigation when the 1853 epidemic occurred.

In 1852 the Lambeth Company relocated its waterworks upstream to Thames Ditton to the west of London where water was not contaminated by London sewage. Snow found that districts partially supplied from this new source had lower death rates from cholera in the 1853 epidemic.[35] As households in the districts where these companies operated could be supplied by either company, even in the same street, he obtained addresses from the Registrar General of people who died of cholera, which enabled him to conduct a survey of households to identify their source of water. He found that the death rate from cholera among people supplied with water from the nearby River Thames by the Southwark and

Vauxhall Company was 14 times higher than that among people supplied by the Lambeth Company from the new source outside London.[36] The results of this epidemiological investigation were reported by the Registrar General, the *Lancet*, and other medical journals as evidence of waterborne transmission of cholera, strengthening the case for construction of new water and sewage systems to avoid fecal contamination of drinking water.

The aims of public health reformers were contrary to the reactionary view that it was a "law of nature" that the weak died off. Some argued that mutual aid interfered with a process of natural selection and survival of the fittest, and there was much laissez-faire, noninterventionist opposition to public health measures.[37] Despite this, pressure exerted by influential philosophical radicals helped to secure enactment of reforms by Parliament between the 1820s and 1870s;[38] however, this did not address the structural inequalities of the social and economic order that contributed to poverty and ill health. Chadwick recognized that environmental action was needed to address the hazards of polluted water, sewage, and animal and industrial waste, and that legislation would be required to support this. Local boards of health required new powers to act against private companies that were supplying contaminated water. The Public Health (Water) Act of 1878 made municipal purchase of private waterworks possible, and following municipalization of separate water companies there was more effective control over the supply of clean water. By the end of the 19th century, about two-thirds of the urban sanitary authorities in England were running waterworks and supplying the majority of people in their area.[39]

The Nuisance Removal Acts of the 1850s and 1860s gave the new medical officers of health powers to control environmental hazards.[40] They were also responsible for investigating outbreaks of infectious disease in schools and factories, searching for cases on house-to-house visits, removing sick people from overcrowded tenements, and vaccinating smallpox contacts. Under threat of a new cholera epidemic, the Sanitary Act was passed in 1866, which greatly extended powers to implement measures for controlling infectious diseases. Riverside sanitary authorities were given responsibility for ships, and the London authority appointed an officer to inspect them.[41] Further measures required legislation, and the Public Health Act of 1872 enabled port sanitary authorities and new urban and rural sanitary authorities to be established. Medical inspection of ships and personnel was rapidly and widely implemented, and this probably played an important role in preventing cholera from being introduced from overseas. The Sanitary Acts of 1866 and 1872 divided the country into sanitary districts, which provided the basis for organizing public health programs, and local authorities were required to provide drainage, sewerage, and an adequate water supply.[42] Partly due to the need for a legal framework, it was not until the late 1860s that municipal governments were empowered to implement many of the public health reforms following elections based on a wider franchise.

The main focus of the public health movement was improvement of water quality and sewerage, initially in response to the threat of cholera.[43] Clearly, the impact on death rates would have varied in relation to the nature of the sewerage and sanitation systems and the timing of implementation, although national-level data indicate that the last major epidemic of cholera was in 1866. A much smaller number of deaths continued to be recorded in the Registrar General's annual reports under the category "simple cholera." However, the British Isles experienced few cases of Asian cholera after the 1860s, mostly linked with infected people arriving from abroad, as in the minor outbreak in the Midlands and North in 1892–93.[44] Although several types of preventive measure are likely to have contributed to the control of cholera, improvements in water quality probably had the biggest impact, reducing mortality from other gastrointestinal and diarrheal diseases in general.

The poorer areas of industrial towns in England were not always covered by the improvements in water and sewage systems, and there is evidence from different towns of area and social class differences in the impact on mortality.[45] Structural poverty and squalid living conditions persisted in working-class areas of northern towns such as Manchester. Only a small minority of people had benefited sufficiently from industrial development to enable them to move out of the filthy and neglected areas where most people worked and lived. Housing in industrial towns was described in the writings of Engels and Dickens as damp, crowded, and poorly ventilated, with pools of stagnant water and piles of stinking refuse in the streets.[46] Although the poorer areas became a focus for sanitary reformers at the end of the 19th century, local legislation was selectively applied, and water closets (WCs), or flush toilets, were only installed in a minority of houses. Most working-class households did not have WCs until new housing was built at the end of the century, and shared use of various forms of "privy" that could not be flushed is likely to have been very unhygienic. WCs were provided in new houses, although evidence from Liverpool at the end of the 19th century indicates that diarrheal disease death rates were no lower in the areas with new housing.[47]

There appears to have been much variation in the implementation of public health measures in different districts of London,[48] and the impact of different measures such as water supplies and sanitation is difficult to assess. Even so, public health measures to prevent cholera and the monitoring of sources of infection probably contributed to the decline in death rates from several diseases. The death rate from the "fevers" group (typhoid, typhus, and "simple fever") declined rapidly in London after the last major epidemic of cholera, as it did nationally (fig. 6.1). Death rates from typhus/typhoid declined dramatically in all registration districts of London between the 1860s and 1870s.[49] Under separate recording, the death rate from typhoid declined considerably in all districts between the 1870s and 1890s, with a great reduction in the differential between the poor and more affluent districts. Improvements were made in water filtration techniques, and strict standards for quality could be imposed on water companies when bacteriological methods for monitoring were developed in the 1880s. Contaminated water supplies are likely to have been the main source of typhoid infection in the city, although poor sanitation and poor hygiene were significant contributors in some areas.[50] Districts in the East End had the highest typhoid/typhus death rates, which peaked in the 1860s. Hardy suggested that the exceptional decline in Shoreditch was due to measures taken by the sanitary department to address soil pollution, inadequate drainage, and polluted wells, and mortality declined slightly in the 1860s as in other parts of London. In general, the decline in typhoid mortality in the city was probably due mainly to safer water supplies and their increasing provision in the poorer areas. Toward the end of the century, attention was focused on other interventions—for example, in Whitechapel where the typhoid death rate remained high due to poor sanitation and domestic hygiene among the immigrant population.[51]

Evidence from Birmingham suggests there was less association between typhoid mortality and domestic sanitary provision than might be expected given the association with poor housing.[52] Differences between households and areas with regard to fecal contamination of water and food might account for this. A study of Bradford found that epidemics of typhoid in the second half of the 19th century had affected people in middle-class households as well as those living in filthy, overcrowded, and poverty-stricken conditions.[53] People who were relatively well-off could afford milk, but dairy products were subject to contamination, while ownership of water closets could be hazardous due to poor plumbing and the risk of fecal contamination of drinking water. The formation of the Sanitary Association and employment of surveyors to inspect sanitation in the 1880s probably helped the better-off to avoid deaths from typhoid.[54] When certain areas had been provided with safer water and improved sewerage, attention during outbreaks could focus on other sources of infection and the less well provided areas.[55] Toward the end of the 19th century, bacteriological laboratory services were introduced, supporting efforts to monitor water, food, and milk supplies. At this stage, higher standards of domestic sanitation may have contributed to a reduction in the incidence of typhoid, while the new public fever hospitals were isolating some of the cases that did occur.[56] However, the earlier decline in typhoid death rates from the 1860s is likely to reflect the public health measures to prevent cholera, particularly improvements in water supplies and sewerage.

The death rate from dysentery and diarrheal diseases, which were mainly caused by fecal contamination of drinking water and food, also declined after the last cholera epidemic in the 1860s. Many diarrheal disease deaths among children and adults were probably prevented by measures introduced to control cholera. Some districts of London were among the first to benefit from improved water and sewage systems, and age-specific death rates from diarrheal disease were generally lower in London than in other towns and the country as a whole. The decline in diarrheal disease death rates among children and adults between the 1860s and 1890s was considerable,[57] and unlikely to be explained by transfer of recording to other categories such as gastroenteritis.[58] The lack of consistent decline in the death rate among infants until after 1900 (figs. 6.2 and 7.5) is considered in chapter 7. The upsurge in diarrheal disease mortality in the 1890s affected all age groups (fig. 6.1), and was probably due to increased incidence of fly-borne and food-borne gastrointestinal infections over a series of hot dry summers.[59] Various changes could have contributed to a subsequent reduction in fly-borne disease, including the removal of refuse and human waste away from inhabited areas, the introduction of covered dustbins in the 1890s,[60] and the gradual reduction of manure in the streets with the replacement of horse-drawn carriages by motor vehicles in the early 20th century. However, the areas in which the poor lived in rapidly growing towns would have been the last to benefit from public health improvements in refuse collection and provision of domestic sanitation.

Improvements in water and sewage systems are likely to have reduced exposure to various pathogens transmitted through fecal contamination of drinking water. Even so, sanitation, hygiene standards, and living conditions in the poorer areas of London and industrial towns would have remained highly conducive to the spread of other fly-borne and food-borne infections that caused diarrhea. Records of sickness treated in London in the second half of the 19th century indicate particularly high diarrheal disease morbidity among young children and older adults;[61] this fact is reflected in the age pattern of mortality (fig. 6.2). A decline in case fatality from diarrheal disease is unlikely to have been due to treatment, and does not necessarily reflect improved resistance to infection. Case fatality would depend on the type of pathogen involved and the age of those infected, as well as current health and nutrition status. The types of pathogens may have been different from those that caused more deaths before the improvement of water quality. In more recent times, very harmful pathogens causing dysentery and diarrheal diseases were replaced by milder species in many countries when water supplies were purified.[62] The milder pathogens would still cause diarrheal disorders, particularly at the extremes of life, in places where hygiene conditions had not improved, although case fatality and death rates would be lower than in earlier times when more harmful pathogens were prevalent.

Although many public health and preventive measures are likely to have contributed to the decline in death rates from gastrointestinal and diarrheal diseases in England, evidence from other countries indicates the particular importance of improvements in water supplies. Waterborne infectious diseases appear to have made a significant contribution to differential mortality decline in France in the 19th century, with mortality declining in three departments where water and sanitation infrastructure was built.[63] Ewald has suggested that development of safe water supplies was critical for the elimination of typhoid, dysentery, and cholera in Western countries, along with other public health and hygiene measures that reduced the risk of transmission. The highly virulent forms of the bacteria causing these diseases had evolved to become dependent on waterborne transmission.[64] The importance of safe water supplies for prevention of cholera is illustrated by the epidemic in Peru in 1991, when the disease spread quickly through Central and South America. The harmfulness of *Vibrio cholerae* was monitored by measuring the amount of toxin produced (toxigenicity). When the epidemic spread to Chile where water supplies were relatively safe, bacteria with high toxigenicity were not found a few years later and the incidence of

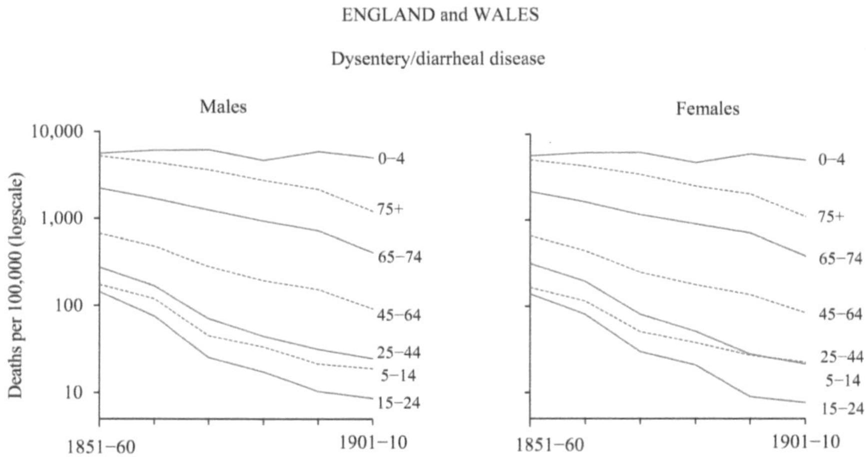

Figure 6.2. Annual average age-specific death rates from diarrhea and dysentery in England and Wales, 1851–60 to 1901–10. *Sources:* Registrar General, *Annual Reports*; *Annual Statistical Reviews*.

cholera was much lower than in Peru. Water quality was poor in Peru, and bacteria with high toxigenicity continued to coexist with bacteria of low toxigenicity for a decade, resulting in much higher incidence of cholera than in Chile.[65]

The benefits of providing safe water in the United States in the 20th century are indicated by a dramatic decline in the typhoid death rate in Philadelphia when filtered water was first provided in 1906, and made available to everyone by 1909.[66] A study of the introduction of water filtration and chlorination systems and death rates over the period 1900–1936 found that provision of clean water was followed by a rapid decline in the typhoid death rates in Philadelphia and other major cities such as Baltimore, Cincinnati, Detroit, and Pittsburgh.[67] Maintenance of public health standards for water and sanitation would have been particularly important in the economic depression of the 1930s when the death rate might otherwise have increased.[68] Much earlier, thousands of deaths from cholera were recorded in New York City in epidemics between 1832 and 1866. Cholera and smallpox epidemics accounted for most of the mortality spikes in the 19th century, but cholera was not a major killer after 1866, and smallpox caused very few deaths after 1902.[69] Given the severity of cholera and smallpox and the high case fatality from these diseases, it is very unlikely that the decline in mortality was due to improved resistance. The recession of these destructive epidemic diseases, which made a significant contribution to overall mortality decline in New York City in the second half of the 19th century, was mainly due to effective preventive measures and public health interventions.

The epidemics of cholera in England in the mid-19th century were part of a worldwide pandemic exacerbated by increased trade and travel. High mortality from cholera is unlikely to have been avoided in England after the 1860s without effective preventive measures and public health interventions. Within four decades of the disease arriving in the country in the 1830s, it had been prevented from becoming a regular cause of high mortality through public health measures backed by legislation, made possible by reformers committed to the political struggle involved.[70] Final control was probably dependent on prevention of reintroduction from overseas and effective measures for containing outbreaks based on new knowledge about the microbial cause of the disease. The epidemiological findings of Snow in the 1850s linking cholera outbreaks with contaminated sources of drinking water had provided a scientific basis for intervention in the public interest, even before the germ theory explained transmission. Bacteriological identification of the bacillus was not achieved until much later in the epidemic of 1883 in Egypt and India.[71] Nevertheless, preventive measures controlled cholera and almost certainly reduced mortality from other gastrointestinal and diarrheal diseases, forming the basis for sustained disease control in the 20th century. Improvements in water supplies, sewage disposal, and personal hygiene; the monitoring of outbreaks of disease; and isolation of cases are likely to have contributed to the prevention of typhoid and other gastrointestinal diseases. The typhoid death rate declined fairly continuously in England after the last major cholera epidemic in the 1860s, and the death rate from dysentery and other diarrheal diseases declined until the resurgence in the hot summers of the 1890s. Exposure to many types of pathogens that caused gastrointestinal infections would have remained high because of poor domestic hygiene, poor food preservation, and fly-borne contamination of food. The fact that infants were particularly vulnerable to diarrheal diseases because of poor weaning practices and the contribution of these diseases to the continuingly high infant mortality rate in the second half of the 19th century are considered in the next chapter.

Chapter Seven

Infant Mortality

In the 18th century there was probably a great deal of fatalism about sickness in the early months of life as deaths among infants were so common. Many deaths in the first two years of life were recorded in a category labeled "infancy" in the London Bills of Mortality. A major category within this was "convulsions," a symptom of many untreated conditions among infants, particularly certain infectious diseases and dietary deficiency.[1] Diarrhea in infants can terminate in convulsions, and many deaths would have been caused by unhygienic or inappropriate weaning foods, water or milk contaminated with fecal matter, and dehydration, as in developing countries today.[2] The summer peaks in "convulsions" deaths probably reflect a seasonal increase in gastrointestinal diseases due to fecally contaminated food and fly-borne germs.[3] Deaths recorded in the category "teething" may also include many deaths from infectious diseases and gastrointestinal infections due to use of contaminated weaning foods.[4] As mentioned earlier, the categories "convulsions" and "fevers" are likely to have included some cases of smallpox among infants, as they could have fever or convulsions but no other distinctive symptoms.[5] The strong correlation (r = +0.6) between "infancy" and smallpox death rates for London based on the Bills of Mortality between 1671–75 and 1831–35[6] and the broad similarity between the trends and major turning points (fig. 3.1) are consistent with this.

This chapter considers the possible causes of the decline in death rates from infant disorders and infectious diseases. Despite the limitations of classification, the simple arithmetic components of mortality change give some indication of the relative importance of the different categories of deaths considered here. The total death rate (for all ages) for London based on the Bills of Mortality declined by about 32% between 1751 and 1801, with "convulsions," "teething," and other "infancy" deaths contributing –0.40 to each unit of change. In the second half of the 19th century, when the death rate for England and Wales declined by 22%, the major contributions to a unit of change were from convulsions/teething (–0.14) and scarlet fever/diphtheria (–0.12). Between 1901 and 1951, the total death rate declined by about 62%; prematurity and congenital and perinatal conditions made a much greater contribution to each unit of change (–0.12), along with convulsions/teething (–0.06), scarlet fever (–0.04), measles (–0.03), and whooping cough (–0.03) (see appendix C1).

The infant death rate declined by 80% between 1901 and 1951, with contributions to each unit of change from measles (–0.02); whooping cough (–0.04);

nonrespiratory tuberculosis (–0.08); respiratory diseases (–0.16); convulsions/teething (–0.16); gastroenteritis/diarrheal diseases (–0.17); and prematurity, debility, atrophy, and congenital conditions (–0.19). Many deaths classified as "convulsions" and other deaths assigned to the vague categories of "debility" and "atrophy" are likely to have been linked with infectious diseases and diarrhea. Under national registration, some deaths from diarrheal disease may have been assigned to the "atrophy" and "debility" categories since the practice of purging often led to rejection of food, emaciation, thirst, and fever.[7] Some epidemic diseases of childhood such as measles also caused diarrhea and respiratory symptoms to which death may have been attributed in the absence of characteristic spots in the very young. The diarrheal diseases and gastrointestinal disorders that killed many infants would have weakened those who survived, making them susceptible to other infectious diseases encountered for the first time. Intercurrent infections would also have increased the risk of death, and only one cause would be recorded depending on the most visible and recognized symptoms.

Wrigley and Schofield's estimates for England suggest that infant mortality declined from the 1740s, contributing to the overall mortality decline.[8] Several other sets of data, with some exceptions, indicate that infant mortality declined in England in the second half of the 18th century.[9] Infant mortality continued to decline before leveling off in the second half of the 19th century, in contrast with the trend for Sweden, where infant mortality declined more consistently (fig. 7.1). The longer series of national registration data for Sweden indicates that infant mortality fluctuated around 200 per 1,000 live births in the second half of the 18th century, then declined sharply after 1810 to around 150 per 1,000. After a brief resurgence in the 1830s, the underlying trend was downward, with fewer spikes in annual mortality from the 1870s onward. Data for Austria, France, the Netherlands, and Norway also indicate that infant mortality declined from the 1870s, in contrast with Belgium and Denmark, where there was no consistent decline between 1850 and 1890 (fig. 7.2), and with England and Wales, where there was a resurgence in the 1880s and 1890s.

The lack of consistent decline in the infant mortality rate for England and Wales in the second half of the 19th century can be seen as a leveling off in a long-term decline from the mid-18th century. Wrigley and Schofield estimated that the annual infant mortality rate for England averaged 195 per 1,000 live births in the first half of the 18th century and 165 per 1,000 in the second half.[10] National registration data indicate that the rate was 155 per 1,000 live births in the mid-19th century (1848–54). Although there was some further decline in the 1870s, the resurgence in the 1880s and 1890s brought infant mortality back to 154 per 1,000 by 1900, after which it declined more rapidly and consistently to reach 30 per 1,000 by 1950.

There were significant geographic and socioeconomic differences in the level and trend in infant mortality in England. Estimates of infant mortality for London in the 18th century based on the Bills of Mortality suggest it was much higher than for England as a whole. However, the decline was probably more rapid in London, from 380 per 1,000 births in the 1740s to 205 per 1,000 in the

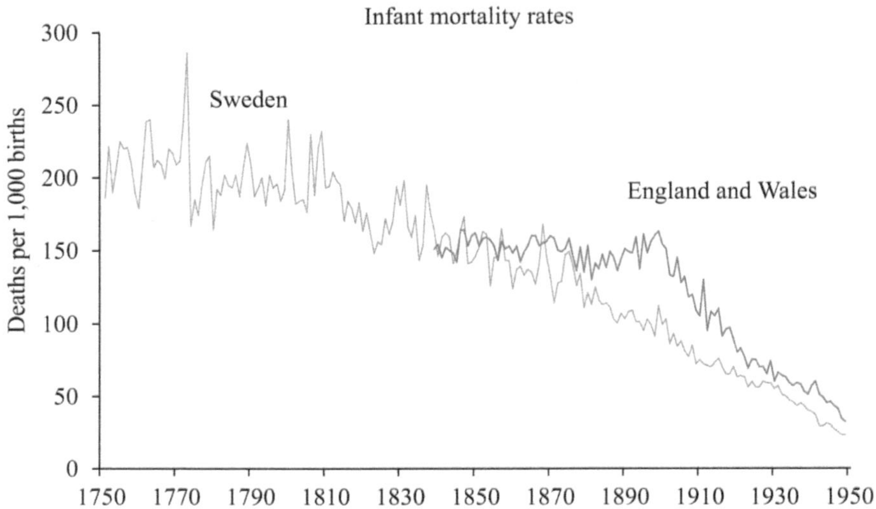

Figure 7.1. Annual infant mortality rates in England and Wales (1839–1950) and Sweden (1751–1950). *Source:* Mitchell, *European Historical Statistics,* 127–33.

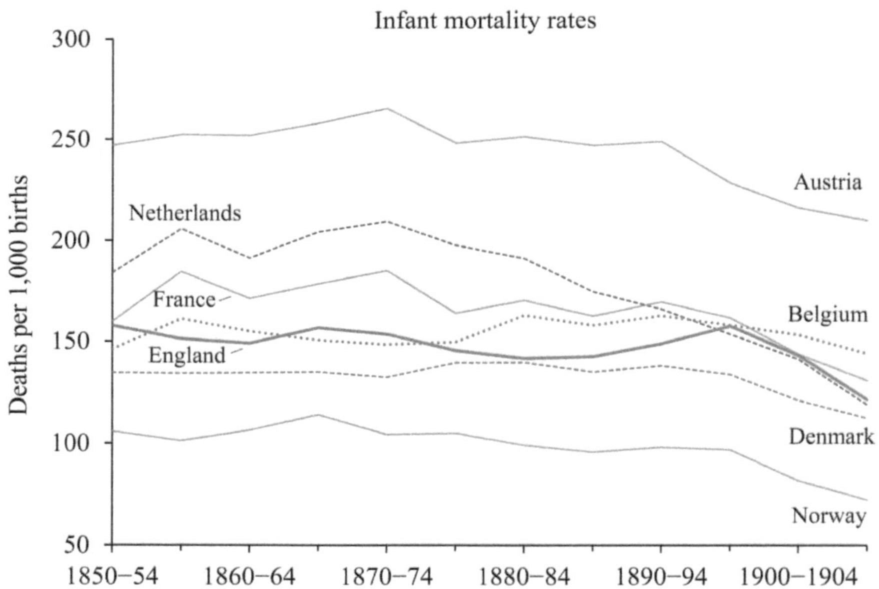

Figure 7.2. Annual infant mortality rates in England and Wales and other European countries, 1850–54 to 1905–9. *Source:* Mitchell, *European Historical Statistics,* 127–33.

1810s.[11] There was a further decline in the first half of the 19th century that was more rapid than in other towns. Data for the British peerage indicate that infant mortality in the 17th century had been about the same as for the population as a whole, but the decline began earlier. The annual average infant mortality rate was estimated at 200 per 1,000 live births in the mid-17th century, 167 per 1,000 in the first half of the 18th century, and 93 per 1,000 in the second half of the century—well below the estimate of 165 per 1,000 for the country as a whole.[12] Many members of the aristocracy lived in rural areas where infant mortality among the general population was lower than in the towns. Registration data indicate that in the second half of the 19th century infant mortality was about 30% higher for counties defined as "urban" compared with "rural" counties.[13] Large differences for particular towns and rural areas were reported by the Registrar General. Infant mortality in 1889–91 was twice as high for three selected towns compared with three rural counties, while the infant diarrheal disease death rate was eight times as high.[14]

Rural areas appear to have experienced declining infant mortality throughout the second half of the 19th century without the resurgence in the 1880s and 1890s in urban areas that affected the national rate.[15] By that time over half the population lived in urban areas, with over half the variation in infant mortality between districts associated with population density.[16] Infant mortality was much higher among children of industrial workers than children of agricultural laborers in the 1890s, and Woods suggested that infant mortality in large industrial towns and cities had come to predominate in the national trend.[17] Against the background of generally declining infant mortality from the mid-18th century, the increase in the national rate in the 1880s and 1890s was anomalous (fig. 7.3). However, the national rate did fall by about 9% between 1865–69 and 1880–84, and in northern industrial towns such as Manchester, Liverpool, and Glasgow the decline was quite dramatic.[18] This coincided with the renewed efforts to vaccinate against smallpox during the Europe-wide pandemic, as discussed in chapter 5. Other infectious diseases also contributed to the decline in the 1870s, including typhoid/typhus/simple fever, scarlet fever, and diphtheria (fig. 7.4). The focus here is on factors specific to changes in infant mortality, including the resurgence in the 1880s and 1890s and the rapid decline in the first decade of the 20th century among all socioeconomic groups.[19] However, it can be noted that the trend contrasts with a fairly continuous decline in the child (1–4 years) death rate from the 1860s, which is considered in chapter 8.

The lack of decline in infant mortality over the second half of the 19th century reflects increasing death rates from measles and "prematurity," an upsurge in respiratory and diarrheal disease deaths in the 1890s, and a lack of decline in death rates from some other diseases (fig. 7.5). The infant death rate from nonrespiratory tuberculosis did not decline much until the 1890s, although the death rate from respiratory tuberculosis was already declining. There was also little decline in the infant death rates from whooping cough and respiratory diseases until the 1890s, while the death rates from measles, diarrheal disease, and prematurity/debility did not decline consistently until after 1900. Premature

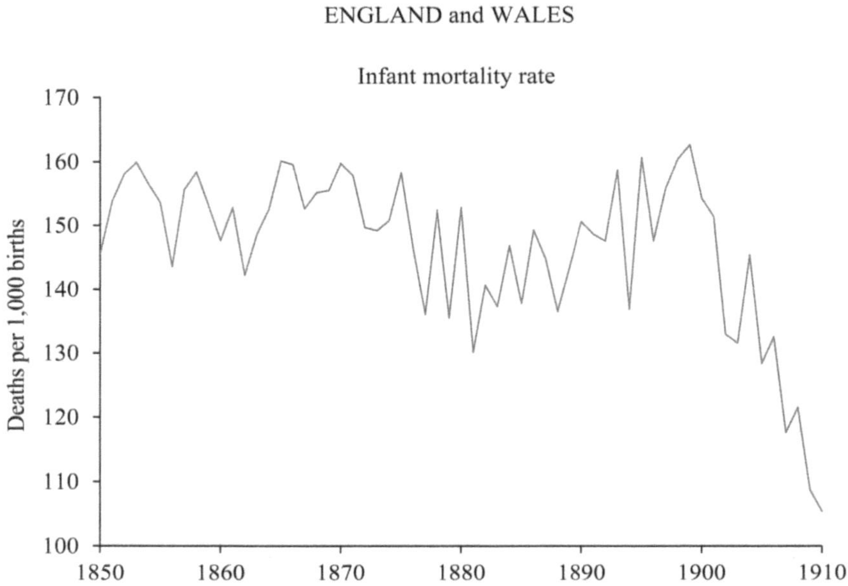

Figure 7.3. Annual infant mortality rates in England and Wales, 1850–1910. *Sources:* Registrar General, *Annual Reports*; *Annual Statistical Reviews.*

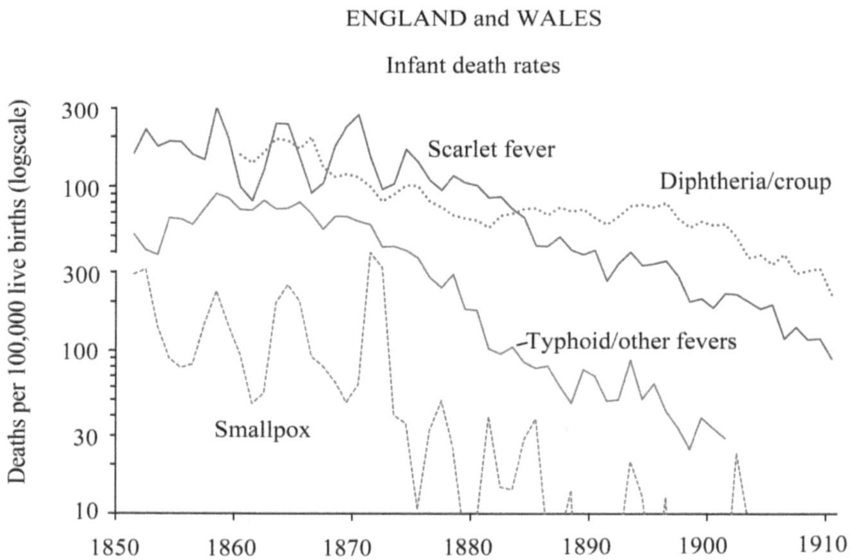

Figure 7.4. Annual infant death rates from scarlet fever, smallpox, diphtheria/croup, and typhoid in England and Wales, 1850–1910. *Sources:* Registrar General, *Annual Reports*; *Annual Statistical Reviews.*

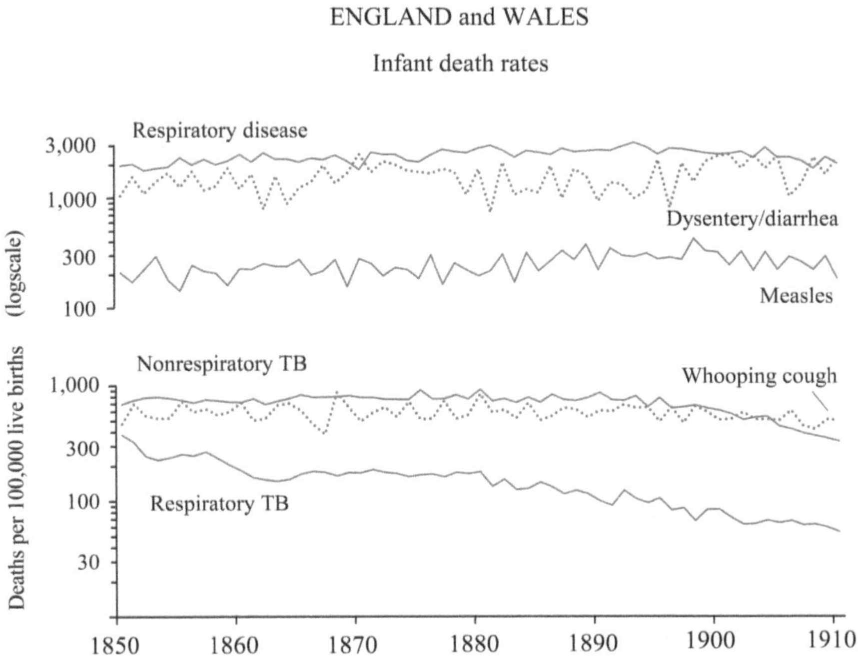

Figure 7.5. Annual infant death rates from tuberculosis, whooping cough, measles, respiratory disease, and diarrheal disease in England and Wales, 1850–1910. *Sources:* Registrar General, *Annual Reports*; *Annual Statistical Reviews*.

birth was recorded as the cause in about 10% of infant deaths in the second half of the 19th century, and the death rate from this increased in the 1880s and 1890s. Deaths attributed to diarrheal diseases accounted for over 40% of all infant deaths in the second half of the 19th century, and the increase in the last two decades, particularly in urban areas, contributed most to the resurgence in the national infant mortality rate. As mentioned, a series of hot dry summers is likely to have contributed significantly to higher diarrheal disease mortality in the 1890s, particularly in the towns and cities where crowded and insanitary conditions persisted.[20]

The relative contribution of different factors to changes in infant mortality is more difficult to assess than the determinants of cross-sectional variation by geographic area and socioeconomic group. Mosley and Chen, in developing an analytical framework for assessing determinants of child mortality in developing countries, pointed out that child deaths are usually a cumulative consequence of multiple disease processes rather than an isolated disease episode,[21] so quantifying the relative contributions to mortality change can be misleading. A mother's health and circumstances during pregnancy can affect the risk of having a premature or low-birth-weight baby, which will be at higher risk of dying in infancy.

Infectious diseases experienced in adolescence and during pregnancy would be debilitating, increasing the risks associated with childbirth along with other factors such as diet and the demands of work. The conditions of female employment and long hours worked in factories would have been detrimental to health and the care that mothers could provide for their children. Pregnancy and childbirth would also have been debilitating, while postponement would allow time to recover, improving survival chances for both the mother and her next child. Longer birth intervals could also result in longer periods of breastfeeding, further improving the child's chances of surviving.[22] Although the decline in infant mortality between 1901 and 1931 does not appear to have been associated with changes in fertility at the national level,[23] there is evidence of an association over the period 1895–1910 for occupational groups with relatively high rates of fertility decline.[24] There was more association between declining fertility and infant mortality in urban areas, and changes in infant mortality at the national level largely reflect changes in urban occupational groups.[25] However, the increase in the national infant mortality rate in the 1880s and 1890s when the birthrate was declining suggests that any beneficial effect of lower fertility did not predominate over adverse influences.

There was also higher maternal mortality in the 1890s, although the level was otherwise fairly consistent in the second half of the 19th century. There is evidence of an earlier decline in the 18th century,[26] and registration data indicate continuing decline in the first half of the 19th century. However, this was followed by a leveling off at 400–500 deaths per 100,000 births until the higher mortality in the early 1890s. Thereafter maternal mortality declined between 1895 and 1910, which reflected a decline in the death rate from puerperal fever and other causes, including hemorrhage and toxemia (fig. 7.6). However, there was no further decline until a sharp drop in 1937, which coincided with the introduction of sulfonamides. As in other Western countries, these proved highly effective against *Streptococcus pyogenes* infection, the main cause of puerperal fever. The proportion of maternal mortality in England and Wales due to these infections declined from 55% in 1872–76 to just 5% in 1976–81.[27]

Puerperal fever had affected the rich and the poor, and lying-in hospitals in the 18th century appear to have been far more dangerous than giving birth at home, which most women did. A link between puerperal fever deaths and the practice of midwives and doctors was suspected in the 19th century. In 1846 Semmelweiss observed that medical students who assisted with autopsies in a hospital clinic in Vienna examined women in labor without washing their hands. His insistence on washing in chlorine of lime demonstrated that cases of puerperal fever could be dramatically reduced, although it was not until the 1880s that the practice was widely accepted.[28] Following Lister's use of antisepsis for surgery in the 1870s, and Pasteur's discovery of the bacterial microorganism responsible for puerperal fever (*S. pyogenes*), antisepsis was introduced in lying-in hospitals.[29] However, most women continued to give birth at home, where the risk of infection would partly depend on the training and practice of midwives. Hygiene practices among women birth attendants

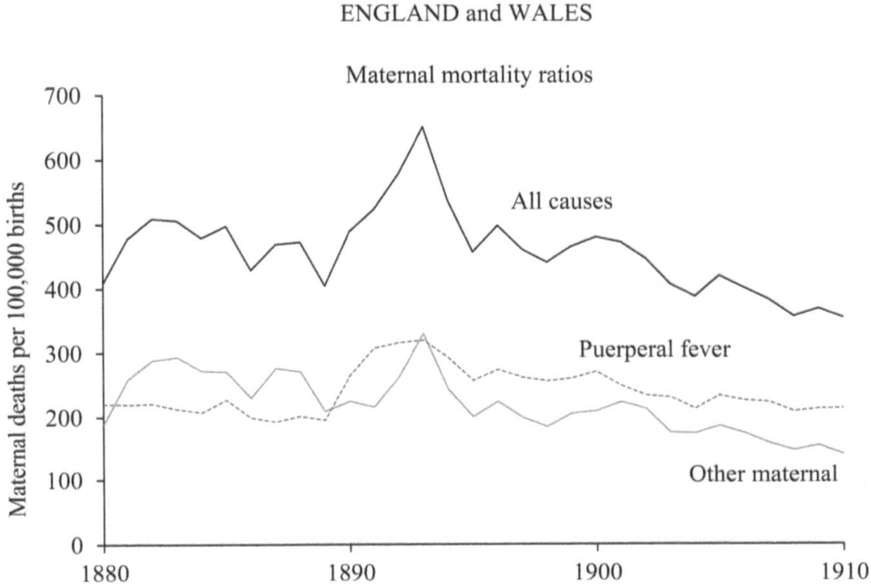

Figure 7.6. Annual maternal mortality ratios for puerperal fever and other causes in England and Wales, 1880–1910. *Sources:* Registrar General, *Annual Reports*; *Annual Statistical Reviews.*

reportedly improved in Scandinavia, Belgium, and the Netherlands at the end of the 19th century. The decline in maternal mortality in England and Wales between 1895 and 1910 may reflect similar improvements, which could also have improved survival chances for babies. However, maternal mortality did not decline in the 1920s and 1930s when training and supervision of midwives reportedly became better organized.[30]

The lack of decline in maternal mortality in the second half of the 19th century and the resurgence in the 1890s parallels the trend in infant mortality. The lack of consistent improvement in the national infant mortality rate in this period is likely to reflect continuingly poor domestic hygiene and infant care as well as the insanitary and crowded conditions in which the majority of people lived in towns and large industrial cities. The diarrheal disease death rate among infants increased between the 1860s and 1890s, in contrast with the trends for older children and adults (figs. 6.2 and 7.5). As discussed in chapter 6, older children and adults probably benefited more from the improvement in water and sewage systems. Some districts of London were among the first to benefit, which could explain the greater improvement in diarrheal disease death rates at these ages in London compared with the country as a whole.[31] However, the death rate from diarrheal diseases among infants was higher than elsewhere, and there was no consistent decline in the second half of the 19th century in London or nationally.

Evidence from developing countries suggests that delay in the decline of diarrheal disease mortality among infants can be due as much to poverty and ignorance about child care as to inadequate public health and preventive measures to control infectious diseases.[32] In the second half of the 19th century in England, many pathogens causing gastrointestinal and diarrheal diseases would have remained prevalent despite improvements in water and sewage systems. A local government survey in 16 towns at the beginning of the 20th century found that infant mortality was associated with poor domestic sanitation in particular.[33] As mentioned in chapter 6, fecal-oral transmission would have been fostered by lack of cleanliness and poor hygiene, with case fatality being determined by the type of pathogens involved, the age of those infected, their health and nutrition status, and other factors. During hot weather, flies would be more abundant and fly-borne infections more prevalent because of lack of sanitation, exposed human excreta, and animal feces in the streets. Although all age groups would have been affected, infants contracting pathogens for the first time would have no immunity. They remained particularly vulnerable to infection from contaminated milk and foods used for weaning, which could not be kept fresh in warm weather. Most infants would experience repeated episodes of diarrhea as in developing countries today, with a high risk of dying from dehydration as mothers are unlikely to have been aware of the need for rehydration.

Working-class households would generally have been the last to gain from public health measures and improved domestic sanitation. The mothers would be the last to benefit from new knowledge about germs, the spread of infection, hygiene, food preparation, and child care. A study of circumstances contributing to continuingly high infant mortality in Bradford at the end of the 19th century concluded that it was not due to their negligence or apathy.[34] While factory work was detrimental to mother-child relationships, infant diarrhea and deaths were as common in mining communities as in towns where women worked in factories, and the total infant mortality rate was about the same for children of miners, textile workers, and unskilled laborers.[35] Dysentery, diarrheal diseases, and other gastrointestinal disorders were almost certainly a greater risk in poor households. In addition to deficiencies in protein and vitamins in weaning foods given to infants, such as bread with milk, domestic circumstances were not favorable to washing equipment used for food preparation, let alone sterilizing it.[36] Many working-class mothers are unlikely to have boiled water to wash bottles, and the benefits of using sterilized milk would have been limited by the hygiene standards in households that could afford to buy it. Use of dangerous or unhygienic pacifiers would also have contributed to infant sickness in poorer families.

The demands on women in the new environment of industrial towns are likely to have had an adverse effect on the relationship with their infants, with detrimental physiological and emotional consequences for their children's development.[37] The ability and opportunity to breastfeed would depend on the mother's nutritional status and health, any work she did outside the home, and other demands on her time. The extent, length, and exclusivity of breastfeeding, and use of supplementary foods, would have affected the risk of diarrheal disorders among infants. Breastfeeding ought to have been preferred because no financial cost was involved, and some women may have known that it reduced the chances of becoming pregnant.[38] Breastfeeding is particularly important for neonates because the mother's first milk, colostrum, contains protective antibodies and other proteins.[39] Early neonatal feeding practices, duration of breastfeeding, and age at weaning can affect the risk of dying in early childhood from gastrointestinal infections and airborne infectious diseases such as measles. Part of the variation in infant mortality between areas, and the lack of increase in the diarrheal disease death rate in some districts in the 1880s and 1890s, may have been due to differences in breastfeeding practices. Data from selected towns in the early 1900s indicate wide variation in the proportion of infants being breastfed (55–85%).[40] However, there is little indication of any major change in breastfeeding practices that could account for the downturn in infant mortality at the beginning of the 20th century, which occurred in all areas and socioeconomic groups.[41] Infants generally are likely to have benefited from improvements in milk supplies, food standards, domestic hygiene, and infant care, while public health improvements in water and sewage systems had contributed to the reduction of diarrheal disease mortality among older children and adults from the 1860s.

The germ theory of infection eventually led to a recognition that the home environment could contain dangers for young children, and that mothers needed to create safe and hygienic domestic conditions and sustain breastfeeding.[42] In the 1890s, concern about high infant mortality became more widespread in England, and voluntary organizations were developed for health visiting, with municipal corporations providing formalized training. Development of the health-visiting movement coincided with the more continuous decline in infant mortality from the beginning of the 20th century.[43] Visits were made to every home with a mother and young child, and nurseries were established where mothers could be instructed in infant care and feeding.[44] The mother-and-child movement in the first half of the 20th century encouraged more careful child-rearing practices in many English-speaking countries. Preston suggested that the new scientific understanding of disease processes led to promotion of measures whereby parents could reduce the risks faced by their children in the home. These included boiling milk and sterilizing bottles, which had been recommended in the 1890s; washing hands; protecting food from flies; and isolating sick family members.[45] Before this, even better-off and better-educated parents had lacked guidance on how to improve their children's survival chances. In the United States, there was less differential in child survival in relation to occupation and education than in England and Wales, but socioeconomic differentials increased as new practices were adopted more quickly by more well-off families.[46]

Mother's education and literacy are strongly correlated with children's survival chances in developing countries today, a relationship that is independent of economic circumstances.[47] Schooling for girls, even of very short duration, seems to empower women to overcome traditional restrictions and enable them to make effective use of basic mother-and-child health services and preventive and curative measures introduced from Western countries.[48] Although such services were not available in Western countries at the end of the 19th century, increasing attendance of girls in schools probably increased their access and openness to new ideas about child care and family planning. Attendance increased in England and Wales after the Education Act of 1870, which made it compulsory. Literacy increased women's access to information about birth control, such as the pamphlet published by Annie Besant and Charles Bradlaugh in 1877. The right to disseminate information about family planning was challenged in a court case in London, but reports of the trial focused attention on the issue and led to a huge increase in the number of pamphlets distributed.[49] This probably contributed to changing attitudes toward the use of birth control, and the birthrate declined after the 1870s. In an analysis of the relationship between female education, fertility, poverty, and infant mortality (nondiarrheal) using data from districts of England and Wales for 1901–10, Woods found that lower infant mortality was associated with female education and there was some association with lower fertility. He concluded that the increase in female education contributed to an improvement in the status of women and gave them greater access to written information and knowledge about preventing pregnancy and how to provide better care for a smaller number of children.[50]

The rapid decline in the national infant mortality rate in the first half of the 20th century, from about 150 per 1,000 live births to 30, reflected reductions across administrative districts and socioeconomic groups.[51] The main cause groups contributing to the decline were prematurity, congenital conditions, and debility, which were associated with maternal health; and respiratory disease, gastrointestinal disease, convulsions, and nonrespiratory tuberculosis. The decline in both infant and child (1–4 years) mortality from respiratory and diarrheal diseases was greater than the decline for certain nutritional deficiency diseases that could reflect improved diet.[52] Although the main determinants of infant mortality decline in England and Wales and other countries are well established, it is difficult to draw conclusions about the relative contribution of female education, smaller families, improved maternal health, child care, hygiene, and safer milk supplies. From the end of the 19th century, improvements in infant and child care and domestic hygiene are likely to have contributed significantly to the downturn in diarrheal disease mortality, while increasing use of pasteurized milk would have reduced the risk of gastrointestinal infections, bovine tuberculosis, and scarlet fever. These beneficial changes for infants, together with the effect of smaller families and less overcrowded living conditions on the transmission of respiratory and airborne infectious diseases, would have contributed to the improvement in child survival, which is considered in the next chapter.

Chapter Eight

Child Mortality

In the mid-19th century, about 60% of deaths among children aged 1–4 years were attributed to airborne infectious diseases and respiratory diseases that were mostly caused by microorganisms. Many of the airborne infectious diseases still common among unvaccinated children in Western countries were frequently fatal in the 19th century. As in developing countries today, children in large families with poor living conditions and inadequate nutrition, would have been at high risk of dying from a series of interrelated or concurrent airborne, respiratory, and other acute infectious diseases. The adverse effect of malnutrition on mortality risk from infectious diseases is well known, and malnutrition can itself be caused by infectious disease as a result of reduced food intake or impaired digestive mechanisms. The association of malnutrition with over half the cases of measles and diarrheal disease in developing countries reflects this two-way relationship.[1] Both measles and whooping cough have independent epidemic cycles, reflecting sociodemographic factors, the immunity gained by survivors, and the time required for replenishment of the "pool of new susceptibles."[2] In the 19th century, the streptococcal disease scarlet fever usually occurred later in childhood, causing particularly high mortality at ages 1–4 years.[3]

Child Mortality Decline

Although infant mortality contributed little to the decline in the overall death rate in the second half of the 19th century in England and Wales, a decline in the child (1–4 years) death rate contributed significantly. Among the childhood diseases, scarlet fever was the biggest arithmetic component of mortality decline, contributing –0.12 to each unit of change in the total death rate (all ages) between 1848–54 and 1901, and –0.04 between 1901 and 1951, while whooping cough contributed –0.02 and –0.03, and measles –0.01 and –0.03, respectively. There was a clear turning point in the child death rate in the mid-1860s, after which it declined consistently apart from fluctuations predominantly caused by scarlet fever epidemics (fig. 8.1).

The main diseases that contributed to the decline in child mortality from the mid-1860s were scarlet fever, typhoid and other fevers, cholera and diarrheal diseases, tuberculosis, whooping cough, and smallpox. The downward trend for these diseases contrasted with the lack of any consistent decline in the measles death

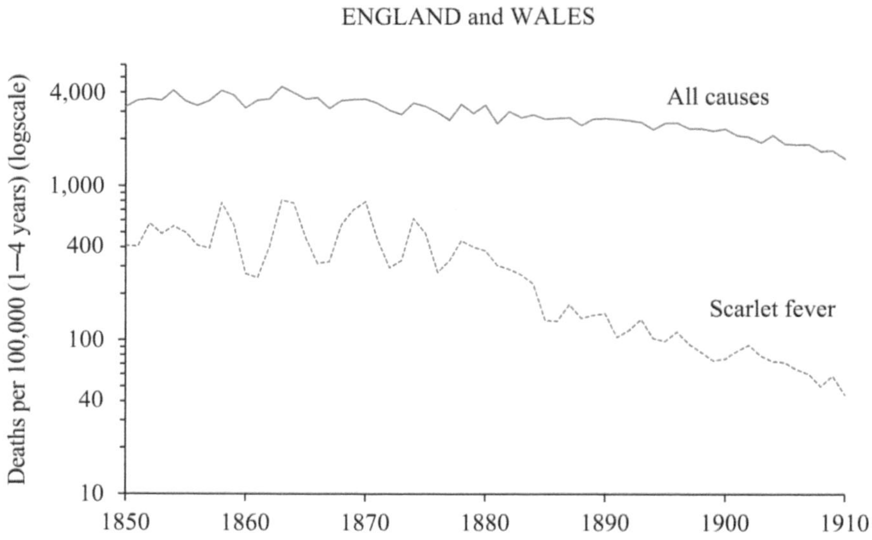

Figure 8.1. Annual child (1–4 years) death rates and scarlet fever death rates (1–4 years) in England and Wales, 1850–1910. *Sources:* Registrar General, *Annual Reports*; *Annual Statistical Reviews.*

rate and an increase in the respiratory disease death rate until the 1890s, indicating the influence of different factors. Scarlet fever can be considered first in view of its predominant influence on the child mortality trend, after which the possible causes of the downturn in death rates from other diseases are considered (figs. 8.2–8.5). The turning point in the 1860s may be particularly significant from a life-course perspective as death rates among adults declined over successive cohorts born after this, as discussed in chapters 12 and 13.

The variable symptoms of clinical scarlet fever, including fever, headache, vomiting, and rash, are caused by a toxin produced by a streptococcal infection usually affecting the throat. The association of hemolytic streptococci with scarlet fever was demonstrated in 1884, although the bacterium was not formally identified as the causal agent until 1924.[4] Streptococci can be contracted through human contact, airborne droplets, or by ingestion and are likely to have been carried by a large proportion of the population as they are today. Several types of streptococci have the toxin-producing capacity to cause scarlet fever, but this only occurs when the bacteria are infected (lysogenized) by an appropriate bacterial virus (bacteriophage). Burnet and White emphasized that the toxin-producing capacity of the bacteria determines the occurrence of clinical scarlet fever.[5] He suggested that the causal agent, *Streptococcus pyogenes,* had persisted as a very common endemic infection in England for at least two centuries. It would have produced repeated subclinical infections of the throat in childhood as no immunity to the bacteria develops following infection. However, if the bacteria produced toxin in an infected child, immunity to the toxin would be acquired and scarlet fever would not be experienced again. The severity of disease is likely to have been affected by the child's health and nutritional status, the dosage of streptococcus contracted, the particular strain, and the mode of infection, which could be through inhaled droplets, transfer of bacteria to the mouth, or by drinking contaminated milk.

Accounts of epidemics of throat infection in the past have suggested that over a very long period the severity of scarlet fever varied. A disease called "febris scarlatina" was described in the 17th century, when it was known as a mild disease.[6] Creighton referred to periodically destructive epidemics of scarlet fever in England in the 18th century. By the end of that century, it seems to have been regarded as the main epidemic disease of childhood, and the malignant form "scarlatina anginosa" was reported to be very prevalent between 1799 and 1802.[7] Even so, scarlet fever was not separately recorded in the London Bills of Mortality in the 18th century, and deaths may have been recorded as "fevers" with some cases mistaken for typhus.[8] However, different manifestations of scarlet fever were already clearly defined, and it was recognized that cases of different severity occurred, even in the same household.[9] For some years after 1803, the disease appears to have become less severe. Records for the period 1804–16 kept by a physician at the Public Dispensary and Fever Institution in London suggest that scarlet fever was still common but a relatively mild disease.[10] This period of apparently less severe infections was over by 1831 when scarlet fever was mentioned in the London Bills of Mortality for the first time and 237 deaths were recorded. National registration data for 1836–39 indicate that many deaths were attributed to scarlet fever, and the number doubled in 1840. Major epidemics were reported in all parts of England and Wales in the 1840s, but the most destructive epidemics occurred in the 1850s and 1860s, when it was the leading cause of child death in the country.

Data from Manchester suggest there may have been some universal influence affecting scarlet fever severity when the resurgence occurred. Death rates from the disease in 1840–42 were similar in different districts of the town, despite all-cause death rates differing by as much as 100%.[11] One possibility is that the resurgence in the death rate could have been due to a more virulent strain of the streptococcus being introduced from abroad. There appear to have been severe epidemics of scarlet fever in Europe and North America between the 1830s and 1880s, although no obvious source of a putative new strain in England has been identified. The reason for the decline in death rates after the 1860s has not been firmly established. At that time, death rates from the acute infectious diseases of childhood were strongly associated with population density. Scarlet fever death rates were four to five times higher in densely populated urban districts compared with the more sparsely populated rural areas.[12] However, it is very unlikely that there were changes in population density that could account for the decline in death rates before the end of the 19th century. Measles and respiratory disease mortality were also strongly associated with population density, and death rates did not decline consistently before the 1890s. A study of epidemics of scarlet fever in England and Wales found an association with fluctuations in wheat prices, which fell rapidly in the 1880s when the death rate declined sharply.[13] However, there is little direct evidence that maternal or child nutrition improved dramatically enough to cause the decline in scarlet fever mortality, and the measles death rate did not decline.

There is evidence that the poorest districts of London had the highest scarlet fever death rates, although the disease caused severe sickness among all social classes.[14] Infection can be transmitted through contaminated milk, which is likely to have been a source in better-off families who could afford it. Contaminated dust and clothing and discharges from the nose and throat are likely to have been a greater risk for severe infection in poorer households. The severe epidemic in 1863–64 probably focused attention on the need for prevention, and an active program of prevention was developed in London from the 1870s with hospitalization of severe cases. This practice had become common by the end of the century despite considerable opposition from families.[15] It is not clear what impact preventive measures had on transmission of severe forms of scarlet fever, although early efforts at disinfection of houses and isolation of the infected seem unlikely to explain the downturn in death rates from the 1860s, particularly as it reportedly occurred first in southwestern counties of England.[16]

The most widely cited explanation for the decline in scarlet fever mortality is that it was due to a change in the virulence of the microorganism. Gale reported that the national death rate from scarlet fever declined after the mid-1860s and suggested it could have been due to a diminution in the virulence of the hemolytic streptococcus.[17] Subsequently, many others have given a similar explanation without suggesting what might have changed the virulence of the microorganism at that particular time. McKeown pointed out that no effective treatment was available until Prontosil was introduced in 1935, and he attributed the decline in the death rate to a change in the "character" of the disease.[18] Others have referred to a milder type or milder form of the disease.[19] The hypothesis is difficult to test but could be stated more specifically: case fatality declined because an increasing proportion of children were infected with a less virulent strain of *S. pyogenes*. The epidemiology of the pandemic in the 19th century suggests that the virulent streptococcal strain continued in circulation along with a putative less virulent strain.[20] There was clearly no sudden change in England and Wales as thousands of children continued to die from scarlet fever in the early 20th century despite the decline in the death rate, and as mentioned, both mild and severe manifestations of scarlet fever reportedly occurred within the same household.[21]

Burnet and White noted the similarity between scarlet fever and diphtheria in terms of the role in both diseases of toxin produced by bacteria. They were more specific about the hypothesis of a change in virulence, suggesting that fluctuations in the virulence of *S. pyogenes* could have been due to changes in the state of infection (lysogenization) of the bacteria by bacterial viruses (bacteriophages) that produced toxin.[22] In the case of diphtheria, it was suspected that there were differences in the virulence of the bacilli in different periods, and in the 1930s research was conducted to identify the different types of bacillus and bacterial viruses involved. The process of natural selection by which a less virulent strain of bacillus could have gained an ecological advantage within the host population is briefly discussed below, and it is plausible that a similar process could account for the history of changes in scarlet fever severity. More recently, when severe forms of scarlet fever began to reemerge in the 1980s in Britain, other parts of Europe, and North America, attention focused on identifying factors that determine streptococcal virulence and how these are distributed in the population.[23]

The issue of whether, how, and why changes in the virulence of *S. pyogenes* infections occurred in the past has contemporary relevance, and comparison has been made between the recent reemergence of severe forms of streptococcal disease and the pandemic of scarlet fever between 1825 and 1885. A recent microepidemiological study analyzed data from outbreaks of scarlet fever in four towns in an agricultural area of Massachusetts in the United States between 1850 and 1910. The highest proportion of deaths attributed to scarlet fever was at ages two to eight years, and deaths from scarlet fever occurred in households of farmers as well as farm laborers, despite the farmers being much wealthier. The communities were not subject to the kind of disruption of food supplies experienced in many urban areas during economic recessions, and the evidence did not suggest that socioeconomic or nutritional factors could explain the distribution of scarlet fever deaths. The study referred to a growing body of evidence from other clinical studies demonstrating that infections in infancy and early childhood, particularly dysentery or enteric infections (typhoid and paratyphoid), affect the ability to absorb key micronutrients, and that deficiencies can leave a child more susceptible to secondary, concurrent, or subsequent infections. Although no specific link was established between dysentery or enteric infections, micronutrient deficiency, and subsequent severe scarlet fever, it was pointed out that such infections were extremely common in Britain and North America in the mid-19th century when scarlet fever mortality was at its highest.[24]

The trend in the scarlet fever death rate in England and Wales over the period 1850–1910 ran closely parallel to the trend in the death rate from enteric/other fevers (fig. 8.2). About half of these deaths were attributed to typhoid when separate recording began in the 1860s, and many deaths classified as "simple fever" could also have been due to enteric infections. The child (1–4 years) death rate from typhoid/other fevers declined from the mid-1860s, which coincided with the successful public health measures to control cholera (fig. 8.3). As discussed in chapter 6, it seems likely that the measures taken to improve water and sewerage systems reduced transmission and incidence of typhoid and dysentery as well as cholera. It is possible that improvements in water quality also had an indirect effect on scarlet fever severity and case fatality, as enteric fevers impair absorption of micronutrients. Many towns in England did not have improved water and sewage systems until the 1890s, and it was probably high typhoid and scarlet fever mortality that eventually led to action in Cambridge, for example. Evidence from West Bromwich in the West Midlands indicates that the introduction of piped water led to a dramatic reduction in scarlet fever deaths when polluted wells were replaced as the main source of drinking water.[25] Most cases of typhoid and dysentery are likely to have been due to drinking water contaminated with infected human feces or to consuming contaminated milk or food. To the extent that public health measures reduced the incidence of typhoid and dysentery, they would reduce a cause of micronutrient deficiency in young children. The severity of scarlet fever experienced by those with no immunity to the toxin would have been partly determined by other recent infections and nutritional status. Any reduction in the incidence of typhoid and dysentery through improved water supplies, sanitation, and hygiene may have indirectly reduced case fatality from scarlet fever, in addition to any direct impact on incidence. The ecological association between typhoid and scarlet fever based on the trends in death rates for England and Wales (fig. 8.2) could be further investigated with any data for local areas and evidence from other countries.

Most severe infectious diseases would have debilitated children, making them more vulnerable to other infections before their health and nutritional status had recovered. Young children vaccinated against smallpox may also have been less likely to die from scarlet fever, because they avoided the debilitating effects of a smallpox attack. The period of reportedly mild manifestations of scarlet fever at the beginning of the 19th century coincided with the introduction of smallpox vaccination. However, there was no close correspondence between annual fluctuations in smallpox and scarlet fever death rates in the second half of the 19th century in England and Wales, and the parallel trends in death rates from typhoid/other fevers and scarlet fever are more strongly indicative of an ecological association (fig. 8.2).

The accelerated decline in the scarlet fever death rate in England and Wales from the 1880s may largely reflect a decline in case fatality, based on comparative evidence from Sweden. National registration data for that country indicate that case fatality for scarlet fever declined rapidly in the 1880s while incidence did not decline (table 8.1). The ratio of deaths to 100 cases declined dramatically from 42 in the 1870s to 23 in the 1880s. While many children may have experienced a less severe attack, which could explain the decline in case fatality, others continued to die from the disease. In England an increasing number of children with severe infectious diseases, including scarlet fever, were admitted to isolation fever hospitals in the 1880s and 1890s. For example, in Birmingham the proportion of reported cases of infectious disease treated in such hospitals increased from 14% in 1882–85 to 83% in 1890–93, and most were cases of scarlet fever and smallpox.[26] Although it is not clear to what extent case fatality among the hospitalized was lower than in the general population, isolation may have reduced transmission from severe cases. At this stage increasing use of pasteurized milk could also have reduced transmission, as scarlet fever has been linked with consumption of contaminated milk in more recent times.[27]

Sore throat was a symptom common to both scarlet fever and diphtheria, and the distinguishing symptom would have been the typical rash of scarlet fever. There may have been some misclassification;[28] for example, if children died

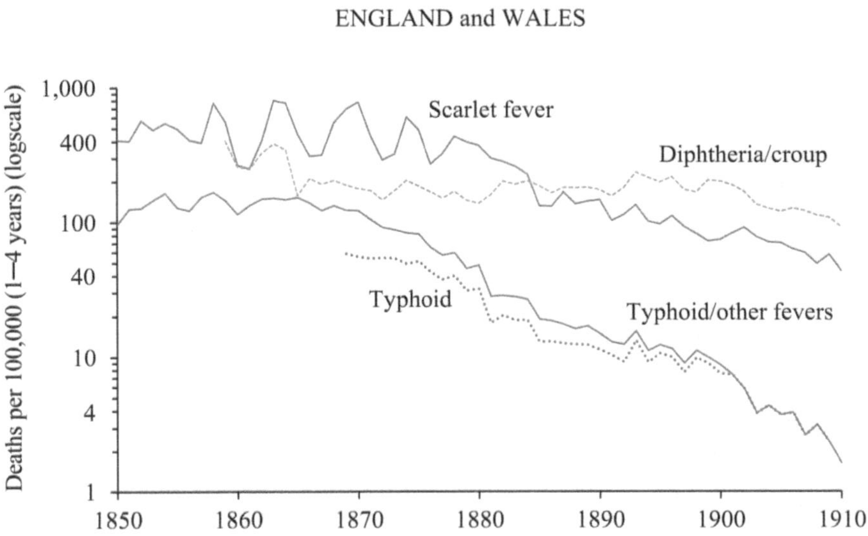

Figure 8.2. Annual child death rates (1–4 years) from scarlet fever, diphtheria/croup, typhoid, and other fevers in England and Wales, 1850–1910. *Sources:* Registrar General, *Annual Reports*; *Annual Statistical Reviews.*

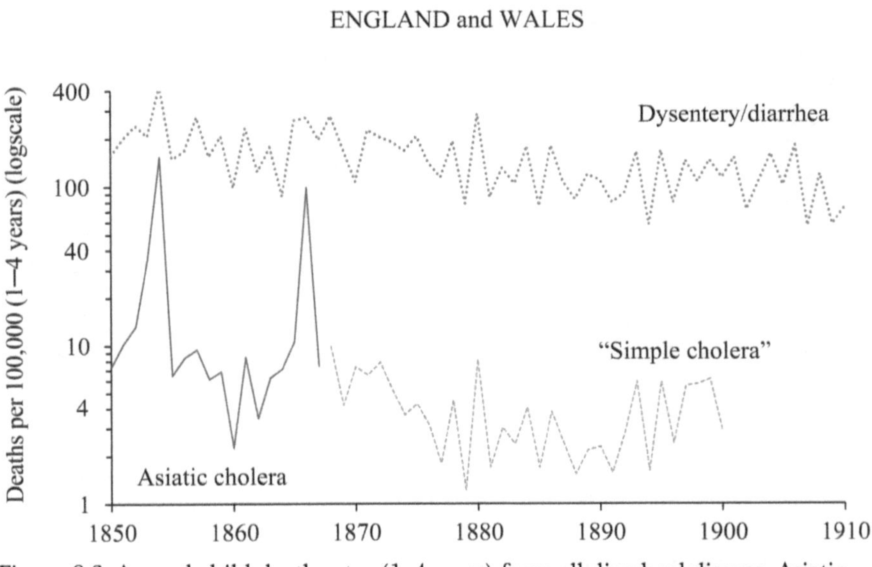

Figure 8.3. Annual child death rates (1–4 years) from all diarrheal disease, Asiatic cholera, and "simple cholera" in England and Wales, 1850–1910. *Sources:* Registrar General, *Annual Reports*; *Annual Statistical Reviews.*

before a rash developed. As there was no upsurge in the diphtheria death rate when the scarlet fever death rate declined (fig. 8.2), the decline in the scarlet fever death rate cannot be explained in terms of transfers of diagnosis and classification. Diphtheria may have been unknown to the medical profession in Britain until outbreaks occurred in several locations in 1855–56, and over 9,000 deaths were recorded in England and Wales in 1859.[29] Before this, the disease may have been much less prevalent than in France, Norway, and Denmark, where there were recognized epidemics in the early 19th century.[30] Burnet and White suggested there were fluctuations in severity as well as incidence of diphtheria, although the causal agent, *Corynebacterium diphtheriae*, had probably been a common and endemic cause of throat infection for many years.

It is not certain what conditions triggered the pandemic of diphtheria in the 1850s and 1860s. Gale reported that the disease had initially affected rural areas of England and Wales more than urban areas, although the differential in the death rate gradually reversed.[31] He showed that the quinquennial death rates from both diphtheria and scarlet fever among children aged 0–14 years declined from a peak in 1861–65. By 1876–78 the diphtheria death rate had fallen by about half before any effective treatment was available. Until the 1890s the trend in the annual death rate was similar to that for croup, a general term for obstruction of breathing. When diphtheria was prevalent, it was probably the commonest cause of croup, and when it was not, parainfluenza viruses are likely to have been responsible as they are today.[32] Because there was no way of identifying the causal agent in croup before the bacteriological discoveries at the end of the 19th century, it is appropriate to combine the death rates for diphtheria and croup. The death rate for diphtheria/croup among children aged 1–4 years leveled off in the 1880s and 1890s before declining continuously in the 20th century (fig. 8.2).

Diphtheria infection is spread by contagion, inhaled droplets, infected dust, and contaminated milk, which would have been a source of infection among people who could afford to buy it. The middle classes may have benefited from advice from medical practitioners about isolation of infected children from the 1880s, and by the 1890s the poorest districts of London had the highest death rates.[33] Diphtheria cases were first admitted to the Metropolitan Asylum Board hospitals in London in 1888. Isolation by hospitalization became increasingly common with the aim of preventing the spread of infection, and case fatality appears to have declined steadily among those admitted between 1888 and 1900. Gale suggested that the use of antitoxin from 1895 could have been the main reason for the downturn in the diphtheria death rate,[34] and this became a widely accepted explanation until inconsistencies in the evidence were reported. Hardy found that the death rate in London reached its peak in 1893, before the introduction of antitoxin in 1895 when it was administered in about 60% of hospitalized cases.[35]

The timing of the decline in the diphtheria death rate in the 1890s could also reflect epidemic fluctuations in incidence or changes in the severity of attacks. The long-term decline in the diphtheria death rate in the United States

Table 8.1. Incidence and case fatality ratios for scarlet fever in Sweden, 1861–70 to 1901–10

Years	Scarlet fever cases	Deaths per 100 cases
1861–1870	7,172	40
1871–1880	8,159	42
1881–1890	10,334	23
1891–1900	8,623	10
1901–1910	8,321	5

Source: Sweden, Statistiska Centralbyrån, *Historisk Statistik 1720–1950.*

began in 1895,[36] but data from Philadelphia suggest a decline in incidence as well as case fatality.[37] In Norway the ratio of deaths to 100 cases declined rapidly from 21 in 1893–95 to 8 in 1902–4, while in Italy it declined from 49 in 1894–96 to 23 in 1903–5 (table 8.2). Although antitoxin was not widely used outside Oslo in 1895, case fatality fell dramatically in Norway as a whole.[38] There was little further decline in case fatality in either Norway or Italy between 1903 and World War I (1914–18). Case fatality in Norway did not decline as much as for other childhood epidemic diseases, and the decline in the death rate in the 1920s and 1930s appears to have been largely due to a decline in incidence (fig. 8.4). A safe antigen for immunization was developed in 1923, and the measure was gradually adopted in Western countries. A dramatic reduction in diphtheria incidence and mortality occurred in England and Wales after 1940 (fig. 8.5), when a national campaign achieved immunization coverage of about 50%.[39]

Studies of diphtheria from the 1920s onward found that many apparently healthy children had bacilli in their throats, and in most cases this did not lead to clinical diphtheria. Burnet and White suggested that children were only likely to develop diphtheria if they contracted a very large dose of bacilli or a particularly virulent strain before they had developed sufficient immunity to the toxin through harmless contact. He suggested that fluctuations in virulence are likely to have been due to changes in the state of infection of the bacteria by toxin-producing bacterial viruses. In the 1930s, research on cultures of bacilli found two distinct types of colony, suggesting that the different types of bacilli could explain the occurrence of mild and severe infections, and hence the pandemic of the 1850s and 1860s.[40] Some indication of how a process of natural selection might contribute to fluctuations in the prevalence of different strains derives from the effect of immunization. Ewald suggested that the harmful *C. diphtheriae* bacilli are selectively suppressed by immunization programs, which can alter the ecological balance in favor of more benign competitors.[41] When toxin-producing bacilli infect a vaccinated person, the toxin is sequestered before it can destroy cells and provide nutrients for the bacteria. He suggested that the extra cost to the bacilli of producing toxin might reduce their ability to compete with the less harmful strains that did not produce toxin. When strains were assessed

Table 8.2. Estimates of case fatality for diphtheria in Norway and Italy, 1870s to early 1910s

Italy		Norway	
Years	Deaths per 100 cases*	Years	Deaths per 100 cases
		1874–1876	14
1888–1890	55	1882	20
1891–1893	54	1890–1892	23
1894–1896	49	1893–1895	21
1897–1899	37	1896–1898	15
1900–1902	29	1899–1901	13
1903–1905	23	1902–1904	8
1906–1908	24	1905–1907	8
1909–1911	24	1908–1910	8
1912–1914	22	1911–1913	7

Sources: Norway, Central Bureau of Statistics, *Health Statistics*; Italy, Central Institute of Statistics, *Cause di Morte, Annuaria di Statistiche Sanitarie.*

* A ratio based on numbers of deaths and cases from separate records. Under-recording of cases may partly account for the higher ratios in Italy.

following vaccination programs, the toxin-producing strains had been replaced by strains that did not produce the toxin that causes diphtheria. The ecological balance between *C. diphtheriae* and its human host population was probably disrupted in the pandemic of the 1850s and 1860s, after which the child death rate from diphtheria remained quite stable until it declined from the mid-1890s (fig. 8.2). The extent to which any decline in severity was due to sociodemographic changes, isolation measures, or a change in the ecological balance between strains of bacillus might be investigated further for countries with incidence data available.

The child death rate from measles in England and Wales also declined from the 1890s (fig. 8.6). This followed an upsurge coinciding with the introduction of compulsory schooling under the Education Act of 1870 that led to an increase in school places and school attendance,[42] which possibly resulted in more rapid spread and high dosage of virus. The rise in measles mortality in Paris in the second half of the 19th century also corresponded with increasing school attendance.[43] In England notification of cases and school closure were proposed for prevention of epidemics, but were not universally accepted or implemented.[44] Measles had an independent cycle of epidemics linked with changing patterns of social contact,[45] sociodemographic factors, and the proportion of "new susceptibles" in the population with no immunity.[46] Analysis of district-level data revealed a strong association between population density and measles death rates,[47] and data from Birmingham indicated an association between high

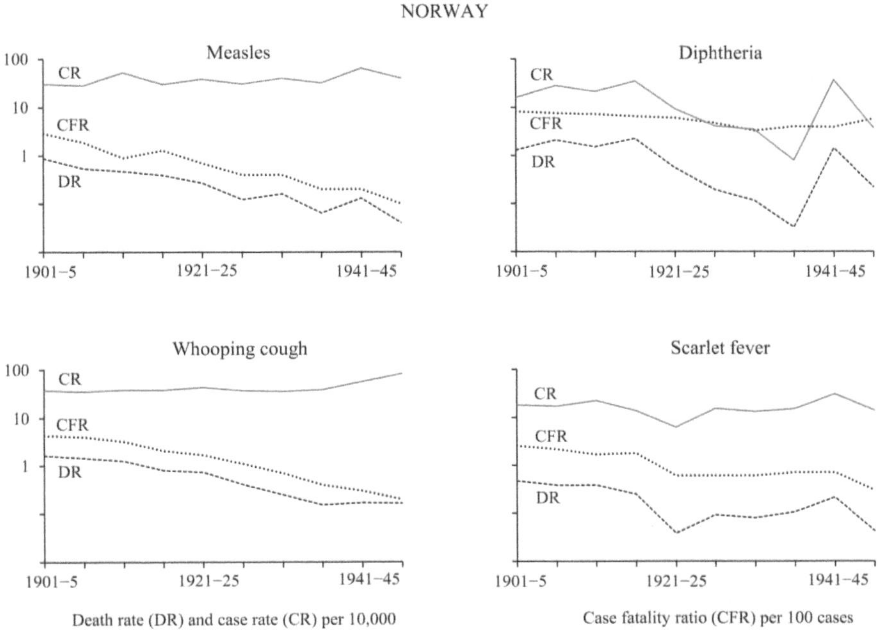

Figure 8.4. Annual average death rates, case rates, and case fatality ratios for childhood epidemic diseases in Norway, 1901–5 to 1946–50. *Source:* Norway, Central Bureau of Statistics, *Health Statistics.*

measles mortality and poor housing in the second half of the 19th century.[48] Data from the national census (persons per room) has suggested that new housing before the end of the century is unlikely to have had much impact on the transmission of airborne infectious diseases that was independent of changes in household composition and family size.[49]

The long-term continuous decline in the measles death rate in England and Wales from the end of the 19th century is likely to reflect a decline in case fatality as in other countries. The ratio of deaths to 100 measles cases recorded in Italy and Norway suggest that case fatality declined from the early 1890s (table 8.3). Other data indicate little decline in measles incidence in Norway in the first half of the 20th century, with the decline in the death rate being largely due to a decline in case fatality. The data from Norway also indicate that the decline in death rates from whooping cough and scarlet fever in the first half of the 20th century was due to a decline in case fatality rather than incidence (fig. 8.4), and data from the United States for 1912–75 support this.[50] It seems reasonable to assume that the decline in child death rates from scarlet fever, whooping cough, and measles in England and Wales in the first half of the 20th century was also due largely to a decline in case fatality (fig. 8.5).

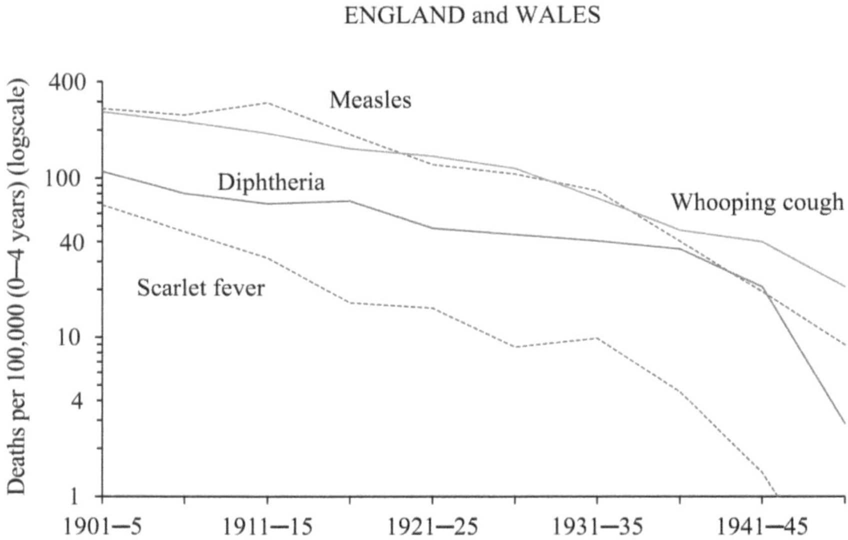

Figure 8.5. Annual average death rates (0–4 years) from measles, whooping cough, scarlet fever, and diphtheria in England and Wales, 1901–5 to 1946–50. *Source:* Registrar General, *Annual Statistical Reviews.*

There is no evidence that the measles virus became less virulent. However, there is considerable evidence that severity of sickness varies with sociodemographic factors,[51] which may explain some aspects of historical trends as well as contemporary variations in measles mortality.[52] The large families and crowded living conditions in England in the late 19th century would have exacerbated the infectious disease environment, particularly among the poor, whose children were already at greater risk because of inadequate nutrition. Historical data from Sunderland for 1885 indicate that measles mortality was higher in households with multiple cases, while severe complications were associated with a large number of siblings.[53] The decline in the annual number of births after 1900 reduced the number of "new susceptibles," and evidence suggests that when there were fewer children in a household, infections occurred at an older, less vulnerable age. The median age at infection increased for measles and other childhood epidemic diseases, and case fatality was much lower at ages three to four years than at one to two. The age distribution of measles infections shifted to older ages in the first two decades of the 20th century, and the decline in the measles death rate at younger ages (0–4) was sufficient to reduce the overall measles death rate despite an increase in the death rate at older ages (5–9).[54]

Evidence from developing countries indicates that severity of measles sickness varies considerably with sociodemographic factors. Aaby and colleagues investigated the relationship between family size, age at infection, nutritional status, living conditions, and the risk of dying from measles in an urban district

Table 8.3. Estimates of case fatality for measles in Norway and Italy, mid 1870s to early 1910s

Norway		Italy	
Years	Deaths per 100 cases*	Years	Deaths per 100 cases
1874–1876	3.4		
1882	3.7	1888–1890	10
1890–1892	4.2	1891–1893	11
1893–1895	3.6	1894–1896	9
1896–1898	2.9	1897–1899	5
1899–1901	3.4	1900–1902	6
1902–1904	2.6	1903–1905	6
1905–1907	2.0	1906–1908	6
1908–1910	2.0	1909–1911	7
1911–1913	2.0	1912–1914	5

Sources: Norway, Central Bureau of Statistics, *Health Statistics*; Italy, Central Institute of Statistics, *Cause di Morte*; *Annuaria di Statistiche Sanitarie.*
* A ratio of deaths to cases using data from separate records. Under-recording of cases may partly account for the higher ratios in Italy.

of Guinea-Bissau. In an epidemic in 1979, case fatality was higher in households where several children had caught the disease. The risk of dying was inversely related to age at infection, suggesting that if contact with measles is delayed, the risk of dying is reduced, even when nutrition has not improved.[55] Research in population biology indicates the importance of the transmission rate (Ro) and the effect of sociodemographic variables on the severity of infectious diseases. Population size, population density, density of susceptibles, family size, birthrate, and behavior patterns in the community can all affect the number of new cases arising from one infected individual. Duration of infectiousness and recovery rates affect transmission, as well as life span of the pathogen and the latency period before the pathogen can be passed on.[56]

While sociodemographic changes affect transmission of infectious disease, severity of infection, and mortality, changes in child survival can have deterministic effects on fertility in a complex two-way relationship. Sociodemographic changes in England from the end of the 19th century probably reduced the severity of airborne infectious diseases, and the improvement in child survival would tend to increase birth intervals as pregnancy is less likely during breast-feeding.[57] There were also voluntary changes in fertility as a result of dissemination of information and increased awareness of birth control methods. Many middle-class women probably adopted methods to reduce the burden of child-bearing, and poorer families are likely to have recognized the benefits of having fewer children to feed when family incomes were grossly inadequate. There was even a decline in the absolute number of births each year from the beginning of the 20th century, which would have reduced the number of "new susceptibles" who could become infected and transmit airborne epidemic diseases. There is also likely to have been a growing awareness that children were more likely to survive than in earlier times, so preventing pregnancies would be less risky in terms of achieving a desired family size. In addition to the health benefits for mothers and children in smaller families, there was probably an increasing awareness of ways to protect children's health. Hardy suggested that diet and nursing care improved, particularly in London where more children's hospitals opened with philanthropic support.[58] Improved access to school and attendance by girls would have increased their access to information and literature about child care. Reduction of family size, together with new housing that alleviated overcrowded living conditions, probably reduced transmission rates, severity, and case fatality for measles, whooping cough, respiratory infections, and possibly diphtheria from the end of the 19th century, contributing to a sustained decline in child mortality. The correspondence of the downturn in the death rates from measles and respiratory disease (fig. 8.6) and the more rapid decline in whooping cough mortality (fig. 8.7) are consistent with a beneficial impact of sociodemographic changes on child mortality from the 1890s.

Child mortality was still very high at the end of the 19th century in the United States, a relatively high-income country, even among well-off families whose children are likely to have been well fed. Physicians and parents lacked information on appropriate health care despite the greater understanding of infectious disease when the germ theory was accepted. However, public health programs were developed based on the new knowledge, and health promotion became vigorous and effective in reaching the general population.[59] Physicians began to play a part in promoting appropriate behavior change, although initially this was mainly among the better-off. Preventive measures in the home are likely to have been the main cause of improved child survival in the United States in the first few decades of the 20th century, while public health interventions improved water supplies and the broader sanitary environment that contributed to reductions in adult mortality.[60] This is consistent with the experience of England and Wales outlined here, while smaller families probably contributed to improved child survival in both countries for the reasons discussed.

Contribution of Improved Child Survival to Overall Mortality Decline

Before considering changes in disease and mortality among adults in the following chapters, it is useful to summarize the changes in infant and child mortality, indicating their relative contribution to overall mortality decline in England and Wales. Death rates at ages 1–4, 5–14, and 15–44 declined continuously from the 1860s, while death rates among infants and older adults (45 and older) did not

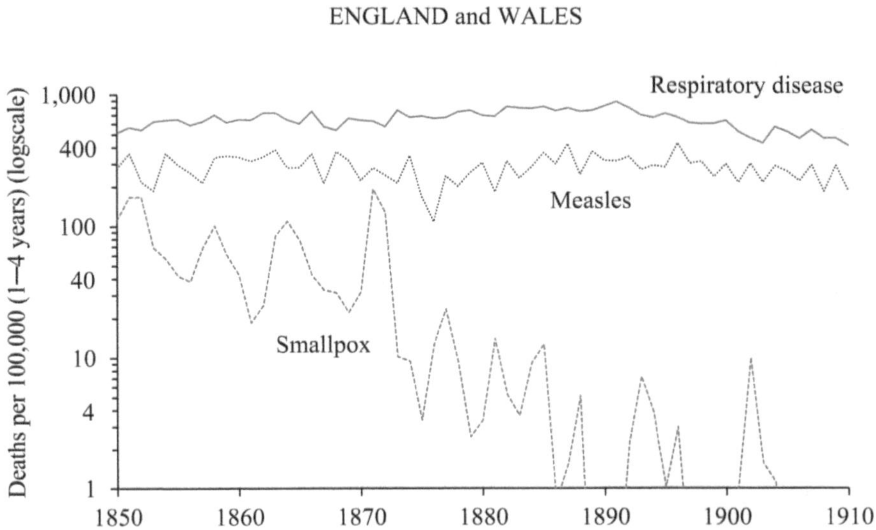

Figure 8.6. Annual child death rates (1–4 years) from all respiratory disease, measles, and smallpox in England and Wales, 1850–1910. *Sources:* Registrar General, *Annual Reports*; *Annual Statistical Reviews.*

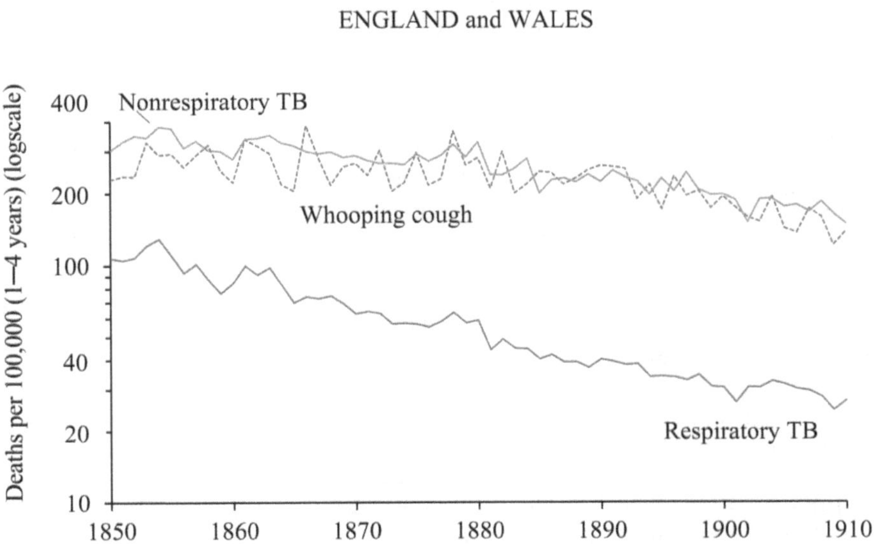

Figure 8.7. Annual child (1–4 years) death rate from respiratory tuberculosis, nonrespiratory tuberculosis, and whooping cough in England and Wales, 1850–1910. *Sources:* Registrar General, *Annual Reports*; *Annual Statistical Reviews.*

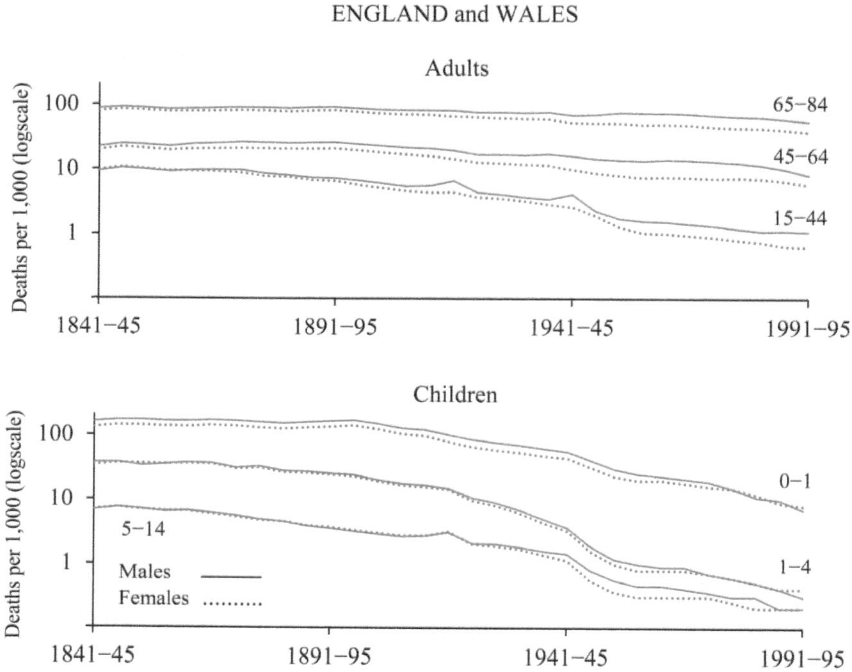

Figure 8.8. Age-specific death rates for males and females in England and Wales in 5-year periods from 1841–45 to 1991–95. *Sources:* Registrar General, *Annual Reports*; *Annual Statistical Reviews.*

decline much in the second half of the 19th century. Although the death rate among older adults declined from the beginning of the 20th century, deaths rates for younger adults (15–44), children (1–14), and infants declined more rapidly, particularly in the 1940s when antibiotics became available (fig. 8.8).

The age-and-sex-standardized death rate in England and Wales declined by 22% in the period 1850–1900, 62% in 1900–1950, and 50% in 1950–2000. The decline in mortality among children (0–4 years) accounted for a significant proportion of the overall mortality decline: 1850–1900 (27%), 1900–50 (51%), and 1950–2000 (27%). In the second half of the 19th century, infant mortality contributed little to the overall decline, and older adult mortality (age 35 and older) accounted for only 20% (appendix D2). In the 20th century, infant mortality made a much greater contribution to the decline, both in the first half (33%) and the second half (30%). The decline in deaths classified as due to "prematurity" and "immaturity" made a particularly significant contribution in the first half of the century, partly reflecting improved maternal health. In the second half of the century, the decline in adult mortality (age 35 and over) accounted for much more of the overall decline (59%). The main contributions to each unit of decline in the overall age-and-sex-standardized death rate in that period came from cerebrovascular disease (–0.12), heart and other circulatory disease (–0.36), cancer (–0.15), respiratory diseases (–0.15), and respiratory tuberculosis (–0.05) (see appendix C1).

The decline in mortality from these and other chronic diseases is considered in the following chapters. The relative contribution of changes in early-life and later-life determinants of adult mortality risk is different for different diseases. Stomach cancer and stroke trends appear to have been responsive to early-life influences; lung cancer to socially related factors in adulthood; and coronary heart disease, chronic obstructive respiratory disease, and breast cancer to influences acting throughout life. On the one hand, diseases for which the predominant influences on mortality risk are those experienced over the life course or in adulthood have become relatively more important as causes of death, including coronary heart disease, breast cancer, and lung cancer. On the other hand, diseases with relatively strong determinants early in life, such as rheumatic heart disease, stomach cancer, and tuberculosis, have become less important.[61] There is a strong inverse relationship between socioeconomic status and tuberculosis mortality risk, which reflects infection in the past as well as recent experience of poor health, under-nutrition, and overcrowded living conditions. The decline of tuberculosis, a major killer in England and Wales in the 19th century, is compared with the very different trends for respiratory disease mortality in the next two chapters.

Chapter Nine

Tuberculosis

Death rates from different acute infectious diseases began to decline at different times in the 18th and 19th centuries, reflecting the relative success of different preventive interventions and other factors. While major killers such as smallpox, typhus, cholera, and typhoid had been nearly eliminated by the end of the 19th century, measles and respiratory disease death rates did not decline. The lack of decline in death rates from respiratory disease in the second half of the 19th century (see chapter 10) contrasts with the decline in death rates from the chronic infectious disease respiratory tuberculosis considered here. This highly visible wasting disease was endemic in London by the 17th century.[1] The death rate from "consumption" recorded in the London Bills of Mortality increased up to the 1740s, leveled off, and then declined after 1800. Because death rates from some other causes declined, "consumption" accounted for an increasing proportion of all deaths, 14% in 1700–49 and 22% in 1750–99. The term "consumption" probably referred to many "wasting" conditions, and Black noted at the time that it was "lax and indefinite" and included many types of emaciation.[2] Deaths from lung diseases other than tuberculosis, such as bronchitis, may have been included, while some deaths involving respiratory conditions were recorded as "asthma."[3] Even so, in the experience of Black and contemporary physicians, a very large proportion of "consumption" deaths in the 18th century were due to pulmonary phthisis, a term used for respiratory tuberculosis. In the 19th century, tuberculosis became a major public health problem exacerbated by rapid population growth in the towns, and it caused much longterm sickness and death, particularly among adults.

Under national registration, other nonrespiratory forms of tuberculosis were recorded separately, including infection of lymph nodes in the neck (scrofula) and abdomen (tabes mesenterica), and tubercular meningitis. There could have been some transfer of recording between phthisis and these categories as well as transfers-in from vague categories such as "atrophy," which may have included some people wasted by tuberculosis.[4] There were probably some transfers between phthisis and the respiratory disease category in the early years of national registration, although the decline of 34% in the death rate from phthisis between 1838 and 1850 is likely to reflect some genuine decline in respiratory tuberculosis mortality. When the death rate from respiratory tuberculosis continued to decline, the Royal Commission on Tuberculosis noted the possibility of transfers to respiratory disease for which the death rate increased until the

1890s.[5] However, respiratory tuberculosis death rates declined for all age groups of males and females, particularly adults aged 15–44, for whom the decline was far greater than the increase in the respiratory disease death rate.[6]

The data from the London Bills of Mortality suggest that the decline in the death rate from "consumption" in the second half of the 18th century contributed –0.09 to a unit of change in overall mortality (appendix C1). National registration data indicate that between 1848–54 and 1901, respiratory tuberculosis contributed –0.33 to a unit of change, which seems too large to be due to changes in classification, particularly as other respiratory diseases contributed –0.10. Nonrespiratory forms of tuberculosis contributed –0.04 to each unit of change. Between 1901 and 1951, the contributions to a unit of change were –0.05 from nonrespiratory tuberculosis, –0.10 from respiratory tuberculosis, and –0.17 from respiratory diseases.[7] In the second half of the 20th century, a further decline in the respiratory disease death rate contributed –0.15 to each unit of change in overall mortality, but by then all tuberculosis contributed only –0.06. Deaths from tuberculosis are now relatively rare in England and Wales as in other Western countries, whereas bronchitis continues to be a major cause of death. Although some acute forms of tuberculosis occur, it is usually regarded as a chronic infectious disease, and bronchitis is also a chronic long-term condition. In this sense, these diseases are distinct from the acute infectious diseases such as smallpox and the epidemic diseases of childhood, although these cause serious respiratory complications and long-term sequelae.

There is a clear contrast between infectious diseases for which death rates declined from at least the beginning of the 19th century, such as smallpox and "fevers," and diseases for which death rates were still not declining in the second half of the 19th century, including respiratory diseases and measles. The lack of decline in the period death rates from measles and respiratory diseases while respiratory tuberculosis mortality was declining casts further doubt on any generalization about improved nutrition causing the decline in airborne infectious disease mortality in this period.[8] As mentioned in chapter 8, sociodemographic changes affecting transmission and severity, prior infections, coinfections, and debilitating sequelae need to be taken into account when considering changes in airborne infectious disease mortality. A whole series of acute infectious diseases were contracted in the early years of life, and there is likely to have been universal contact with smallpox, measles, and tuberculosis in England in the 19th century. The decline in smallpox mortality was due to preventive measures, as discussed in chapter 5. As a result of vaccination, the proportion of children suffering an attack of smallpox declined considerably in the first quarter of the 19th century, and after the pandemic of 1870–71 when renewed efforts to vaccinate were supported by other preventive measures. In this chapter, the possible effects of these dramatic changes can be borne in mind when comparing trends in death rates from tuberculosis, respiratory diseases, and the airborne epidemic diseases of childhood that often caused respiratory complications.

Cockburn suggested that tuberculosis is unlikely to have affected hunter-gatherers, except in recent times when they contract an infection from people living in more densely populated and settled communities. Human beings were more likely to develop tuberculosis when the introduction of agriculture encouraged a more settled way of life and eventually the growth of towns.[9] In England in the 17th century, the majority of people still lived in rural areas where tuberculosis was probably less prevalent. However, there would have been increasing contact with town dwellers by people from rural areas who had no previous exposure to the microorganisms prevalent in the towns.[10] Dubos and Dubos emphasized the social context of tuberculosis and its association with the process of industrialization, urbanization, migration, and increased social contacts between people in the increasingly crowded towns.[11] Large population movements are known to have contributed to the spread of tuberculosis. For example, increases in the tuberculosis death rates in the 19th century in parts of the United States such as the southern states and New York have been linked with the movement of people during the Civil War,[12] and with immigrants arriving from areas of high prevalence in Europe such as famine-stricken Ireland. The tuberculosis death rate was still increasing in Ireland in the second half of the 19th century,[13] possibly reflecting a later process of urbanization and contact between people living in rural areas and towns compared with England.

The main causal agent of tuberculosis, *Mycobacterium tuberculosis,* known earlier as tubercle bacillus, is usually transmitted in droplets exhaled by infected people when they cough, which are then inhaled by others through the nose or mouth. Another strain of bacillus, *Mycobacterium bovis* has a wide range of hosts although it has usually transmitted to humans via contaminated cow's milk. Nearly all clinical cases of bovine tuberculosis were extrapulmonary, and those infected were not likely to infect others. A study in England in 1927 isolated *M. bovis* in 29% of patients with nonrespiratory tuberculosis and in just 1% of patients with respiratory tuberculosis.[14] In the usual case of a child being infected with *M. tuberculosis* for the first time by inhalation of infected droplets, inflammation develops around the primary infection in the lung where bacilli multiply slowly compared with other bacteria. Over a period of a few weeks, the body's immune system develops a degree of cell-mediated immunity to *M. tuberculosis* antigens. On contact with the corresponding antigens, the T cells (immunocytes) are damaged, releasing toxic chemical substances that damage other cells in the infected organ. In a complex process the body becomes sensitized to the by-products of the immune reaction in a type of allergy, particularly to the toxic product, tuberculin. New cells are produced rapidly to maintain the integrity of tissues, and a process of containment usually results in the bacilli being "walled off" in granules (tubercles) that harden and calcify.[15]

Even when the bacilli have been contained within a hard nodule, they can remain virulent for weeks or years and an internal source of reinfection if the nodule is disrupted, which was apt to happen in adolescence or early adulthood. When relatively large numbers of bacilli enter the lung of someone sensitized by an earlier infection, whether from an internal latent source such as this or a new infection from outside, the reaction is much more violent than in someone who is not sensitized.[16] Primary infection in childhood would often produce mild symptoms that could go unnoticed and not be recognized as tuberculosis, but the infection had the potential to progress sooner or later to clinical tuberculosis. Many cases are likely to have been the result of a reactivation of a latent infection rather than reinfection.[17] Failure of the containment process in a minority of cases as a result of high dosage of bacillus, poor health, and nutrition status, or other factors affecting resistance and immune response, would result in proliferation of tubercles in the lung (or other infected organ) leading to its destruction. A minority of children with a primary infection would succumb to generalized tuberculosis as a result of bacilli escaping into the blood from the original focus before containment, leading to infection in other parts of the body such as kidneys, bones, spine, or brain. In newborns and very young children, infection could progress in the primary site, or in metastatic foci, causing spinal deformity, miliary tuberculosis, and tuberculous meningitis.[18]

The destructiveness of tuberculosis at the beginning of the 19th century should be viewed in the context of the infectious disease environment at that time, and the series of epidemic diseases to which all children would be exposed in large families and overcrowded living conditions. Most people living in the towns of England in the 18th and 19th centuries would have contracted airborne infectious diseases and a tubercular infection early in childhood. Recent episodes of acute infectious disease and coinfections are likely to have contributed to the risk of clinical tuberculosis developing. Infections with microorganisms that convey immunity and produce rashes (exanthems), such as measles and scarlet fever, can temporarily suppress tuberculin sensitivity. Although this may not increase the risk of tuberculosis developing,[19] respiratory complications can occur and coughing could reactivate a latent infection. Physical disruption of the lungs might affect the process of containment of primary infection or reactivate a latent infection leading to clinical tuberculosis. Coughing and respiratory complications during smallpox, measles, whooping cough, and respiratory infections could all have caused reactivation of latent tubercular infections among children, adolescents, and young adults.[20]

Links between smallpox and consumption were recognized by physicians in the 18th century.[21] Black reported medical opinions about different causes of death recorded in the London Bills of Mortality in 1778, and referred to smallpox in the following terms: "It attacks the same person but once in life. . . . One of every seven infected die of natural disease [smallpox]. . . . To the former deadly catelogue [*sic*] may be superadded a frightful train of mangled constitutions and countenances, of consumptions, abscesses, ulcers, ophthalmics, blindness."[22] The Royal Commission on Vaccination at the end of the 19th century referred to the secondary effects of smallpox among those who survived, particularly "scrofula," a term used at that time for both respiratory and nonrespiratory forms of tuberculosis: "all writers on smallpox attest the frequency with which scrofulous affections [*sic*] follow in its [smallpox's] train and that in such measure as vaccination is less impoverishing and less depressing than smallpox, in just such measure does its substitution for smallpox act in prevention of scrofula."[23] This perception of a link between the destructive disease smallpox and consumption was borne out by later studies that indicated smallpox exacerbated the effects of tubercular infection leading to potentially fatal clinical tuberculosis. Smallpox also produced secondary respiratory complications such as bronchitis and bronchopneumonia. In the 1960s Dixon reported that disruption of the lungs could occur with smallpox infection, and that vaccination would have prevented this potential trigger for the development of clinical tuberculosis.[24]

A hypothesis that the debilitating effect of smallpox increased the risk of clinical tuberculosis and death from that disease is supported by evidence of ecological association between smallpox and tuberculosis mortality in the 18th and early 19th centuries. The quinquennial death rates from smallpox and consumption recorded in the London Bills of Mortality over the period 1701–6 to 1831–36 were quite strongly correlated even with the underlying trend removed ($r = +0.6$). If smallpox vaccination reduced the risk of dying from tuberculosis, it would be expected that young children and adolescents benefited most. While there are no data by age for England at the beginning of the 19th century, data from Sweden indicate that the death rate from tuberculosis at ages 0–9 years fell in the first three decades when smallpox vaccination was introduced, while the tuberculosis death rate among adults continued to increase.[25] Most clinical tuberculosis in older adults would have been due to reinfection or reactivated infection. Adult deaths appear to have predominated as the tuberculosis death rate at all ages increased from the 1760s to the 1860s.[26] After this, it declined quite sharply as in England and Wales (fig. 9.1). Data from Paris also indicate that the death rate from tuberculosis at ages 0–19 declined in the 19th century, while age-specific death rates for those 20 and over continued to increase.[27]

In England and Wales, period death rates from tuberculosis were declining for all age groups in the second half of the 19th century (figs. 9.1 and 9.2). This continued in the 20th century apart from temporary setbacks during the two world wars, which occurred in other European countries,[28] particularly at ages 10–19 and 20–29. At those times, conditions were conducive to transmission and lower resistance to tubercular infection. In the second half of the 19th century, the majority of tuberculosis deaths among adults were due to respiratory tuberculosis, and age-specific death rates declined at a similar rate for males and females (fig. 9.1). This consistent improvement in death rates is anomalous considering the deleterious living conditions and work environments. Even more remarkable is the decline in cohort death rates from respiratory tuberculosis for adults born in successive decades throughout the 19th century (fig. 9.3), when there is unlikely to have been any consistent improvement in the economic standard of living, diet, or living conditions of most people.

The lack of significant decline in the period death rates from nonrespiratory tuberculosis for both sexes before the 1880s (fig. 9.1) probably reflects continuingly poor food quality and infected milk. The most likely causes of the downturn in the death rate from the end of the 19th century are increasing use of sterilized milk and public health monitoring to prevent the sale of contaminated food.[29] Children in particular were affected by nonrespiratory forms of the disease, while death rates from respiratory tuberculosis were much

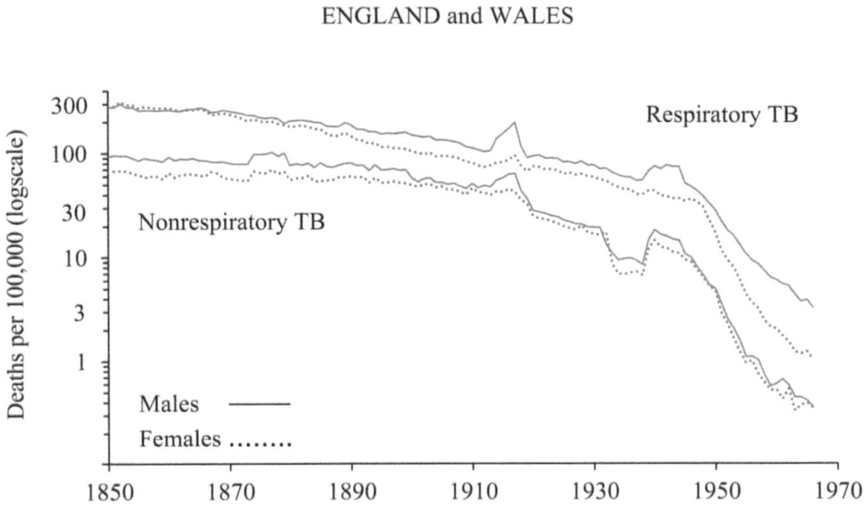

Figure 9.1. Annual age-standardized* death rates from tuberculosis for males and females in England and Wales, 1850–1970. *Sources:* Registrar General, *Annual Reports*; *Annual Statistical Reviews.* * Standardized to the age structure of the population (persons) of England and Wales in 1901.

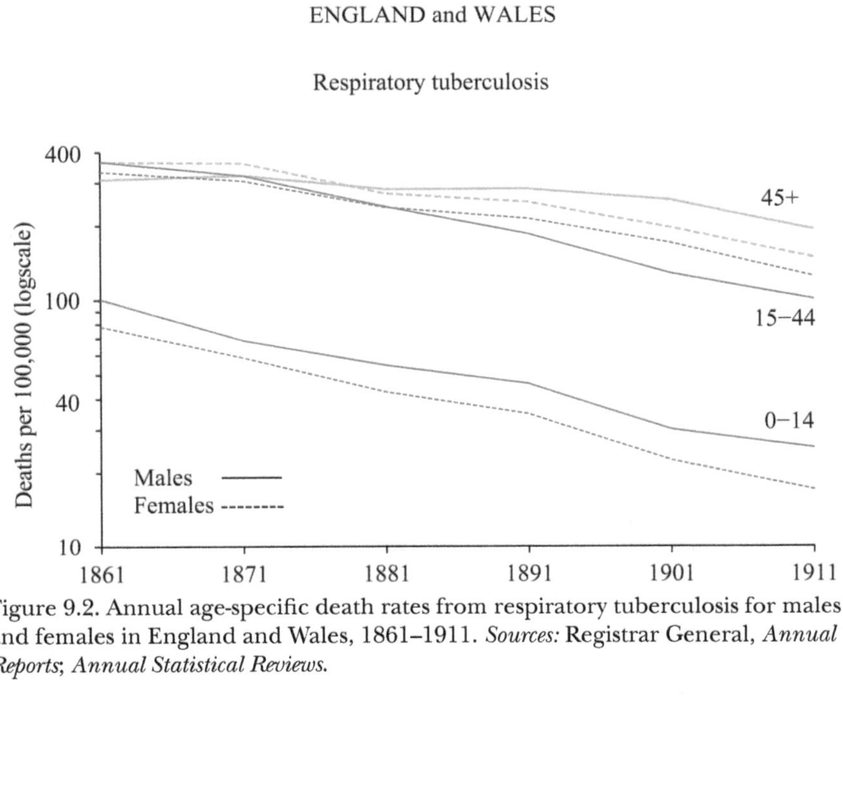

Figure 9.2. Annual age-specific death rates from respiratory tuberculosis for males and females in England and Wales, 1861–1911. *Sources:* Registrar General, *Annual Reports*; *Annual Statistical Reviews.*

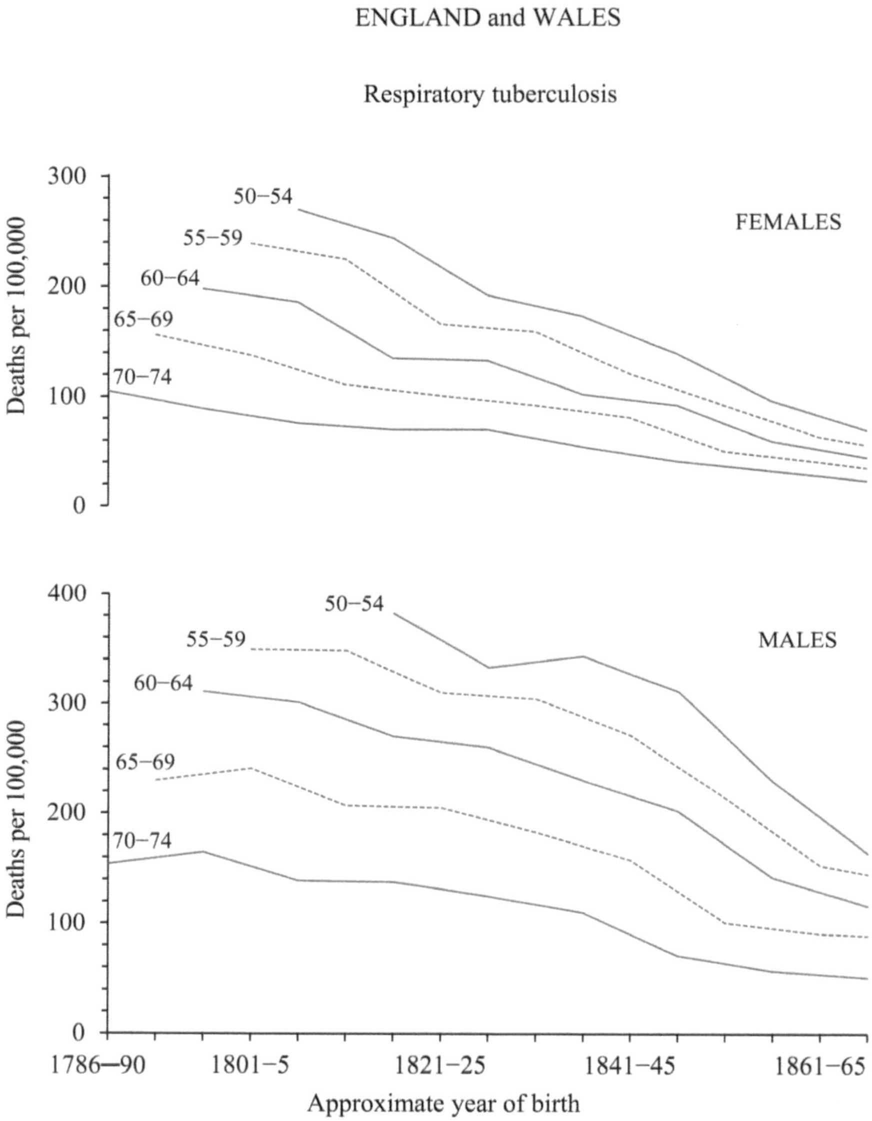

Figure 9.3. Annual age-specific death rates from respiratory tuberculosis for males and females in England and Wales by year of birth, 1786–90 to 1866–70. *Sources:* Registrar General, *Annual Reports*; *Annual Statistical Reviews.*

higher among adults than among children. There were differences in the respiratory tuberculosis death rates in different parts of the country, and although rates declined throughout England and Wales in the second half of the 19th century, there were differences in the rate of decline.[30] Death rates were particularly high in major industrial areas such as the northern textile towns, the northeast coalfields, Birmingham, the West Midlands, South Wales, London, and the metropolitan counties. The disease affected all socioeconomic groups, although the poor in heavily industrialized towns were particularly at risk. There were marked differentials in mortality at the county level, with the death rate in Lancashire being about 50% higher than in Worcestershire, most likely reflecting worse economic circumstances and living conditions in the more industrial county.[31] Woods found that death rates from phthisis declined by more than 50% between the 1860s and 1890s in many districts, including parts of the rural north, the south Midlands, and East Anglia. Death rates appear to have declined in nearly all districts, whether characterized as "urban" or "rural."[32]

When people in towns became very sick, it is likely that some returned to the village they came from, and transmission could explain high death rates from tuberculosis in rural areas.[33] Exposure to tuberculosis infection is likely to have remained universal, with men in the towns being particularly exposed to high dosages of bacilli in the overcrowded factories, workshops, and public houses that were conducive to transmission. Crowding and poor ventilation in housing and workplaces, together with poor diet, contributed to high respiratory tuberculosis mortality, and there is little convincing evidence of major improvements that could affect incidence of clinical disease before the end of the 19th century, and treatment is unlikely to have reduced case fatality. Although better ventilation of public places was advocated much earlier, action may have been limited to prisons, hospitals, and meeting halls, rather than the crowded workplaces, houses, and tenement buildings where most people spent their time. As early as 1796, the Manchester Health Board was aware that infection was spread by children and adults working in the crowded cotton factories, and this affected the neighborhoods where they lived. However, the decline in respiratory tuberculosis mortality began long before the Factories and Workshop Acts and the Housing and Crowding Acts, and before enforcement of building regulations and bylaws that might have had some impact later.[34]

In the early 19th century, activists concerned with public health knew that tuberculosis was likely to spread among people who lived and worked in close proximity to those infected, and that defective ventilation of workplaces, houses, and shops was a major problem compounded by dust in the textile, clothesmaking, and other factories.[35] The writings of those concerned about working conditions suggest they had not improved by the mid-19th century. Engels described workers in the factories of Manchester and the manufacturing towns looking like "hollow-eyed ghosts, riddled with scrofula (tuberculosis) and rickets."[36] Despite having obvious clinical symptoms, infected people would have had little choice but to continue working in the crowded conditions conducive to the spread of tuberculosis, or be unable to feed themselves and their dependents. Contacts with people from other social classes would have fostered transmission of infection from the crowded impoverished communities that were typical of this phase of rapid industrialization. Factory owners with little concern for the well-being of machine operators enforced long working hours in crowded and unhealthy conditions.[37] Before passage of further factory legislation and the rise of the trade union movement in the early 20th century, employees themselves had little influence over the working conditions that prevailed. Conditions in many industrial towns contributed to a miserable and exploited existence for many people who lived in fear of not having work when the alternatives were the workhouse, begging, or stealing.

Living conditions in slums and in the streets allowed little respite from what William Blake, in his poem "Jerusalem," referred to as "dark satanic mills." Charles Dickens's portrayal of "Coketown" in *Hard Times* conveys an impression of conditions for working people living in "an ugly citadel where nature was as strongly bricked out as killing air and gases were bricked in."[38] Poorly fed people living in crowded, unheated rooms would be unlikely to open windows for ventilation allowing cold air to enter. As population grew in the towns exacerbating the demand for housing in inner-city areas, private landlords were able to charge high rents, forcing many people to share rooms. Housing for the urban working class ranged from squalid cellar dwellings, lodging houses split into single rooms where several people slept on the floor, and tenement houses where the average number per room in London could be as many as 12 according to contemporary reports.[39] The external environment in rural areas may have been more salubrious than in the rapidly growing industrial towns, although most farm laborers and their families lived in dilapidated, single-room, "wattle and daub" buildings with no drainage or sanitation. Improvements made by a few landowners are unlikely to have had a significant impact on death rates in rural areas in the 19th century.[40] New buildings in the towns to accommodate people in working-class occupations tended to be brick "back-to-back" terraced houses in the Midlands and the north of England, and single rows of terraced houses in London and the south of the country.

High tuberculosis mortality in England in the 19th century owed much to rapid urbanization and industrialization, with some occupational groups being particularly vulnerable due to overcrowded housing as well as poor working conditions. An association between high tuberculosis mortality and urbanization has been observed in developing countries in more recent times. Given the poor housing conditions and work environment for most people in the growing industrial towns of England, the decline in age-specific death rates from respiratory tuberculosis across successive birth cohorts in the 19th century is remarkable. It is extremely unlikely that there was an improvement in conditions that might have reduced the dosage of bacillus being contracted or the risk of dying from tuberculosis over successive birth cohorts in the first half of the 19th century when population growth was at its most rapid. On the contrary, living conditions in towns are likely to have become even more crowded and unhealthy as a result of in-migration from rural areas. The housing stock may have grown at a slightly faster rate than population in the second half of the 19th century;[41] however, it is unlikely that changes in the quantity and quality of housing were sufficient to have had much impact on overcrowding and infectious disease transmission until the building of terraced houses that complied with local bylaws toward the end of century.[42]

From the mid-19th century, some local authorities attempted to control the standard of new housing. Local housing acts in some towns in the 1860s linked housing and sanitation policies, which together with later acts extended slum clearance to more cities, including London.[43] However, in Manchester, for example, demolition did not lead to new housing being built for the occupants, and there was little direct municipal involvement in house building until the 1890s.[44] The Royal Commission on Housing of the Poor in 1885 recognized that overcrowding was by then a more serious problem than sanitation. Following the 1890 Housing Act, some municipal housing was built to minimum standards regarding crowding and sanitation, which provided new accommodation for a few tens of thousands of families in major cities such as Manchester, Liverpool, and London. Toward the end of the 19th century, municipal authorities and philanthropic organizations began to provide new housing for the poor on a larger scale,[45] overcoming opposition from those regarding this as interference with the workings of a "free market."

There is evidence that average real incomes increased in England and Wales in the second half of the 19th century, and rising real wages for some occupations after the 1870s may have improved the economic standard of living of many working people.[46] Cheaper imports and cooperative societies provided better value food for the working poor, but there was still widespread poverty and under-nutrition up to World War I.[47] The diet of many of the urban poor probably still consisted mainly of carbohydrates.[48] As mentioned in chapter 4, evidence of increased average height between the 1860s and World War I[49] could reflect the reduced impact of acute infectious diseases in childhood as much as any improvement in nutrition. In the first half of the 19th century, there were almost certainly periods when the economic standard of living and diet for most people in England did not improve.[50] Malnutrition can contribute to the risk of dying from infectious diseases, and tuberculosis is particularly lethal in poorly fed and crowded communities;[51] however, it is very unlikely that the decline in tuberculosis mortality throughout the 19th century in England can be explained by improvements in living conditions, or better nutrition as McKeown suggested.[52]

There appears to be no reported evidence to support a natural selection hypothesis that might explain the very long-term decline in tuberculosis mortality. Any women with lower natural resistance to tuberculosis may have died earlier and left fewer children than other women,[53] so it might be expected that high mortality could eventually select out those most susceptible. It is not clear, though, to what extent partial resistance can be conveyed genetically. Studies in England in the 1940s and 1950s found that the degree of exposure to infection is the predominant factor for development of tuberculosis. Only when the degree of exposure to infection was high did incidence of tuberculosis among those with no sign of previous contact with *M. tuberculosis* exceed that of those who were tuberculin positive based on a Mantoux test.[54] The degree of infectivity and closeness of contact with cases appear to be more important than blood relationship per se. A study of tuberculosis in blood relatives, spouses, and non-relatives found that age-standardized death rates did not indicate any hereditary influence.[55] Earlier studies that included twins found an association between the risk of tuberculosis and how closely related a person was to someone with clinical disease;[56] however, this could have been due to more frequent and closer contact rather than shared genes. The role of genetic factors seems to be less significant than socioeconomic and environmental factors, which predominate as determinants of morbidity and mortality. Historically, the impact of adverse living conditions, such as those occurring in times of war, appear to be particularly significant with the death rate only falling when conditions improve again.

It seems unlikely that an immunogenetic explanation could account for the decline in tuberculosis death rates in England and Wales in the 19th century. The decline throughout the century is very unlikely to have been due to nutrition as there is little evidence of a consistent improvement. The suggestion that the long-term decline in tuberculosis mortality might reflect a decline in virulence of the microorganisms[57] has not been supported by any evidence. In fact, a study of tuberculosis in England in the period 1923–40 found that case fatality was still extremely high (50%) among cases of clinical tuberculosis.[58] There was also no decline in case fatality over this period, the decline in the death rate reflected a decline in the incidence of clinical tuberculosis, and infection with *M. tuberculosis* continued to be universal (fig. 9.4).

There was no national tuberculosis prevention policy in England before the late 1880s, although there were some public health initiatives to reduce mortality from the 1860s. Hardy found that sanitary authorities in many districts of London were enforcing improvements in ventilation during visits for inspection, cleansing, and maintenance of tenements and other buildings where the poor lived. Some medical officers of health made appropriate recommendations to prevent transmission, although these did not lead to widespread action and there was opposition to notification of cases. Sanitary authorities in some districts offered disinfection of premises and linen in households with tuberculosis cases, but take-up appears to have been very low.[59] These initiatives are unlikely to have had much impact on exposure to infection or on the dosage of bacillus contracted as crowded housing and working conditions persisted. Men in common lodging houses and people living on the streets were particularly vulnerable to tuberculosis.[60] Confinement of the destitute poor in workhouses probably increased their risk of developing clinical tuberculosis, although it may have restricted the spread of infection in the community as a whole. By 1890 one-third of phthisis deaths in London occurred in workhouses, and in England as a whole the proportion increased from 8% to 24% between 1870 and 1920.[61]

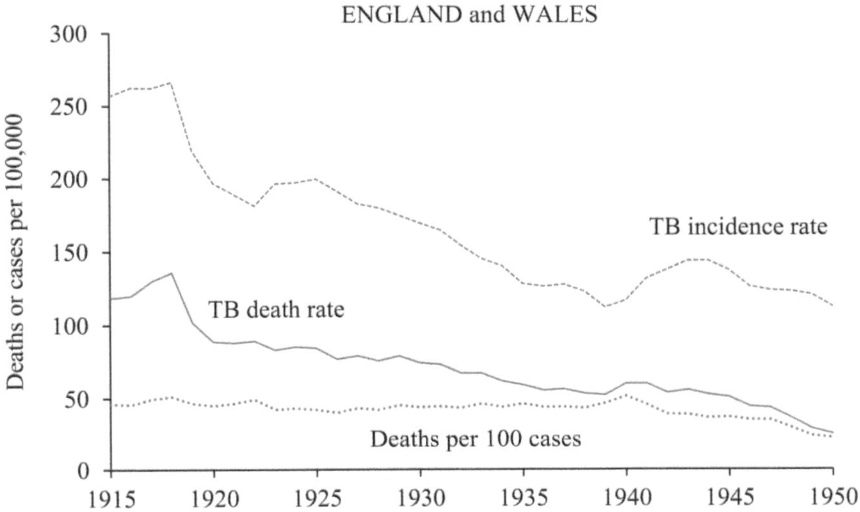

Figure 9.4. Annual incidence rates, death rates, and case fatality ratios for tuberculosis in England and Wales, 1915–1950. *Source:* Registrar General, *Annual Statistical Reviews.*

A more scientific rationale for isolation of infective cases and other preventive measures came with Robert Koch's identification of *M. tuberculosis* in 1882, acceptance of contagion theory, and an increased understanding of transmission. A few prevention officers were active at the local level in the late 1880s, and a coordinated antituberculosis scheme was proposed for Britain as a whole. The National Association for the Prevention of Tuberculosis was established in 1898,[62] and an international conference in London in 1901 addressed by Koch stressed the importance of educating the public about the disease and how it spread.[63] Antituberculosis movements, health education, and control programs had begun to develop in other Western countries, and prevention programs in Philadelphia and New York City in the 1890s were among the first.[64] The control program in New York adopted a systematic approach based on mass education, mandatory notification of cases, free sputum examinations, nursing follow-up, and isolation of infective cases.[65] In England an article in the journal *Public Health* in 1900 referred to tuberculosis as a disease of poverty. It was recognized that the disease was most prevalent among the poor and that education and public participation would be essential components of a national program focused on early diagnosis and isolation of cases. Municipal and local authorities were to be responsible for services, and a system of diagnostic centers and residential institutions was developed. Notification of tuberculosis was made compulsory in 1913 on the recommendation of the Royal Commission on Tuberculosis.[66] The number of sanatoriums in Britain increased from 3 in the 1900s to over 300 by the 1930s, and the number of dispensaries increased from 1 to about 500.[67]

Long before these beneficial measures in the 20th century, there is evidence of a decline in the period death rate from "consumption" in London from about 1800, and registration data indicate a decline in age-specific death rates from respiratory tuberculosis over successive cohorts born in England and Wales in the 19th century. This phase of the long-term decline in tuberculosis mortality is unlikely to be explained by either reduced exposure or improvement in living conditions, work environments, or nutrition. A plausible explanation for declining tuberculosis death rates throughout the 19th century is that smallpox vaccination prevented many children and young adults from a severely debilitating disease that increased the risk of tubercular infection developing into clinical tuberculosis. From the end of the 19th century, several factors are likely to have reduced the risk of a high dosage of bacillus being contracted, including improved ventilation in new housing and in the workplace, reduced domestic overcrowding, smaller families, and isolation of the sick. Care in sanatoriums for those diagnosed early and procedures for collapsing the lung in more advanced cases may have contributed to recovery in some cases,[68] although case fatality is unlikely to have been reduced much before streptomycin was introduced in 1947.[69]

Such measures as educating the public, building new housing, and isolating the infected are likely to have reduced rapid transmission and high dosage of bacillus, although infection appears to have been unavoidable. As late as the 1950s, most children in England were tuberculin positive from natural infection, and before BCG vaccination was introduced most people in Western countries were naturally sensitized to tuberculin by age 30.[70] However, preventive measures, reduced overcrowding, and sociodemographic changes from the end of 19th century probably reduced the risk of contracting the high dosage of bacillus that was more likely to result in clinical disease. A study of pulmonary tuberculosis in England and Wales in the 20th century estimated that each infectious case had "effective contact" (enough to lead to infection), with an average of 22 individuals in 1900; but this number had declined to 10 by 1950 and to 1 by 1990. This reduction probably made a major contribution to the decline in incidence of clinical tuberculosis. The main factors involved are likely to have been reduced domestic crowding; smaller households and families; improved diet; the decline of acute infectious diseases that had increased susceptibility to clinical tuberculosis; better hygiene behavior with regard to sneezing, coughing, and spitting; and the isolation of increasing numbers of infected people in sanatoriums.[71] Such improvements, together with the use of pasteurized milk and BCG vaccination from the 1920s, probably account for most of the decline in tuberculosis incidence and mortality in the 20th century. Although the relative contribution of different factors would be difficult to estimate, prevention of clinical disease is likely to account for most of the decline in tuberculosis mortality.

Chapter Ten

Respiratory Diseases

The continuous decline in the period death rate from respiratory tuberculosis in the second half of the 19th century contrasts with an increase in the death rate from other respiratory diseases (mainly bronchitis and pneumonia) from the 1840s to the 1870s. The respiratory disease death rate then leveled off in the 1870s and 1880s until the influenza pandemic of 1889–91, which affected all age groups (figs. 10.1 and 10.2). Apart from this epidemic, the general trend over the period 1875–1915 reflects changes in the bronchitis death rate, which declined from the 1890s, while the long-term decline for pneumonia began around 1905 (figs. 10.3 and 10.4). Trends for subcategories are likely to have been affected to some extent by changes in classification of the primary cause of death. The trend in the respiratory disease death rate at ages 45–64 was relatively unaffected by transfer of recording from the "old age" and "ill-defined" categories, although there may have been some transfer of diagnosis from respiratory tuberculosis in the second half of the 19th century. Although the death rate among adults declined, the downturn in the death rate at all ages from the 1890s reflects a decline among young children (0–4 years) in particular (fig. 10.2). After the 1890s, the total respiratory disease death rates declined for males and females, apart from World War I years and in the major influenza pandemic of 1918 (fig. 10.1). After World War II, the death rate for females leveled off while that for males increased, most likely due to higher prevalence of cigarette smoking.

A review of trends in death rates from respiratory disease in the 20th century focused on three categories because of changes in classification: asthma, pneumonia, and chronic obstructive pulmonary disease or COPD (chronic bronchitis, emphysema, bronchiectasis, bronchial catarrh, and other obstructive airway diseases). The COPD death rate at ages 15–74 declined steadily with a more rapid decline after the 1960s, which probably reflects the decline in cigarette smoking among older men. The risk of chronic respiratory disease is affected by smoking and other irritants, as well as recent severe acute respiratory infections; however, it is also partly determined by experiences earlier in life. The study found that the long-term trend in period mortality was superimposed on a declining trend over successive cohorts born in the second half of the 19th century.[1] Several factors could have contributed to a reduced risk of bronchial damage in childhood that could impair development of the lungs, including the absence of influenza epidemics from the 1850s to the 1890s, avoidance of the respiratory complications of smallpox by being vaccinated, and reduction in severity of airborne

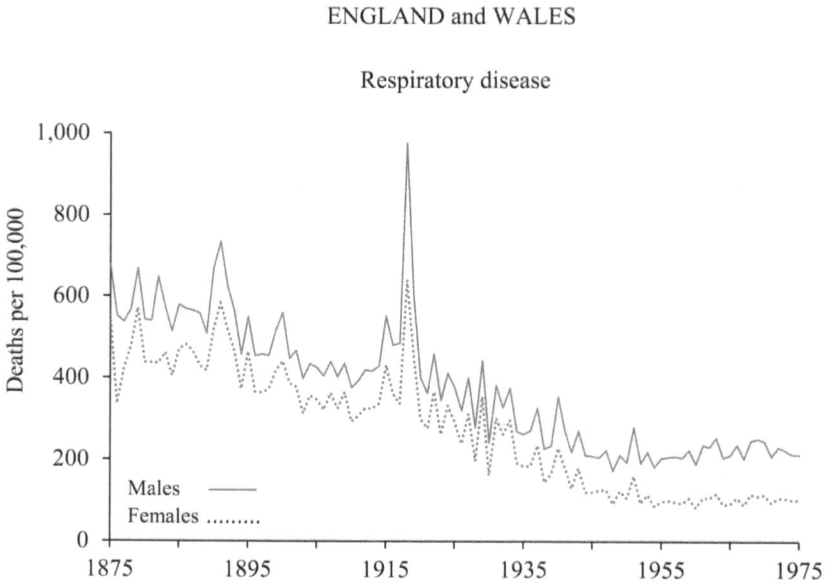

Figure 10.1. Annual age-standardized* death rates from respiratory disease for males and females in England and Wales, 1875–1975. *Sources:* Registrar General, *Annual Reports*; *Annual Statistical Reviews.* * Standardized to the age structure of the European standard population (persons).

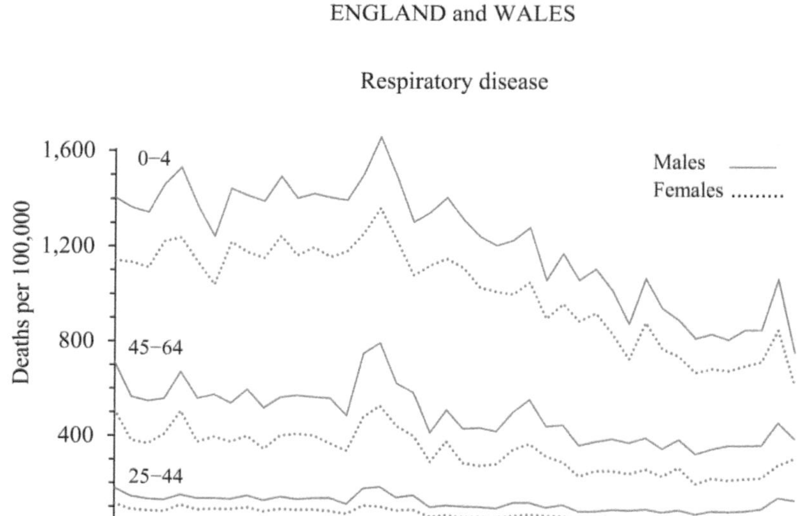

Figure 10.2. Annual death rates from respiratory disease among males and females aged 0–4, 25–44, and 45–64 in England and Wales, 1875–1916. *Sources:* Registrar General, *Annual Reports*; *Annual Statistical Reviews.*

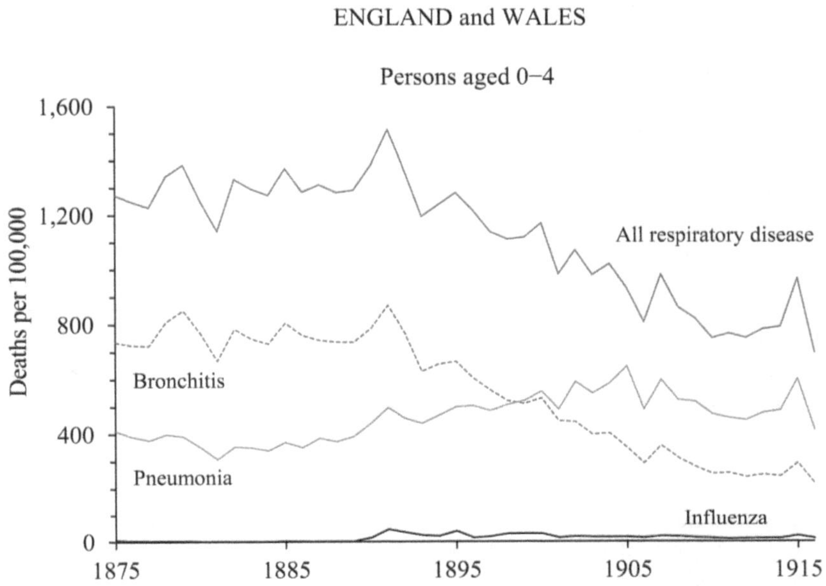

Figure 10.3. Annual death rates from all respiratory disease, bronchitis, pneumonia, and influenza among children aged 0–4 in England and Wales, 1875–1916. *Sources:* Registrar General, *Annual Reports*; *Annual Statistical Reviews.*

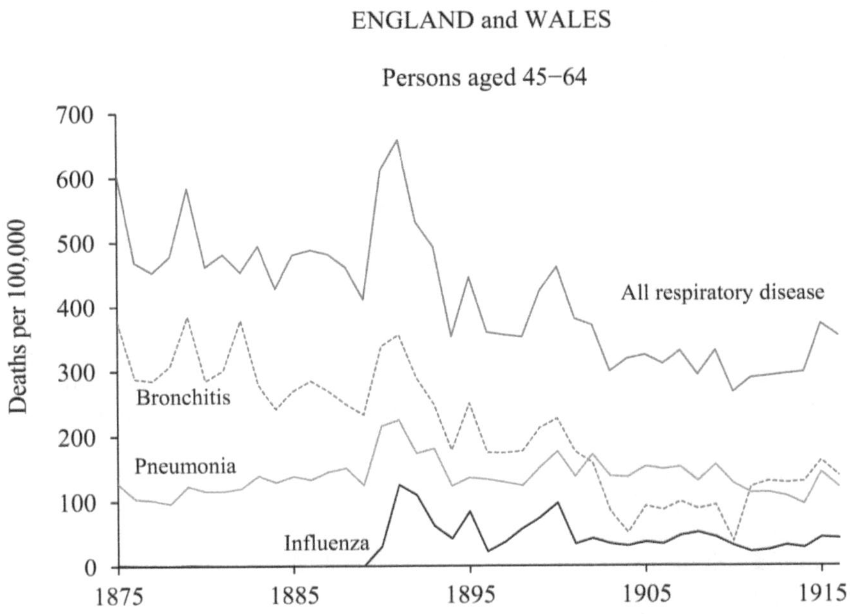

Figure 10.4. Annual death rates from all respiratory disease, bronchitis, pneumonia, and influenza among persons aged 45–64 in England and Wales, 1875–1916. *Sources:* Registrar General, *Annual Reports*; *Annual Statistical Reviews.*

infections from the 1890s. A decline in age-specific death rates from pneumonia over successive cohorts born in the second half of the 19th century may also have been due to such cohort-related effects. Nevertheless, influences in later life probably predominated in the gradual decline in the period death rate from pneumonia in the 20th century. The decline in death rates from both lobar and pneumococcal pneumonia for all age groups from the 1930s coincided with a decline in the influenza death rate.[2] The decline in the total pneumonia death rate became much more rapid when antibiotics were introduced in the 1940s. The asthma death rate remained relatively low and steady until a decline in the 1950s, which may have been linked with controls on air pollution. However, other irritants such as infections and allergens may have a greater role in provoking acute attacks and aggravating chronic asthma, while an "epidemic" in the 1960s was probably due to use of certain types of aerosol.[3]

Despite the long-term decline in death rates, all respiratory disease still accounted for over 14% of deaths in England and Wales at the end of the 20th century, while tuberculosis accounted for only 0.1%. The contribution of respiratory disease to overall mortality decline in the 20th century was less significant than in some other European countries.[4] Relatively high respiratory disease death rates may partly reflect climatic conditions and increased mortality in cold winters. The combination of damp, poorly ventilated housing and industrial air pollution could explain higher respiratory disease mortality compared with European countries that have colder winters, such as Norway.[5] Many of the adverse living conditions associated with respiratory tuberculosis, such as overcrowded housing and workplaces, large families, and under-nutrition, would have contributed to high respiratory disease mortality throughout the 19th century. New housing built from the end of the century probably alleviated some of the harmful effects of overcrowding, dampness, indoor smoke, and poor ventilation. However, smoke from domestic coal fires and industrial emissions, and working conditions for factory workers, continued to cause serious respiratory problems.

Male textile workers, who were a large proportion of all factory workers in the 1890s, had a death rate from respiratory disease that was two and a half times higher than that of agricultural workers, despite having higher pay.[6] Mortality from chronic bronchitis is associated with heavily industrialized and polluted areas, and marked urban-rural and area differentials persisted into the 20th century.[7] Studies in the 1950s found high mortality associated with air pollution,[8] and later studies identified effects on children's health.[9] Comprehensive measures to address the problem were not implemented nationally until after the Clean Air Act of 1956.[10] Evidence from local studies indicates the respiratory benefits of considerable reductions in atmospheric smoke and sulfur dioxide,[11] although at the national level the steady decline in the bronchitis death rate continued with no acceleration in the 1960s and 1970s.[12] In view of this, it seems unlikely that the decline in respiratory disease mortality between the 1890s and 1950s was due to an improvement in air quality.

Children from poorer backgrounds in areas with high levels of air pollution were likely to develop worse lung function following lower respiratory tract infections.[13] Evidence from both urban and rural areas in the 1960s indicated a socioeconomic gradient in the frequency of chronic cough and incidence of bronchitis among children of presmoking age. The gradient was similar to that for adult men and women, and much higher bronchitis incidence and mortality among lower socioeconomic groups was not explained by air pollution.[14] Differences in childhood experience, particularly the severity of respiratory infections, contribute to the risk of developing chronic respiratory disease later in life when cigarette smoking and dusty working conditions as well as air pollution also contribute to adult bronchitis. Although public health measures improved air quality and the work environment in England and Wales in the second half of the 20th century, cigarette smoking and infection persisted as major contributors to bronchitis morbidity and mortality.[15] The Whitehall Study of male civil servants found that nearly all deaths from chronic bronchitis at ages 40–64 were among cigarette smokers, although the strongest predictor of mortality was reduced lung function.[16] Factors other than cigarette smoking have clearly been involved in socioeconomic differentials in respiratory function and mortality, as indicated by the differential among children of presmoking age,[17] and the steep social class gradient in bronchitis mortality in the 1920s when smoking habits were more uniform.[18] Longitudinal investigation has suggested that cigarette smoking has the greatest effect on the prevalence of symptoms in young adults (age 20), followed by a history of respiratory tract illness in the first two years of life.[19]

Childhood social circumstances contribute to lifetime risk of fatal respiratory disease through the effects of poor intrauterine development, childhood infections, and impaired growth, as well as exposure to risks in adulthood associated with poor housing, indoor smoke, outdoor air pollution, and tobacco smoke.[20] There is evidence from long-term follow-up studies that respiratory infections in childhood can lead to long-term damage and a greater risk for respiratory disease in adulthood. Lower respiratory tract infections and more overcrowded living conditions in childhood were independently associated with chronic cough in adulthood, as well as cigarette smoking and socioeconomic status.[21] Bronchitis and pneumonia in the first two years of life were found to be associated with impaired adult lung function.[22] There is also a geographic association between adult mortality from bronchitis/emphysema and past infant mortality from bronchitis and pneumonia.[23] The downturn in the infant respiratory disease death rate around 1891 corresponds with a downturn in the respiratory disease death rate at ages 45–64 for adults born around 1891 (fig. 10.5).

The irritant effects of common respiratory infections such as influenza, common cold, and other viral and bacterial respiratory infections can damage the lungs, eventually leading to chronic and deteriorating symptoms such as disabling cough and breathlessness. Unlike many airborne infectious diseases, bronchitis is not known to convey immunity, although lobar pneumonia produces an important immune response. The bacterial causal agents, different types of pneumococci, are differentiated by the type of antigen (specific soluble substance) surrounding the microorganism. Pneumococci continue to

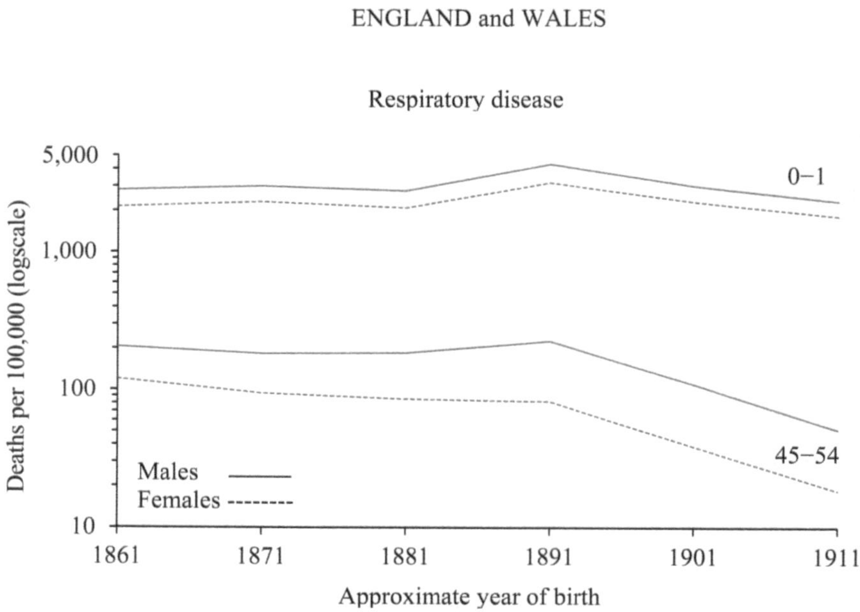

Figure 10.5. Respiratory disease death rates at ages 0–1 and 45–54 in England and Wales by year of birth, 1861–1911. *Sources:* Registrar General, *Annual Reports*; *Annual Statistical Reviews.*

multiply and eventually kill the infected person unless sufficient antibodies are produced to control the specific soluble substance that protects the bacteria.[24] Lobar pneumonia is an extremely severe disease with high case fatality, and there was no effective treatment before the introduction of sulfapyridine in 1938 and antibiotics in the late 1940s. Vaccination for children under two years of age was added to the routine childhood immunization program in 2006, although the impact has been limited because the decrease in pneumococcal cases caused by the vaccine serotypes was largely offset by an increase in cases caused by nonvaccine serotypes.[25]

Some other common epidemic diseases of childhood can also result in secondary respiratory complications, particularly in large families with inadequate food and poor living conditions. Pneumonia is the most common severe complication of measles in developing countries, accounting for most measles-related deaths.[26] During measles outbreaks, pneumonia incidence rises due to primary measles virus pneumonia or secondary bacterial pneumonia.[27] At least one of the common bacterial pathogens—pneumococci, streptococci, staphylococci, or *Haemophilus influenzae*—can usually be found in cases of childhood measles with respiratory complications, and viruses are also a significant cause of measles-related pneumonia.[28] A study in Nigeria found that bronchopneumonia was a complication in 47% of hospitalized measles cases and that 28% of those children died.[29] A similar study in Uganda found that half of the deaths among hospitalized measles cases involved bronchopneumonia, 13% bronchitis or pulmonary tuberculosis, and 18% diarrhea and vomiting.[30] Measles virus causes a specific inflammatory reaction in the tracheobronchial system, and bronchopneumonia was a common secondary complication of measles in the past. Records for Glasgow from the period 1893–1912 indicate that bronchitis, pneumonia, and bronchopneumonia were complications in 54% of measles deaths.[31]

Respiratory infections, measles, and whooping cough can result in lasting damage to the respiratory system. Fifty cases of collapsed lung among children in a London hospital in the 1940s involved pneumonia (34%), bronchitis (26%), whooping cough (14%), and measles (8%).[32] Among 1,894 children admitted to a Manchester hospital between 1948 and 1955 with whooping cough or measles, 50 (3%) died and 52 (3%) had detectable damage to the lungs on radiographic follow-up in 1954–55, half of them involving bronchitis and recurrent cough.[33] The susceptibility of very young children with whooping cough to pneumonia and lung damage is well recognized. The main causal agent, the bacillus *Bordetella pertussis*, produces an acute tracheobronchial inflammatory reaction, which can be a specific primary cause of bronchitis. There is evidence that immunity gained through whooping cough infection or immunization in childhood probably wanes later in life, and whooping cough has been identified among adults working in hospitals.[34] Without confirmation of the causal agent, the disease in adults can be mistaken for bronchitis, and this may have resulted in some misclassification in the past. The evidence of secondary respiratory complications of whooping cough and measles among children suggests that these infections led to much chronic pulmonary disease and possibly permanent damage before high coverage of immunization was achieved in the 1960s. By the 1970s there were relatively few hospitalized cases of measles in England, although about half of the deaths were the result of respiratory complications.[35]

As mentioned in chapter 8, the decline in death rates from measles and whooping cough from the end of the 19th century may reflect a decline in the severity of infections due to sociodemographic changes, particularly fewer births and smaller families. These changes are also likely to have reduced transmission rates and severity of respiratory infections among both children and adults.[36] Children attending school can infect younger siblings with the common airborne diseases of childhood and frequently expose them to streptococcal, pneumococcal, and respiratory infections. Children appear to be the main source of influenza and other respiratory infections introduced into households.[37] In the past they would have been the most likely household members to spread respiratory infections within the family, with older adults being particularly vulnerable. Prospective studies in the 1970s found that the likelihood that any household member would catch influenza was almost twice as high in households with children than in those without.[38] Much of the association of high infectious disease death rates with poor housing could be explained by large families. The number of children in a family appears to be more important than the level of crowding, either within the household as measured by persons per room, or in the community. The risk of contracting primary respiratory infections is partly determined by contacts in the community and within the household, and incidence has been found to increase with the number of siblings and family size.[39] The incidence rate for bronchitis and pneumonia among a cohort of children born in north London in the period 1963–65 who were followed up for five years was almost twice as high for those with three or more siblings compared with those with one sibling. Although rates of infection were lower among breast-fed children, they increased with the number of siblings, both for those who were breast-fed and those who were not.[40]

Successive birth cohorts from the end of the 19th century benefited from an improved airborne infectious disease environment in childhood due to reduced overcrowding, smaller families, and less severe infections. There was a decline in death rates from these diseases in the 1890s, and a decline for respiratory diseases after the major pandemic of influenza in 1889–93. Influenza had been a significant cause of death in Europe for centuries, and epidemics were clearly recognizable because many people were infected within a period of a few weeks, displaying the familiar symptoms of fever and catarrh lasting a few days. Epidemics occurred regularly at intervals of a few years, mainly causing deaths among infants, and among old people who are prone to develop pneumonia. However, major pandemics occurred at longer intervals, such as those in 1847–48 and 1889–93 when many deaths were recorded. Between the 1850s and the 1890s, very few deaths from influenza were recorded in England and Wales, although the disease is known to have been prevalent in Europe.[41] When the pandemic reached England in 1890, a second and third wave caused high mortality in 1891–92, which was the peak in the respiratory disease death rate. Adults were particularly affected as shown by the death rates from influenza and all respiratory disease at ages 45–64 (fig. 10.4). A further impact on adult cardiovascular mortality is discussed in the next chapter, although it can be noted here that the epidemic of influenza in England in 1890–92 marked a major turning point in the death rate from cardiovascular disease as well as respiratory disease.

After the 1889–93 pandemic, "seasonal influenza" continued to cause significant numbers of deaths in "normal" seasonal epidemics up to World War I. At the end of war, the most destructive pandemic of any kind in history occurred in 1918–19, when an estimated 25–50 million people died worldwide. As in the previous pandemic, there were waves of infection in England with a peak in mortality in November–December 1918, and a second peak of about 150,000 deaths in February–March 1919. Burnet and White emphasized the striking difference in the age distribution of fatalities compared with previous pandemics.[42] In 1918–19 the highest proportion of deaths was among adults aged 15–44, while in the 1889–93 pandemic it was among older adults aged 45–74. In the 1920s the age distribution of deaths from influenza once again became skewed toward older people. The death rate remained quite high until a decline in the 1930s and 1940s, after which it remained fairly constant despite a major pandemic in 1957.

The influenza pandemic of 1957 may have been the most widespread of any kind in history,[43] although less destructive of life than the one in 1918–19. The conditions at the end of World War I made the 1918–19 pandemic exceptionally destructive. The first cases indicating high case fatality were recorded among American soldiers at the western front in the autumn of 1918.[44] Those who fell sick at the front were typically transported to triage hospitals behind the lines where infection would have spread rapidly in the grossly overcrowded conditions. Deaths from secondary invasion of bacteria were common, and the bacterium *H. influenzae* was frequently isolated from fatal cases.[45] Bacterial infections were rife in army camps, barracks, in the trenches, and in places where civilian life was seriously disrupted, and there were no effective drugs for treatment. From the front, many of the sick were transported to other hospitals, and the interaction of massive troop movements and upheavals in civilian life provided further routes for rapid transmission around the world. It is likely that food shortages following the war and undernourishment contributed to high mortality. By contrast, at the time of the 1957 influenza pandemic, most of the world was relatively peaceful and more prosperous, and antibiotics were widely available to treat bacterial infections.[46]

Pandemics of influenza have occurred about every 10 to 40 years when a major genetic change in the virus produced a new strain to which most people had no immunity. This probably explains the epidemics in the 18th century, including that in 1743 when the disease was given its Italian name as well as the destructive pandemic affecting England in 1890–92. Different antigenic types of influenza have been implicated in more recent pandemics. Influenza viruses differ in respect of several antigens, and strains have been classified into three "types": A, B, and C. Within these types, there are several strains that have different surface antigens, which provide no cross-immunity to other strains. Burnet and White suggested that influenza A was always prevalent in large populations, and three conditions contributed to the occurrence of an epidemic—climatic conditions (winter), large numbers of people with no immunity, and the strain of virus.[47] If the virus passing regularly between different regions mutated, it would be more likely to spread than a previous strain to which some people had gained immunity. This theory of "antigenic drift" producing a competitive advantage for a mutated virus seemed to provide an explanation for periodic pandemics. However, the pandemic of "Asian influenza" in 1957 involved a type-A virus (A2) with such a marked antigenic difference that it was unlikely to have arisen by a simple mutation. As the strain in the 1918 pandemic was thought to have come from pigs in North America, the idea developed that "Asian influenza" in 1957 may have come from an animal reservoir.[48]

Following the 1957 pandemic, research focused on trying to identify new strains that resembled the viruses involved in the 1918 pandemic, in terms of protein molecules on the surface of the virus to which the immune system develops antibodies, since a similar combination of proteins (H1N1: hemagglutinin type 1 and neuraminidase type 1) might indicate potential for another severe pandemic. In the 1970s there was growing concern because many people would have no immunity to the H1N1 combination as they were born after 1918, and H1N1 was identified on prevalent viruses in 1976. However, Ewald argued that there was no reason to suppose that the H1N1 combination was the factor that made the virus virulent and potentially as harmful as that in 1918.[49] He suggested that investigations should also focus on the process of natural selection that could favor more virulent or less virulent strains of influenza virus within the competitive environment of the human body in which viruses seek food.

Since 1918, the emergence of four pandemic viruses descended from the 1918 pandemic virus has been documented, but there is no evidence that this occurs through direct viral mutations alone.[50] Among the combinations of 17 hemagglutinin receptor bindings and 10 neuraminidases known to exist, only a few subtype combinations, such as H1N1, H2N2, and H3N3, have been observed in human-adapted or pandemic influenza A viruses. More common avian influenza subtypes, such as H4 and H6, have not been found in human-adapted viruses. A recent update on pandemic influenza emphasised the uncertainty as to whether the novel avian influenza A (H7N9) virus that emerged in China in 2013 could evolve into a human pandemic virus. H7N9 is similar in many respects to H5N1, a highly pathogenic avian virus that kills domestic poultry. An important difference is the low pathogenicity of H7N9 compared with H5N1, which means it is less likely to be observed until a rare case of human infection occurs, although both viruses result in high case fatality when humans are infected. Fortunately, there is no evidence to-date of person-to-person transmission, although the importance of preparedness is recognised in view of the unpredictable nature of influenza viruses.[51] For individuals, protection against pandemic influenza is likely to depend on effective vaccination. Vaccination against "normal" seasonal influenza could have a role in prevention of cardiovascular accidents as well as influenza in view of possible links between the diseases discussed in the next chapter.

Chapter Eleven

Cardiovascular Disease

The main focus in the next three chapters is on changes in death rates from major chronic diseases in the context of a greatly changed infectious disease environment. Although major epidemic diseases such as smallpox, typhus, typhoid, and cholera had ceased to cause high mortality and were largely eliminated from England by the end of the 19th century, many other acute infectious diseases of childhood and the chronic infectious disease tuberculosis remained prevalent. The main epidemic diseases of childhood and common respiratory and gastrointestinal infections continue to be prevalent today, although most are generally not life threatening in industrialized countries or case fatality is extremely low. Some of the acute infectious diseases convey immunity, and a specific immune response will occur whenever the microorganism is contracted throughout life. This might tend to be overlooked as the immune response prevents acute infection, although there can be biophysiological consequences that are potentially harmful, either in the short run or cumulatively. Many common viruses and bacteria are now known to be associated with particular forms of chronic disease, including the cardiovascular diseases considered in this chapter.

Bearing in mind the dramatic reduction in death rates from major epidemic diseases that had already occurred by the 1870s, cardiovascular diseases became increasingly predominant as death rates from acute infectious diseases, tuberculosis, and respiratory diseases declined (fig. 11.1). Together with the increase in the death rate from cancer, this constitutes much of the shift in cause of death that has occurred in the epidemiological transition. Cardiovascular disease and other chronic diseases are more likely to occur at older ages, and their growing predominance was linked with increased longevity resulting from the decline in infectious disease death rates. A study of the transition in Italy recognized that the distinction between communicable and noncommunicable disease is not clear-cut as infections are involved in the pathogenesis of many chronic diseases.[1] Evidence of association between microorganisms and chronic diseases previously regarded as noncommunicable, with causality established in some cases, clearly has implications for any theory of epidemiological transition.

A key feature of the transition from acute infectious diseases and tuberculosis to other chronic diseases is the dramatic change in the proportion of deaths attributed to these diseases at different ages. The changing balance of causes,

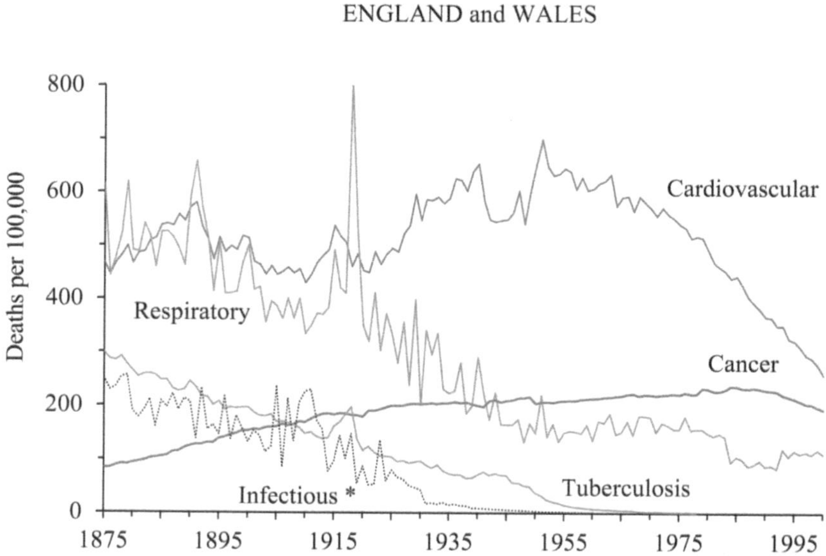

Figure 11.1. Annual age-and-sex-standardized† death rates from cardiovascular disease and other major cause groups in England and Wales, 1875–2000. *Sources:* Registrar General, *Annual Statistical Reports*; Office for National Statistics, *Twentieth Century Mortality*. * Infectious includes smallpox, measles, scarlet fever, dysentery/diarrhea/cholera, diphtheria, and whooping cough.† Standardized to the age structure of the European standard population (persons).

from acute infectious diseases among children and tuberculosis among younger adults to cardiovascular disease, cancer, and other chronic diseases in middle and older adult age groups, is the most striking feature of the transition. This is illustrated by the change in cause-of-death structure between 1851 and 2001 in England and Wales (fig. 11.2). The idea that contact with infectious microorganisms in early life, and also throughout life, can be a significant determinant of morbidity and mortality from chronic disease is a major theme in the remaining chapters. In this chapter, phases of increase and decrease in the cardiovascular disease death rate are reviewed along with evidence concerning well-established socioeconomic, lifestyle, and behavioral risk factors. The possible role of microorganisms is considered with regard to the long-term effects of childhood infections on mortality risk in adult life, cumulative effects of infection encountered throughout life, and more immediate links between recent infections and cardiovascular events.

Cardiovascular disease, the largest category of chronic disease, includes cerebrovascular disease, heart disease, and other diseases of the circulatory system. The underlying process of atherosclerosis appears to have affected humans for thousands of years,[2] which raises the question of what could have been the

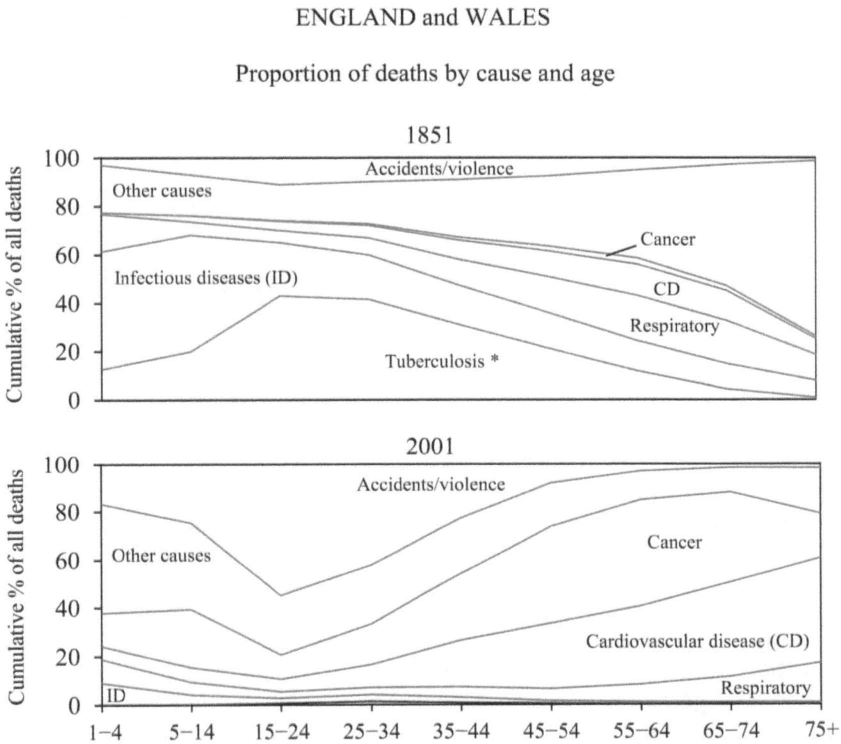

Figure 11.2. Percentage of deaths attributed to the main groups of causes at different ages in England and Wales in 1851 and 2001. *Source:* Registrar General, *Annual Statistical Report, 1851*; Office for National Statistics. *Mortality Statistics: Cause, Series DH2.* * There were very few deaths from tuberculosis in 2001.

causal factors in earlier times. In the relatively modern era, deaths in the 18th century in England were recorded in categories that suggest cardiovascular accidents were included. The category "sudden death" in the London Bills of Mortality probably included deaths due to heart attack or stroke, while many deaths recorded as "apoplexy" and "palsy" would have been due to stroke (cerebrovascular accidents). Black noted that the terms often "alternated" in 18th-century records. He suggested that paralysis, hemiplegia and paraplegia, "polypi" (coagulations of the blood), internal aneurysm (distension and weakness of the arteries), palpitation of the heart, and syncope (fainting due to a drop in blood pressure) were included in the crude categories "apoplexy" and "sudden death."[3] The term "apoplexy" had been used since the time of Hippocrates in ancient Greece (460–370 BC). As a result of the practice of postmortem dissection toward the end of the 19th century, apoplexy caused by obstruction or hemorrhage was linked with degeneration of the arteries, and the term cerebrovascular disease came into use. The traditional lay term "stroke" was widely adopted by the medical profession as systems of care were developed in the second half of the 20th century,[4] although the terms cerebrovascular accident and cerebrovascular disease are still used in the medical literature.

Trends in Cardiovascular Disease Mortality

In the mid-19th century (1848–54), the national registration records indicate that 5% of deaths in England and Wales were attributed to cardiovascular disorders, and the proportion rapidly increased to 15% in 1901 and 48% in 1951, before decreasing to 40% in 2001. Most of the increase was due to an increase in the heart disease death rate, as the age-and-sex-standardized death rate from cerebrovascular disease declined fairly consistently from the 1890s (fig. 11.3). The death rates from heart disease and other circulatory disease increased between 1851 and 1901, contributing +0.20 to each unit of change in the overall death rate. Cardiovascular disease as a whole contributed –0.05 to each unit of change for the years 1901–51, and –0.48 for 1951–2001 (appendix C1), reflecting a declining death rate for females in particular and a decline in cerebrovascular death rates for both sexes throughout the century. This is consistent with international data indicating that female mortality from cardiovascular disease fell along with overall mortality, except at very old ages affected by transfers-in from the "old age" category.[5] At ages 45–64 no deaths in 1848–54 were attributed to old age and only 1.5% were classified as "ill-defined," suggesting that more specific recording over time would not have distorted cause-specific mortality trends for this age group.[6]

Recent research on cardiovascular disease mortality trends in Western countries has tended to focus on subcategories, such as heart disease (referred to as coronary or ischemic heart disease in different studies) and cerebrovascular disease. However, the death rate for the group as a whole may be more reliable when considering long-term trends. Trends for subcategories have been affected by changes in classification, diagnostic practice, and preferences for attributing death to one specific primary cause rather than another, which are more likely to have affected subcategories of cardiovascular disease.[7] Despite both "intergroup" and "intragroup" diagnostic error, there is evidence that for the major cause groups—cardiovascular disease, respiratory disease, and cancer—errors tend to cancel each other out. A study comparing antemortem and postmortem diagnoses for 1,200 patients in England and Wales in 1975–76 found that 16.1% of deaths ascribed to cardiovascular disease by clinicians were attributed to a different ICD order group after autopsy, and 23.8% of deaths attributed to cancer by clinicians. Less than half of the deaths in the three main order groups were attributed to the correct subcategory before autopsy. However, the difference in the proportion of deaths in each of the main order groups after transfers-in and transfers-out was only +3.2% for cardiovascular disease (40.8% vs. 44.0%), –2.1% for respiratory disease (10.7% vs. 8.6%), and –0.4% for cancer (21.7%

vs. 21.3%).[8] These three large groups together accounted for 73.2% of deaths before autopsy and 73.9% on reclassification after autopsy.

A review of disease classification studies conducted between 1917 and 1970 found no convincing evidence that the proportion of errors had changed, although the types of disease and mistakes in diagnosis had altered.[9] A more recent review of studies based on 53 different series of data on autopsies from several countries, mostly for the period 1970–99, found that total error rates had decreased. The proportion of cases in which the principal underlying disease or primary cause of death was missed had declined considerably; however, the study did not report on diagnostic error rates for the main categories of disease after transfers-in and transfers-out.[10] A recent study in five selected areas of England and Wales in 2010–11 compared the underlying cause of death certified by a doctor with an independent nonautopsy assessment and found the net difference was only +1% for neoplasms (1,455 vs. 1,474), +6% for diseases of the circulatory system (1,375 vs. 1,454), and −7% for diseases of the respiratory system (879 vs. 821), which was similar to the findings of the study of autopsies conducted in 1975–76.[11]

When considering trends in chronic disease death rates, multiple causes of death also need to be borne in mind. Certification of the underlying cause is problematic when any one of several disorders could eventually have proved fatal.[12] This could have affected recording of cardiovascular disease deaths in particular, because of changes in the practice of stating respiratory disease as a secondary, rather than a primary, cause of death.[13] Bearing in mind the possibility of transfers of recording from one category to another, it is important to consider relative trends. Major turning points in death rates for the broad groups of chronic disease can be identified and distinguished from changes due to recording practice that produce a noticeable "step" in the trend. Relatively few studies have focused on total cardiovascular disease mortality, although this can overcome some of the problems of classification change.[14] This approach has a further advantage as underlying disorders such as arteriosclerosis, hypertension, and embolism can lead to different cardiovascular events (heart attack, stroke, or pulmonary thrombosis), such that death will be classified in one subcategory rather than another.

The national registration records for England and Wales allow consideration of the long-term trend in the age-standardized death rate from all cardiovascular disease since the mid-19th century. Despite the lack of specific diagnosis at that time and many subsequent changes in component subcategories, this is a useful indicator in conjunction with age-specific death rates. The trend over the period 1875–2000 was essentially the same for males and females with regard to both short-term fluctuations and major turning points, apart from a greater increase in male mortality between 1920 and 1950 (fig. 11.3). Death rates for both males and females increased between 1875 and 1891, but this was followed by a decline until 1910. During the period 1891–1910, the specified subcategories were much the same, with 31% of deaths attributed to apoplexy and hemiplegia and 17% to endocarditis, pericarditis, angina, syncope, aneurysm, and

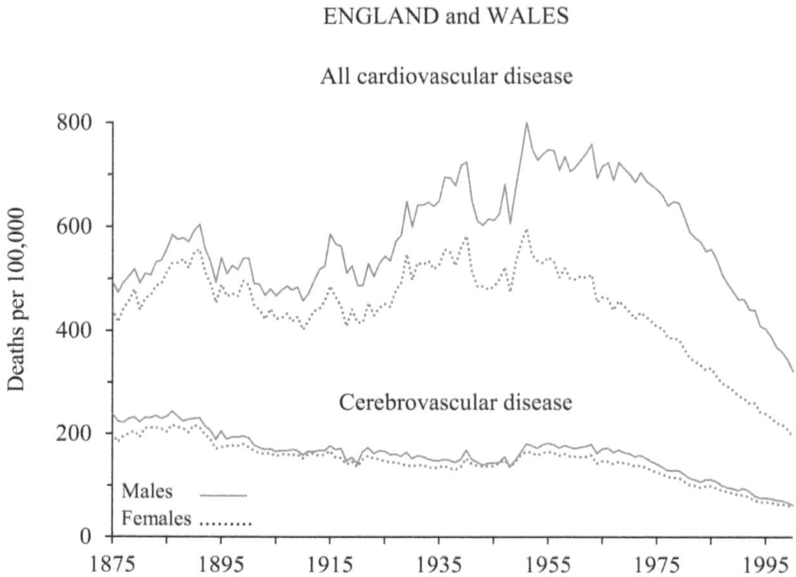

Figure 11.3. Annual age-standardized* death rates from all cardiovascular disease and cerebrovascular disease for males and females in England and Wales, 1875–2000. *Sources:* Registrar General, *Annual Statistical Reports*; Office for National Statistics, *Twentieth Century Mortality*. * Age- and sex-specific death rates applied to the age structure of the European standard population (persons).

thrombosis. Because of changes in the predominant subcategories over a long period, it is useful to consider three phases of the long-term trend within which classification was reasonably consistent: 1875–1915, 1920–40, and 1940–2000. Because over 80% of cardiovascular disease deaths were at ages 45 and over, it is useful to focus on the middle-age group, 45–64, which was little affected by transfers from the "old age" and "ill-defined" categories.

The close correspondence of short-term fluctuations and major turning points in the age-standardized death rates from cardiovascular disease for males and females throughout the period 1875–2000 (fig. 11.3) suggests that they were exposed to a common "risk environment," which would include the domestic and local environment, climate, air pollution, and infectious diseases. This is even more the case with cerebrovascular disease for which there was no divergence of death rates when cigarette smoking among men and women increased at different times, and thus the long-term downward trend in death rates was much the same (fig. 11.3).

The long-term trend in the death rate from cardiovascular disease, with major turning points around 1891 and 1951, is unique among causes of death. However, the earlier turning point around 1891 also occurred for respiratory diseases for which the main underlying causes were airborne infections, as

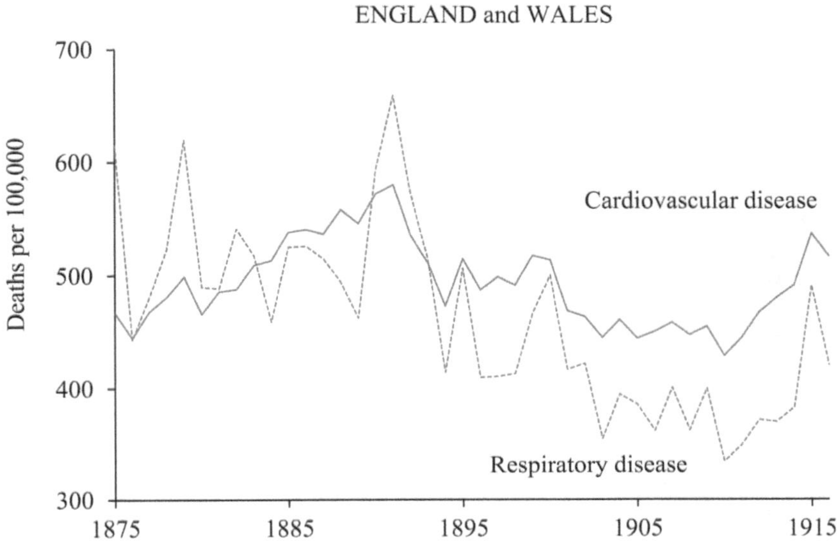

Figure 11.4. Annual age-and-sex-standardized death rates from cardiovascular disease and respiratory disease in England and Wales, 1875–1916. *Source:* Registrar General, *Annual Statistical Reports*; Office for National Statistics, *Twentieth Century Mortality*.

discussed in chapter 10. The correspondence between trends for cardiovascular disease and respiratory disease over the period 1875–1916 (fig. 11.4) suggests some kind of ecological association between these types of disease. The coefficient of correlation between the series was high ($r = +0.84$) and statistically significant ($p < 0.05$), even with the long-term underlying trend removed ($r = +0.68$). After the major turning point in the age-standardized death rates from cardiovascular disease and respiratory disease around 1891, the respiratory disease death rate generally declined, apart from the decade of the 1910s and the major spike in 1918 during the influenza pandemic (fig. 10.1). Although fluctuations in the cardiovascular disease death rate have generally corresponded with fluctuations in deaths due to "seasonal influenza," no spike in cardiovascular disease deaths occurred in the 1918 influenza pandemic, which suggests that deaths among older adults were recorded as due to influenza rather than cardiovascular disease.

In the interwar period, 1920–40, the death rates from cardiovascular and respiratory disease diverged as the death rate from cardiovascular disease increased. However, short-term fluctuations in the cardiovascular disease death rate continued to correspond with those for respiratory disease, which reflected fluctuations in the death rate from "seasonal influenza" (fig. 11.5). Clearly, climatic variation, including cold winters, could contribute to spikes in cardiovascular, respiratory, and influenza deaths. However, epidemiological and other evidence discussed below suggests that influenza and other common respiratory infections may have a causal role in cardiovascular accidents and underlying disorders.

The long-term trend in the cardiovascular disease death rate, with a decline from around 1891, belies earlier notions of a "modern epidemic," although death rates for males and females increased again in the interwar period and between 1945 and 1950 (figs. 11.5 and 11.6). The death rates from heart disease among males also increased at ages 25–44 and 45–64 in the 1950s and 1960s (fig. 11.7), although this did not result in an increase in the age-standardized death rate from all cardiovascular disease (fig. 11.6). The early peak around 1891 reflects the death rates at ages 45–64 and 65 and over, among whom most cardiovascular deaths occurred (fig. 11.8). The death rate among younger adults aged 25–44 had been declining long before the 1890s, probably reflecting different types of cardiovascular disease. The similarity between trends in death rates at ages 45–64 and 65 and over, along with the earlier decline at younger adult ages, suggest that any cohort-related influence did not predominate, and there is no apparent turning point in age-specific death rates in relation to year of birth. Nevertheless, a life-course perspective is important for understanding coronary heart disease, since risk of the disease in adulthood is associated with maternal health, intrauterine development, and health in childhood, as well as socioeconomic and lifestyle-related influences throughout life.[15]

Low birth weight is associated with an increased risk of heart disease later in life, and high ischemic heart disease death rates were found in areas of England and Wales that had high neonatal mortality earlier in the 20th century. Retardation of fetal development and contributing maternal factors may affect the risk for heart disease later in life,[16] although differences in breastfeeding or in the experience of childhood infectious diseases could also affect the development of underlying cardiovascular disorders. A recent study found similarities between the trend in infant mortality and the all-cause death rate at ages over 70, using mortality data from France from the mid-18th century onward presented by year of birth. As the long-term decline in infant mortality from that time mainly involved a reduced impact of acute infectious diseases, it was suggested that the corresponding reduction in death rates at older ages for the same years of birth might be due to a reduced burden of infection-related inflammation, delaying the development of atherosclerotic and thrombotic conditions.[17]

Barker suggested that certain causes of cardiovascular disease operate through the mother and infant experience while others operate in adult life,[18] in which case declining period death rates following the immediate postwar increase (1945–50) would only partly reflect earlier improvements in maternal and child health. The determinants of coronary heart disease are likely to operate over the whole life course, through intrauterine development, growth and health in childhood, social conditions, occupational status, diet, physical activity, smoking, and other risk factors in adult life including infections. In addition to long-term effects of childhood infectious diseases, infections such as influenza may have a more immediate impact triggering cardiovascular accidents in adulthood.[19] The long-term trends in age-specific death rates in England and Wales,

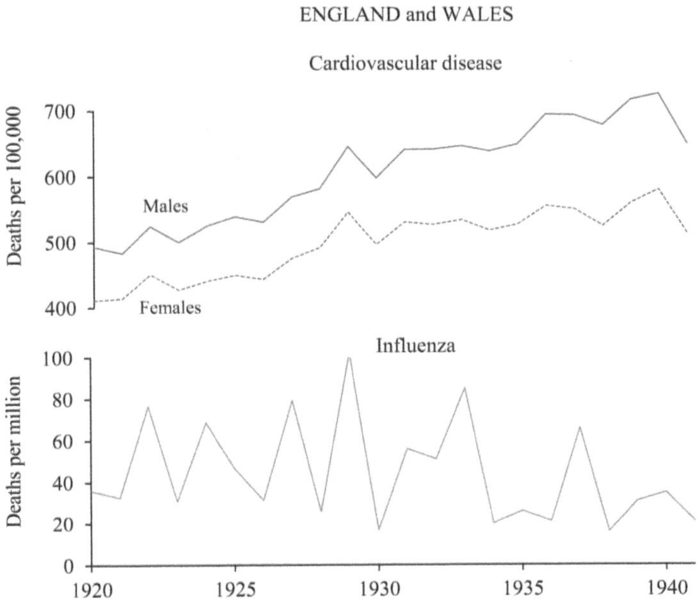

Figure 11.5. Annual age-standardized death rates from cardiovascular disease and influenza in England and Wales, 1920–41. *Source:* Registrar General, *Annual Statistical Reviews.*

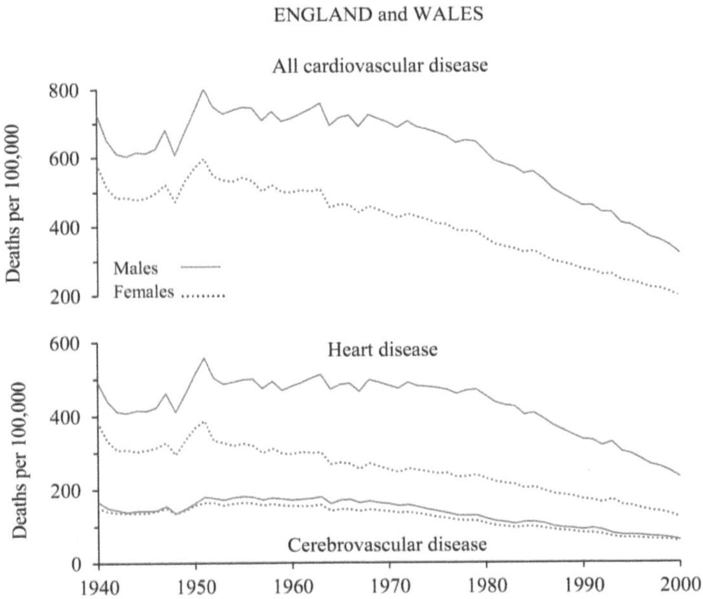

Figure 11.6. Annual age-standardized death rates from all cardiovascular disease, heart disease, and cerebrovascular disease for males and females in England and Wales, 1940–2000. *Sources:* Registrar General, *Annual Statistical Reports*; Office for National Statistics, *Twentieth Century Mortality.*

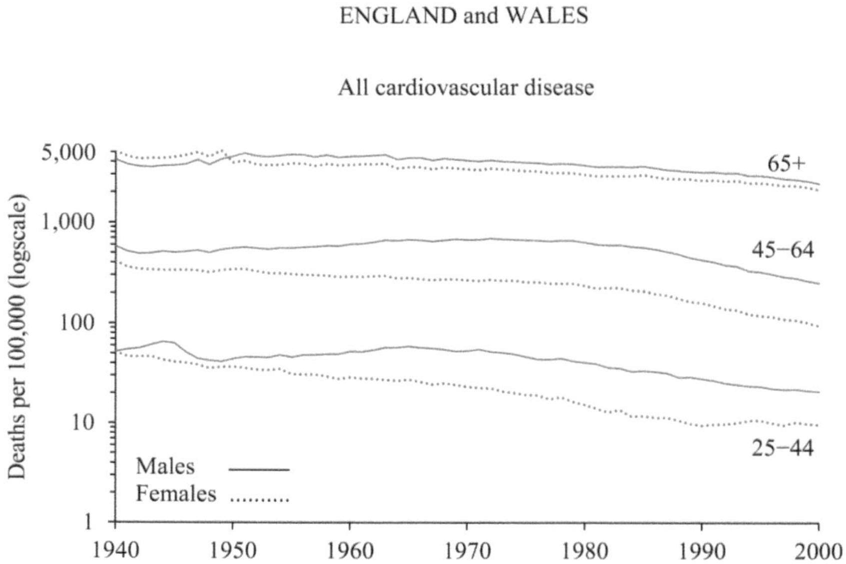

Figure 11.7. Annual death rates from cardiovascular disease for males and females aged 25–44, 45–64, and 65+ in England and Wales, 1940–2000. *Sources:* Registrar General, *Annual Statistical Reports*; Office for National Statistics, *Twentieth Century Mortality*.

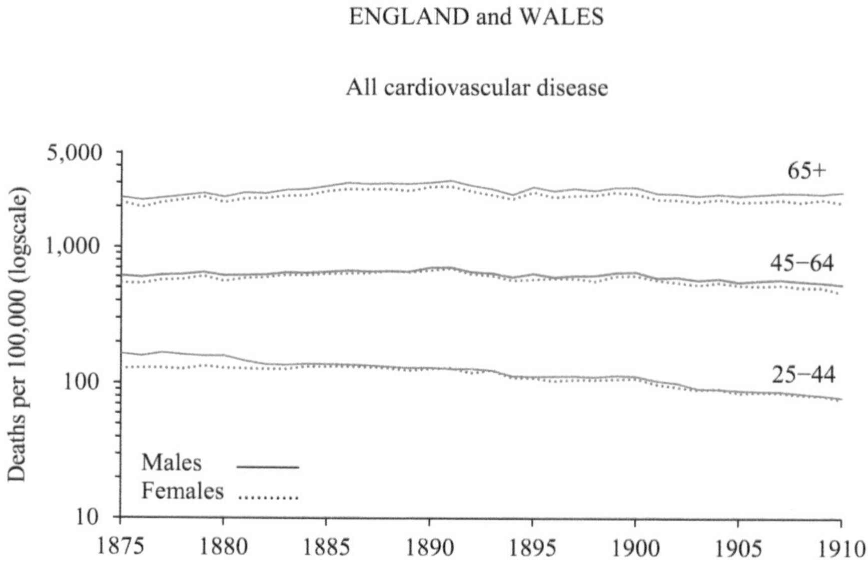

Figure 11.8. Annual death rates from cardiovascular disease for males and females aged 25–44, 45–64, and 65+ in England and Wales, 1875–1910. *Sources:* Registrar General, *Annual Statistical Reports*; Office for National Statistics, *Twentieth Century Mortality*.

and the lack of any clear cohort-related turning point, suggest that exogenous risk factors in adult life have been the predominant influence on trends in mortality from cardiovascular disease. The rise and fall of coronary heart disease mortality occurred at much the same time at all ages. Age-period cohort analysis, which attempts to distinguish the influence of factors operating over the life course from those nearer the time of death, has indicated a small cohort-related influence on trends, although period-related effects explain most of the change in death rates over time.[20] Cohort influences are more predominant in the mortality trends for other chronic diseases, particularly cancer among females and peptic ulcer, as discussed in chapters 12 and 13.

The age-standardized death rate from cardiovascular disease declined quite sharply after 1891 among both males and females, as did the cerebrovascular disease death rate (fig. 11.3). At this early peak in cardiovascular mortality, 35% of the deaths were attributed to cerebrovascular disorders, including 21% recorded as "apoplexy." Most of the apoplexy deaths were among adults and are likely to have been due to stroke. The decline became even more rapid from 1951, although cerebrovascular disease still accounted for 36% of all cardiovascular deaths. The more specific subcategory cerebral hemorrhage was reported to be the main component of cerebrovascular mortality decline between 1932 and 1965.[21] A study of autopsies found a decrease in mortality from cerebral hemorrhage between 1932 and 1999 and an increase in cerebral infarct mortality until the 1970s.[22] A study in the United States found that the decline in the death rate from cerebral hemorrhage between 1930 and 1960 was partly offset by an increase in the death rate from cerebral thrombosis.[23] Although these trends probably reflect some transfer of diagnosis between subcategories, the decline in cerebral hemorrhage mortality outweighed other increases. The death rate from all forms of cerebrovascular disease declined for most of the 20th century in the United States,[24] as in England and Wales (fig. 11.9), with much of the decline occurring long before effective treatments became available.

Despite sharing some contributing factors and underlying disorders, trends in stroke and heart disease mortality display significant differences such as a weak ecological association between international death rates from the two diseases, and different long-term trends in England and Wales. When the death rate from stroke declined in the first half of the 20th century, the death rate from heart disease increased. Changes in diagnostic specificity and preference for assigning primary cause of death may have affected death rates from heart disease to some extent. With the greater awareness of the role of hypertension in ischemic heart disease, there may have been some transfer of recording.[25] When the death rate attributed to ischemic heart disease increased rapidly in England and Wales between 1945 and 1950, the death rates attributed to hypertension, and "myocardial insufficiency" or "myocardial degeneration," declined. Even so, a study of original death certificates from Ontario, Canada, for 1931–51 suggested that the increase in ischemic heart disease mortality was genuine.[26] The final downturn in the death rate from ischemic heart disease in England and Wales occurred from the 1970s (fig. 11.6), a few years later than in the United States.[27]

However, the death rate from all heart disease, which takes into account transfers between subcategories, declined from 1951. This is reflected in the trend in the death rate from all cardiovascular disease, which declined from 1951 as in the United States (fig. 11.9).

Risk Factors and Differentials in Cardiovascular Mortality

In view of changes in diagnostic and recording practice affecting subcategories, trends in death rates from all cardiovascular disease combined were considered in a study of long-term changes in age and sex differentials. The long-term increase in excess male mortality (fig. 11.3) is unlikely to have been greatly affected by revisions of the ICD codes, as change was steady year by year, with no pronounced "step" in years when the classification changed. Over the period 1861–1992 in England and Wales, and 1900–1991 in the United States, close similarities were found in the levels and trends for death rates from all cardiovascular disease among males and females aged under 25 years and over 75. This contrasted with a growing sex differential in cardiovascular death rates at ages 35–74 between the 1920s and 1960s.[28] With little sex differential in cerebrovascular disease mortality, heart disease was the main determinant of the increasing sex differential in total cardiovascular disease mortality. Other studies in England and Wales attributed the widening gap between male and female death rates from ischemic heart disease to the more rapid increase in cigarette smoking among males after World War I.[29] Increasing excess male mortality in the United States was also found to be due mainly to differences in cigarette smoking, although higher ischemic heart disease death rates for males than females among nonsmokers indicated that other factors were also involved.[30]

In view of common risk factors and underlying pathogenic processes, it is not surprising that heart disease and stroke mortality have a similar association with socioeconomic status. Most studies of risk factors for stroke identified physiological and behavioral factors acting predominantly during adult life, such as hypertension, obesity, smoking, physical inactivity, high blood cholesterol, and diabetes.[31] Differential changes in cigarette smoking were involved in a reversal of the socioeconomic gradient in cardiovascular disease mortality, although changes in diet, leisure activity, and work-related factors may also have contributed.[32] The death rate from heart disease was much higher for women in socioeconomic groups IV–V based on husband's occupation than in groups I–II, over the period 1931–71. On the other hand, the death rate for men had been higher in groups I–II between 1931 and 1951, but by 1961 it was higher among men in groups IV and V.[33] The increase in the heart disease death rate was more rapid and continuous among men in the lower socioeconomic groups.[34] Those of working age had been more affected by the decline in pneumonia and tuberculosis mortality and the transition to other chronic diseases.[35] This raised the question of whether the widening socioeconomic differentials in mortality based on occupational groups were the result of health selection effects, or

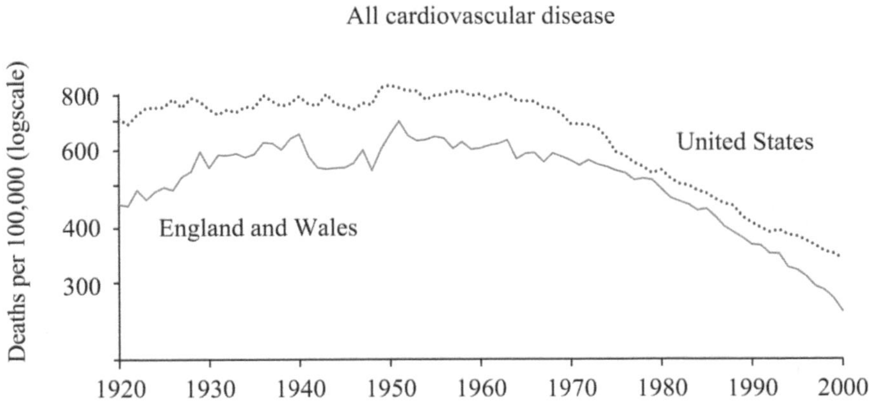

Figure 11.9. Annual age-and-sex-standardized death rates from all cardiovascular disease in England and Wales and the United States, 1920–2000. *Sources:* Registrar General, *Annual Statistical Reports*; Office for National Statistics, *Twentieth Century Mortality*. Centers for Disease Control and Prevention, *Mortality Database.*

possibly changes in occupational structure.[36] However, research using other indicators of socioeconomic status showed that increasing differentials were not due to changes in the structure of the labor force. Using census data to identify socioeconomic groups of women and men based on housing tenure (owner or renter) and car ownership (owner or no car) and death registration data, mortality differentials between socioeconomic groups were identified that were as great as those between groups I and V based on men's occupation.[37] The socioeconomic differential was based on a large relatively disadvantaged group (renting/no car), rather than a small and diminishing group of unskilled manual workers. A combination of indicators of socioeconomic status identified a step-by-step mortality gradient, with the highest mortality among men who had an unskilled manual occupation, rented accommodation, and no car.[38]

Particular occupational groups have been used in many studies of specific risk factors for cardiovascular disease. The studies by Doll and Peto and their colleagues on a cohort of British doctors followed up from 1951 provided strong evidence of association between cigarette smoking and heart disease. One-quarter of the excess mortality among cigarette smokers was due to ischemic heart disease, and the excess risk of dying was particularly high for adult males under 45 years of age.[39] Comparative studies of occupational groups indicated the possibility of risks associated with sedentary work. Bus conductors were found to have lower incidence of coronary heart disease and hypertension than the more sedentary bus drivers,[40] although choice of a less active job could reflect a propensity to become overweight. The Framingham study in the United States found that the risk for cardiovascular disease from being overweight was independent of other well-established risk factors.[41] Prevalence of obesity among adults has increased in Western countries as the prevalence of other risk factors has declined, and prevalence among children in England also increased rapidly between 1974 and 2003.[42] Obesity is associated with hypertension, insulin resistance and diabetes mellitus, hypertriglyceridemia, potentially harmful cholesterol levels, and some cancers.[43]

Multivariable studies controlling for confounding effects have contributed to a vast body of evidence linking increased risk of cardiovascular disorders and death with dietary factors, lack of physical exercise, and cigarette smoking. A study of British civil servants (Whitehall study) found that men in the lowest grade had a higher prevalence of established risk factors, and three times the mortality rate from coronary heart disease compared with those in the highest grade (administrators). However, less than half of this socioeconomic differential was explained by the well-established risk factors—obesity, high blood pressure and blood cholesterol level, and cigarette smoking.[44] It was suggested that part of the association between socioeconomic status and cardiovascular disease might be due to differences in psychosocial work conditions.[45] It had long been suspected that stress contributed to the risk of cardiovascular disease and heart attacks, with different types of stress affecting different occupations. Further research in the Whitehall and other studies has suggested that the demands of work are less important predictors of risk than other sources of work-related stress.

In a second phase of the Whitehall study, the socioeconomic gradient in morbidity and mortality among both women and men was investigated in relation to work circumstances, social support, and well-established risk factors. To assess psychosocial factors, self-reports and independent assessments were used to measure job demands, support from colleagues, and the degree of control people had over their work. In a follow-up of the civil servants in different grades, it was found that psychosocial factors could account for some of the missing predictive power of smoking, blood cholesterol levels, diastolic blood pressure, body mass index (weight [kg]/height $[m]^2$), and high blood pressure. On the one hand, higher risk for coronary heart disease was found among women and men who had low control over their jobs—an effect that was independent of employment grade and the established coronary risk factors. On the other hand, high job demands or lack of colleague support were not related to coronary outcomes.[46] Evidence of higher fibrinogen concentrations in men and women with independently assessed low job control suggested a possible psychophysiological mechanism linking low job control with coronary heart disease as fibrinogen increases the risk of blood clots.[47]

Subsequent research indicated that both low job control and a further indicator of work-related stress, "effort-reward imbalance," are independently associated with coronary heart disease.[48] A twofold increase in the risk for cardiovascular mortality was found in a prospective cohort study of industrial workers in Finland based on similar indicators of work stress.[49] The evidence points to some role for work-related psychosocial factors in the development of cardiovascular disease, although the relationship with material circumstances has to be taken into account. Among the general population, income is a hard indicator of socioeconomic status that has a direct bearing on both material and social aspects of life outside work that can affect health, such as diet, housing, and leisure. One study based on a representative sample of the population of Sweden found a strong association between income and cardiovascular disease mortality, but only 10% of this was attributed to low job control.[50] A study of middle-aged men in Finland found a raised risk for acute myocardial infarction and death associated with indicators of work-related stress, but this was concentrated in the low-income groups.[51] The relationship with health outcomes is even more complex in view of changes over time in jobs and income. Not having work is a source of stress and material deprivation, and unemployed men and their wives have a higher risk of heart disease.[52] A life-course perspective suggests that both current and past circumstances affect the development of cardiovascular disease. Powerful economic, political, and social forces affect opportunities for individuals in different socioeconomic groups to find work and change jobs to improve their workplace circumstances. It seems unlikely that there has been any significant reduction in work-related stress that might have contributed to the recent decline in cardiovascular mortality.

Risk Factors and Trends in Cardiovascular Mortality

Long-term follow-up investigations such as the Whitehall study in England and the Framingham study in the United States have greatly increased knowledge about risk factors and socioeconomic differentials in cardiovascular disease morbidity and mortality. However, some aspects of long-term trends in cardiovascular mortality cannot be easily explained by changes in the prevalence of established contemporary risk factors. The increase among men and women in the second half of the 19th century predated significant increases in cigarette smoking and sedentary lifestyles. Although increasingly more specific certification of cause of death probably affected trends, it is unlikely to explain the decline in total cardiovascular disease death rates in England and Wales between 1891 and 1910.

Many studies have examined mortality trends in the 20th century focusing on middle aged groups unaffected by transfer of recording from the "old age" category of deaths. When death rates from heart disease were seen to increase in England and Wales in the 1920s and 1930s, it was recognized that people were living longer because they were less likely to die from infectious diseases in childhood and early adulthood.[53] A higher proportion of people were reaching ages at which cardiovascular disorders and events occurred, although this in itself would not explain the "modern heart disease epidemic." Since then much has been learned about the risk factors that contribute to cardiovascular disease. Follow-up studies of "no risk" and "at risk" groups have estimated that over 75% of coronary heart disease deaths could be avoided if people did not smoke and adults were in low-risk categories for blood cholesterol and diastolic blood pressure.[54] Although genetic factors may influence the propensity to high blood pressure and high serum cholesterol, it is clear that modification of lifestyle and health-related behavior can significantly reduce the risk of cardiovascular disorders, heart attacks, and strokes.[55] Recent evidence-based recommendations have focused on avoiding excess alcohol; not being overweight; exercising; not smoking; eating fruit, vegetables, and low-fat protein; and reducing intake of salt, total fat, saturated fats, and dietary cholesterol.

There is a tendency for some risk factors to become more prevalent with urbanization, although harmful aspects of lifestyle can be prevalent in rural areas or diffuse to them. Persistent urban-rural differences in cardiovascular disease mortality are likely to reflect economic, sociocultural, and occupational factors, as well as the prevalence of physiological risk factors such as high blood pressure.[56] In developing countries, the prevalence of hypertension and coronary heart disease increases as people move to the towns and adopt new lifestyles, including high fat consumption, cigarette smoking, and more sedentary occupations.[57] In some developing countries, a higher proportion of cardiovascular disease can be due to rheumatic heart disease and other heart disorders known to be linked with infection or nutritional deficiency. However, even in the 1970s death rates from all cardiovascular disease among men and women in middle-aged groups in Trinidad were nearly double those in England and Wales.[58] The idea of an epidemic of the "industrial way of life" is misleading, and the different epidemic patterns of heart disease in developing countries indicate that local strategies are required to address this global problem.[59]

International, geographic, and socioeconomic differences in the timing of the decline in coronary heart disease death rates suggest a process of diffusion of preventive measures and treatment.[60] Trends in cardiovascular disease mortality since World War II have varied considerably in Western countries, which can be partly explained by different responses to knowledge about major risk factors. However, the effects of these factors can be cumulative, and establishing the contribution of changes in health-related behavior to changes in cardiovascular mortality is complicated by delayed effects. Beneficial changes in lifestyle can lag behind science-based knowledge about risk factors, and there is often a lag before such changes have an impact on coronary heart disease mortality. Different assumptions about the length of a lag period can affect conclusions about the nature of the relationship, as recognized in studies of changes in economic conditions and mortality rates.[61] Studies of time series found contradictory evidence, such as a decline in cardiovascular disease mortality among women in Switzerland between 1951 and 1976 that was unequalled in other European countries, despite increasing consumption of cigarettes and animal fats.[62] Subsequent analysis of data from several countries indicated beneficial changes in consumption of food products between 1954 and 1965 and cigarette consumption between 1969 and 1973 were associated with a decline in coronary heart disease mortality between 1969 and 1975.[63]

A consistent fall in male and female death rates from cardiovascular disease after 1950–51 was reported for Canada, the United States, France, and the United Kingdom, as well as Switzerland, while the downturn occurred later in

Norway (1960s) and Ireland (1970s).[64] The decline in total cardiovascular mortality in the 1950s predated a reduction in the prevalence of well-established risk factors for heart disease such as cigarette smoking.[65] While influenza vaccination could have affected trends in total cardiovascular mortality, the decline in the United States between 1963 and 1983 was found to be associated with a decline in cigarette smoking, reduced prevalence of high blood cholesterol, and beneficial changes in food consumption.[66] The onset of the decline in coronary heart disease mortality coincided with the peak in prevalence of cigarette smoking in 1964, and with public health warnings about tobacco, saturated fats, and cholesterol.[67] The decline in coronary heart disease mortality between 1968 and 1981 has been attributed to prevention strategies resulting in beneficial changes, such as reduced smoking, increased physical exercise, improved diet, and decreased levels of blood cholesterol, particularly among higher socioeconomic and educational groups.[68]

Between 1970 and 1985, total cardiovascular disease death rates declined in most Western countries, but not among males in Greece and some Eastern European countries where only female death rates declined.[69] Relatively high death rates from cardiovascular disease in countries undergoing economic transition in the 1990s have been attributed to the lack of improvement in health-related behaviors and adverse effects of deteriorating social and economic conditions.[70] For example, in Russia, increased alcohol consumption was implicated in a reduction in male life expectancy of about six years between 1990 and 1994.[71] Cardiovascular disease death rates in several Eastern European countries reached a peak at this time and then declined.[72] Death rates from coronary heart disease were declining in most Western countries by the 1980s and in some Eastern European countries in the 1990s.[73] Studies in different countries found that reductions in the prevalence of three major risk factors—high blood cholesterol, high blood pressure, and cigarette smoking—could explain up to three-quarters of the decline in coronary heart disease mortality; for example, in Finland between 1972 and 1992.[74] A reduction in the prevalence of these risk factors in Iceland over the period 1968–88 corresponded with changes in the death rate from ischemic heart disease, which leveled off between 1968 and 1985 before declining quite sharply. There was some lag between changes in health-related behaviors and incidence of ischemic heart disease among men, although changes in lifestyle could explain up to three-quarters of the decline in mortality as in other countries.[75]

A study in England and Wales concluded that 58% of the decline in ischemic heart disease mortality from 1981 to 2000 was attributable to reductions in lifestyle-related risks, particularly tobacco smoking, while 42% could be due to medical interventions.[76] In the United States, 44% of the decline in the coronary heart disease death rate from 1980 to 2000 was attributed to reductions in total blood cholesterol, systolic blood pressure, smoking, and an increase in physical exercise, and 47% to treatment particularly for acute myocardial infarction, unstable angina, and heart failure.[77] The results of studies of aspirin, thrombolysis, drugs for reducing hypertension and blood cholesterol, and coronary artery bypass surgery were used to estimate the effect of treatment. Studies in several Western countries have reported similar proportions of the decline associated with reductions in lifestyle-related risks (40–60%) and medical interventions (35–50%),[78] although some of these are preventive rather than curative and extrapolation of trial results may overestimate the effects of treatment at the population level.

A review of trends in heart disease mortality in the 20th century in England and Wales concluded that treatment is unlikely to account for a large proportion of the decline from the 1970s, although by the 1990s more widespread use of thrombolysis and aspirin following myocardial infarction probably contributed by reducing case fatality.[79] The increase in ischemic heart disease death rates in the 1920s and 1930s and subsequent decline occurred among men and women in all age groups, which indicated predominantly period-related influences. The review considered lifestyle-related factors, particularly evidence of a decline in cigarette smoking among men and women, and declining average per capita consumption of butter and lard from 1970.[80] Reduced consumption of these saturated fats was consistent with lower ischemic heart disease mortality, although epidemiological evidence does not indicate an independent association. Raised low-density and low high-density lipoprotein are risk factors, and a combination of lack of exercise and a diet high in saturated fat may contribute to increased body fat and harmful blood cholesterol levels. It was suggested that key factors such as saturated fat, blood cholesterol, and cigarette smoking may have interacted, rather than trends in mortality being due to single risk factors.

Between 1950–51 and 1996, the total cardiovascular disease death rate in the United States declined by more than 50%, despite an increase in the death rate from coronary heart disease until 1963.[81] The decline between 1950 and 1963, when coronary heart disease mortality was increasing, reflected declining death rates from stroke and other circulatory disorders. The Framingham Heart Study found an increase in the prevalence of hypercholesterolemia between 1950 and 1960, and a decline in the prevalence of high blood pressure.[82] However, the decline in stroke mortality began long before the 1950s and effective treatment for hypertension.[83] The cerebrovascular disease death rate fell by about 50% in most Western European countries between 1950 and 1990,[84] and the decline in stroke mortality in England and Wales became more rapid from the 1950s.[85] The decline in the United States from that time has been linked with the introduction of treatment for hypertension, the main risk factor for cerebrovascular disease.[86] However, some evidence suggests that antihypertensive medication accounted for less than 25% of the decline in the United States and New Zealand in the 1970s.[87] Clearly, the long-term decline in cerebrovascular disease mortality since the beginning of the 20th century predated effective treatment for hypertension by many years, and factors other than treatment are likely to account for much of the decline in mortality.[88]

In England and Wales, the age-standardized death rate from cerebrovascular disease declined by 43% between 1891 and 1920, long before anticoagulant and antihypertension treatments. The death rate from stroke was generally declining throughout the 20th century, although a sharp increase occurred in the immediate postwar period, 1945–50 (fig. 11.3). During the course of the century, there may have been some transfer of recording from stroke to heart disease, although this is unlikely to account for the large decline in mortality in different countries. Similar rates of decline at different ages suggest that period-related influences predominated, although people born around the turn of the century appear to have benefited from some cohort-related influence.[89] Reductions in cigarette smoking and in other lifestyle-related risks, particularly as a result of dietary changes, are likely to have had a period-related effect on cardiovascular disease mortality trends. These changes can explain much of the decline in the second half of the 20th century, although neither preventive measures nor treatment were involved in the decline in the period death rate between 1891 and 1910 in England and Wales (fig. 11.4). For those born around this time, there was also a decline in the relative risk for stroke mortality later in life.[90] The decline in period death rates from stroke from the 1890s coincided with the decline in respiratory diseases, measles, and diphtheria, and there is considerable evidence of association between specific respiratory infections and different forms of cardiovascular disease from epidemiological and other studies that may help to explain this ecological association.

Microorganisms and Cardiovascular Disease

Some aspects of the long-term trends in age-standardized death rates from cardiovascular disease are not readily explained in terms of well-established risk factors. It is widely recognized that high blood pressure, high blood cholesterol, tobacco smoking, certain dietary elements (particularly cholesterol, fat, and sodium), physical inactivity, and obesity are major risk factors for cardiovascular disease.[91] Many studies have contributed to a greater understanding of the social determinants of health and disease, and lower socioeconomic status and low control over work have been established as significant risk factors for cardiovascular disease.[92] However, none of these are proximate determinants of disease, and most lifestyle- and behavior-related factors are intermediate determinants rather than primary causes of underlying cardiovascular disorders such as atherosclerosis and embolism. A comprehensive understanding of cardiovascular disease requires an understanding of pathogenesis, and the role of infection has been suspected for many years.[93] There is now considerable evidence that microorganisms are associated with the underlying pathogenic processes and with potentially fatal cardiovascular accidents, suggesting that changes in the infectious disease environment may have been an important determinant of changes in cardiovascular disease morbidity and mortality in the past.

Common viruses have long been implicated in heart disease, such as Coxsackie viruses linked with pericarditis and myocardial disease. Many viruses have been found to produce myocardial disease, and common coinfections with bacteria could have synergistic effects.[94] An association between group-A streptococcal infection and both rheumatic fever and rheumatic heart disease has been found in many studies.[95] Several laboratory studies in the 1950s and 1960s investigated the effect of the presence of viruses in the blood. Influenza and mumps viruses were found to produce agglutination of platelets in human and animal blood.[96] Mustard compared the formation of platelets in response to viruses with the process of blood clotting in response to a cut vessel. The research suggested that blood clotting during antigen-antibody reactions might be a cause of embolism and a "trigger" for potentially fatal cardiovascular accidents.[97] It also suggested that the underlying cardiovascular process of atherosclerosis might be a cumulative effect of immune responses to viruses encountered throughout life, leading to arteriosclerosis and an increased risk of cardiovascular accident.[98] A key finding was the monoclonal nature of cells in arteriosclerotic plaques, which is consistent with it being the product of cell mutations caused by infectious microorganisms.[99]

The lifelong process of atherogenesis adversely affects the functioning of the arteries. Atherosclerosis is now regarded as an inflammatory disorder, and not simply a result of lipid deposits accumulating on the inner walls of the arteries.[100] The clinical manifestations of atherosclerosis include coronary artery disease, stroke, abdominal aortic aneurysm, and peripheral vascular disease.[101] The pathogenesis of coronary heart disease involves interaction of atheroma and thrombosis. There is little evidence that the rise and fall of heart disease mortality has been associated with changes in the prevalence of atherosclerosis, and changes in thrombotic tendency may have been influential.[102] The potential consequences of narrowed or blocked arteries (arteriosclerosis) depend on which vessels are most affected. Diseased cerebral vessels potentially cause stroke, diseased coronary vessels can lead to angina or heart attack, while diseased kidney vessels can lead to kidney failure. Since the 1980s, many studies have identified and investigated association between cardiovascular disorders and infection, particularly with *Chlamydia pneumoniae, Helicobacter pylori,* and cytomegalovirus.[103] A prospective study found that chronic infections significantly increased the risk of carotid atherosclerosis developing in the future, independently of other well-established cardiovascular risk factors.[104] Several studies have identified common microorganisms that are associated with atherosclerosis, and the evidence of association appears to be strongest for *Chlamydia pneumoniae.*[105] This is one of the commonest pathogens known to cause community-acquired pneumonia worldwide, and it may infect nearly everyone at least once.[106] As *C. pneumoniae* and other microorganisms associated with atherosclerosis might be just "passive bystanders" with no role in cardiovascular disease pathogenesis, studies are seeking to clarify the relationship between infection, inflammation, atherosclerosis, and thrombosis.[107] *C. pneumoniae* could cause damage through inflammation, the immune response, or more directly. There is also evidence of its association with Alzheimer's disease as well as atherosclerosis, based on its presence in the brains of Alzheimer's patients but not controls. This suggests that these very distinct chronic diseases might be linked to a common underlying infectious disease process.[108]

Association between both *C. pneumoniae* and *H. pylori* infections and coronary heart disease was found to be independent of well-established risk factors.[109] An association was found between different forms of cerebrovascular disease and infection with *H. pylori* and other pathogens, which suggested a possible prothrombotic effect. The association was independent of well-established risk factors and socioeconomic status.[110] However, doubts have been raised concerning the limitations of small studies, potential confounding by socioeconomic status, and the possible role of other inflammatory processes.[111] Infections are less common in higher socioeconomic groups, and a large prospective study found that ischemic heart disease was not associated with *C. pneumoniae* infection in professional men.[112] Nevertheless, much of the evidence from epidemiological studies, clinical investigations, and pathophysiological observations indicates that acute infections may have a role in inflammatory responses, activation of blood platelets, coronary artery disorders, disruption of atherosclerotic plaques, development of thrombi, and cardiovascular accidents.

Infections and the immune response to them could have a generic role in underlying cardiovascular disorders and different manifestations of cardiovascular disease,[113] acting within a complex causal web of lifestyle-related, socioeconomic, and environmental risk factors. Lifestyle-related factors such as high levels of total blood cholesterol and low-density lipoproteins (LDL), hypertension, obesity, and smoking cannot fully explain the underlying disorders.[114] Repeated infections with many pathogens over the life course could contribute cumulatively to atherosclerosis, which increases the risk of cardiovascular accidents. Bacterial and viral infections and coinfections are common, and multiple infections may be involved in atherothrombosis, which could partly explain the lack of effectiveness of targeted antibiotic treatment for prevention of acute cardiovascular events.[115] Acute infections with certain specific microorganisms may be more significant in triggering cardiovascular accidents than chronic infection, with immunization offering the possibility of reducing the risk.[116]

A recent review of evidence found that large, well-designed studies have consistently reported a two- to threefold increase in the risk for acute coronary syndromes within one to two weeks of respiratory infection. It was concluded that acute infections, especially respiratory infections, have a role in triggering strokes and acute coronary events within a multifactorial causal web.[117] A further review focusing on influenza[118] found that the evidence from many observational studies generally supported the hypothesis that seasonal influenza can "trigger" acute myocardial infarction and fatal heart attack, as suggested in earlier studies of temporal association.[119] A review of the biological basis for a causal mechanism suggested that when infection increases inflammation of the arterial walls, this may destabilize and rupture atherosclerotic plaques, leading to embolism and thrombosis.[120] Clinical trials could determine whether vaccination against influenza protects against cardiovascular accidents. A few studies have found that vaccination reduces the risk of acute coronary syndromes among people with underlying cardiovascular disorders, and further large-scale investigation could assess the effect.[121] The relative absence of spikes in the trend for annual cardiovascular disease death rates in England and Wales after the 1960s (fig. 11.6) is consistent with a possible protective effect of influenza vaccination at the population level.

In view of associations and evidence of links between acute respiratory infections and cardiovascular disease, the similarity between the trends in death rates over the period 1875–1915 (fig. 11.4), and the correspondence of short-term fluctuations in cardiovascular disease and influenza mortality between 1920 and 1941 (fig. 11.5), are not surprising. Excess mortality from both respiratory disease and cardiovascular disease has been reported in peak years for deaths from seasonal (nonpandemic) influenza. Although weather conditions may account for some of the association,[122] the earlier evidence of blood coagulation during antigen-antibody reactions,[123] together with considerable evidence from observational studies, suggests that influenza infection can be a direct cause of embolism, thrombosis, acute myocardial infarction, and fatal cardiovascular accidents.[124] The role of influenza as a trigger for heart attacks has been less well publicized than lifestyle-related risk factors, although the need to increase vaccination rates for older adults and those with underlying cardiovascular disorders is recognized.[125]

Evidence concerning the role in cardiovascular disease of other specific respiratory pathogens, including *H. influenzae*, *C. pneumoniae*, and *Streptococcus pneumoniae*, could also come from immunization studies,[126] which can be conducted in developing countries as well as industrialized countries. Targeted research linking specific vaccine-preventable diseases with specific cardiovascular outcomes could provide more definitive evidence concerning the causal role of specific microorganisms. With regard to influenza, clinical trials in different parts of the world could determine whether influenza vaccination provides significant protection against cardiovascular accidents for those most at risk. As children are frequently the source of respiratory infections affecting adults, as discussed in chapter 10, the experience in Japan with a program of vaccinating children against influenza warrants further investigation. Excess winter deaths from influenza, pneumonia, and all causes were considerably reduced in the population as a whole,[127] and further investigation might reveal an impact on cardiovascular mortality. Prevention will be particularly important in low-income countries as most people will not gain access in the foreseeable future to expensive treatments for heart disease available in more affluent countries. This consideration also applies to the growing burden of cancer morbidity in low-income countries and among the aging populations of high-income countries, as discussed in the next chapter.

Chapter Twelve

Cancer

Cancer is not exclusively a modern disease, and paleopathological evidence of many of its forms has been found in ancient human remains. Even so, the evidence from thousands of prehistoric and ancient remains, such as fossils, mummies, and skeletons, suggests neoplasms were not common until after the medieval period in Europe.[1] Investigation of Egyptian mummies suggests malignancies were rare,[2] although multiple melanoma cases have been well documented, and also nasopharyngeal carcinoma, which is readily identifiable through damage to the skull.[3] Hippocrates made the distinction between malignant and benign cancers in the fifth century BC.[4] Although malignant cancers are now usually referred to as malignant neoplasms, the term cancer is used here as it has a longer history in the research literature. At the end of the 18th century in England, there were early references to cancer as a form of "tubercle," and only a few deaths were recorded in the "cancer" category in the London Bills of Mortality. In some cases the wasting may have been difficult to distinguish from the effects of tuberculosis for the purposes of recording cause of death. When national registration began in England and Wales, the term malignant tumors was already in use, although "carcinoma" was not formally distinguished from "genuine crude tubercle" until 1855.[5] Pathologists sought to define the difference between cancer and tuberculosis, which occur in many of the same sites in the body, and the idea of an inverse relationship developed despite both occurring at the same time in a few cases.[6] It is now usual to regard cancers as a group of diseases, differing widely in etiology, frequency of occurrence, and site of manifestation.

The underlying processes in cancer have long been regarded as linked with the cumulative effects of irritants and carcinogens. Burnet suggested that errors in the repair of DNA could explain associations between carcinogens and particular sites of cancer, such as radiation and skin cancer, cigarette smoking and lung cancer, naphthylamines and bladder cancer, radium salts in paints and bone sarcoma, and many others. The molecular-level process in "environmental cancer" could involve a carcinogenic agent entering cells and causing damage to the DNA, which can be repaired but with an increased risk of informational error and abnormal cells that can replicate out of control.[7] In recent years, research in molecular biology has contributed to greater knowledge about the malignant transformation of a cell through accumulation of mutations.[8] Two classes of gene play a role by promoting growth (proto-oncogenes) or suppressing growth (tumor suppressor genes). For a cancerous tumor to develop, several mutations must occur in the original cell's growth-controlling genes, which normally takes many years. During the course of life, genes are damaged by environmental carcinogens, infections, or chemicals produced in the cells of the body. Errors may occur in the cell's genes when the enzymes replicating DNA make copying mistakes, and the damage becomes a permanent mutation if the repair system fails. The effectiveness of the proteins that repair damaged DNA can be impaired by inherited defects, and gene mutations that would normally accumulate over many years occur more frequently, including mutations of genes involved in controlling cell proliferation.[9]

There are now two main theories of carcinogenesis: somatic mutation theory, which focuses on the cellular level and regards carcinogenesis as a problem of cells proliferating beyond control; and tissue organizational field theory, which views carcinogenesis as a problem of tissue organization. Mutation theory has long viewed cancer as being the result of a single somatic cell that has undergone DNA mutations on genes that control cell proliferation. Carcinogens either cause the propagation of already mutated cells or cause mutation of genes that control proliferation. The more recent alternative theory suggests that cells would normally proliferate, and although interactions between cells in a particular system usually maintain tissue organization and repair, carcinogenic agents can disrupt this process.[10] Ewald and Swain Ewald emphasized that a general theory of oncogenesis should incorporate the role of infection, as microorganisms may enhance the mutation-driven process or compromise barriers that prevent oncogenesis. In developing an evolutionary theory based on the distinction between barriers and restraints that inhibit but do not prevent oncogenesis, they suggested that prevention strategies will need to be based on a better understanding of infectious causation and multiple causes.[11] In addition to infections, established carcinogens and risk factors include tobacco, dietary components, industrial products, air pollution, and alcohol. Such factors probably explain much of the large variation in site-specific cancer death rates internationally.[12] Doll found that cancer incidence or mortality was higher in urban compared with rural areas for 23 out of 26 types of cancer in a study of 13 countries, which he attributed mainly to differences in personal behavior (cigarette smoking, alcohol consumption, sexual promiscuity, exposure to ultraviolet light, diet, and family size) and other factors including atmospheric pollution, occupational hazards, and genetic differences in susceptibility.[13] Despite the different theories of carcinogenesis, there is a general consensus that exposure to carcinogens is preventable, and that infections linked with cancer can be controlled by antibiotics (bacterial infections) and vaccines (viral infections).

Long-Term Trends in Cancer Mortality

The registration records for England and Wales provide the longest series of national mortality statistics for cancer. In the mid-19th century (1848–54) only 1% of deaths were attributed to cancer, but the proportion increased to 5% in

1901, 16% in 1951, and 26% in 2001. The increase in the proportion of deaths due to cancer between 1951 and 2001 occurred despite a decline in the cancer death rate as the decline was less rapid than for other causes of death. The decline in the cancer death rate contributed significantly (–0.15) to each unit of change in total mortality (appendix C1). Despite a decline in the death rates from cancer over successive birth cohorts of females, their lifetime probability of dying from cancer increased as death rates from other causes declined faster. Men have also been increasingly likely to die from some form of cancer since the mid-19th century. On the basis of incidence rates for 1992–94, it was estimated that 35% of males and 33% of females would eventually be diagnosed with some form of malignancy,[14] although survival rates for cancers of most sites have been improving in recent decades.[15]

Some aspects of trends in site-specific death rates in the 20th century have been linked with changes in the prevalence of established risk factors such as cigarette smoking, although earlier trends are more difficult to explain. The age-standardized cancer death rate for both males and females increased in the second half of the 19th century before cigarette smoking became widely prevalent (fig. 12.1). The "aging" of the population, with an increasing proportion of older people, does not in itself account for increasing cancer mortality as death rates increased at different ages. After World War I, period death rates for males continued to increase, while death rates among females leveled off or declined. This divergence continued after World War II, when death rates among males aged 55–64 and 65–74 in particular increased more rapidly (fig. 12.2). The increase continued until the 1960s, when the death rates leveled off before declining from the mid-1980s. For females, there was a more continuous decline in period age-specific death rates from the 1930s and a more rapid decline in the 1990s.

Interpretation of long-term trends in period death rates from cancer is complicated by the interplay of "generation effects" and "period effects." The more recent decline in the period death rate from all forms of cancer in the 1980s and 1990s reflected a simultaneous decline in age-specific death rates for adults (fig. 12.2). This indicates the predominance of period-related influences, which can include improvements in treatment, earlier diagnosis, and changes in certification practice as well as risk factors.[16] For cancers with poor prognosis, declining period death rates are more likely to reflect declining incidence. In the past, cancer survival rates were extremely low and did not change much over time, so trends in period death rates before the mid-20th century are more likely to reflect changes in incidence, diagnosis, and certification.[17] A decline in incidence can reflect changing exposure to carcinogens and, more recently, effective prevention programs leading to changes in behavior, such as antismoking campaigns. Some of the decline in period cancer death rates in the 1980s and 1990s is likely to be due to earlier diagnosis and more effective treatment. Survival rates in England and Wales have improved steadily since the 1970s for most types of adult cancer, although less rapid improvement for those less well off has widened the socioeconomic differential.[18] The relative contribution of

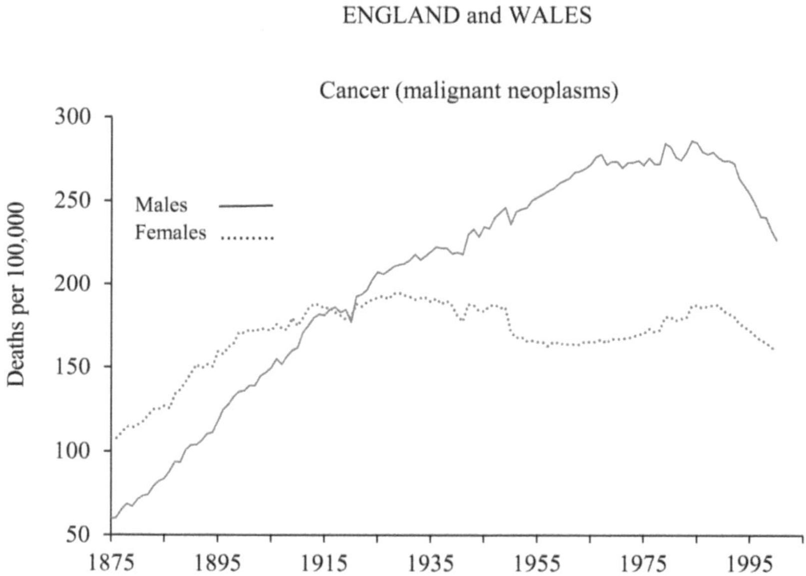

Figure 12.1. Annual age-standardized death rates from cancer for males and females in England and Wales, 1875–2000. *Sources:* Registrar General, *Annual Reports*; *Annual Statistical Reviews*; Office of Population Censuses and Surveys, *Mortality Statistics: Cause, Series DH2.*

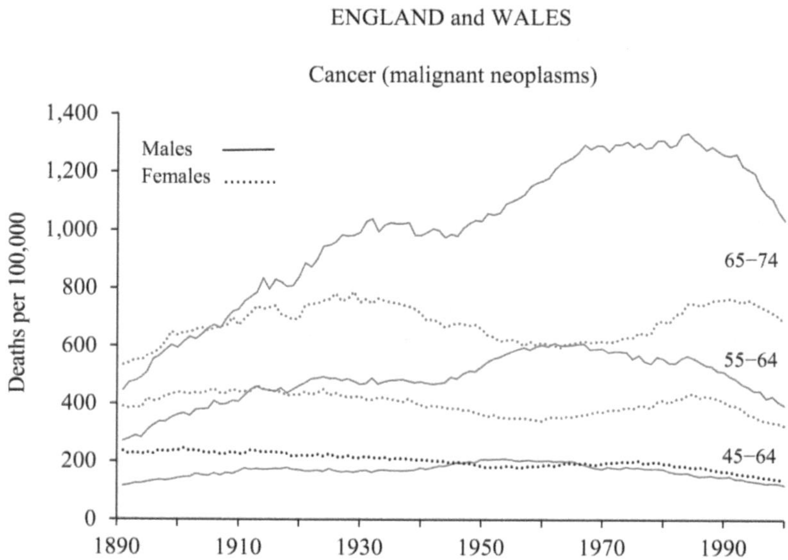

Figure 12.2. Annual age-specific death rates from cancer for males and females in England and Wales, 1891–2000. *Sources:* Registrar General, *Annual Reports*; *Annual Statistical Reviews*; Office of Population Censuses and Surveys, *Mortality Statistics: Cause, Series DH2.*

different influences on trends in period death rates from cancer such as treatment, prevention, lifestyle changes, and generation effects would be difficult to quantify.

Some kind of generation-related influence probably underlies the decline in the age-standardized period death rate for females between 1925 and 1965 (fig. 12.1). A study of deaths from all forms of cancer in the period 1951–80 found that the death rate for females had declined for those born after the 1920s, while the rate for males had declined for those born after about 1900.[19] An association between height and cancer suggested the possible influence of health-related experiences in childhood, which may affect growth-related factors linked with cancer in adult life.[20] Long-term trends in female cancer mortality also suggest predominant generational effects linked with childhood circumstances, so that each generation has to some extent carried its own risk of cancer mortality into later life. Age-specific death rates from all forms of cancer plotted in relation to year of birth indicate a turning point in mortality for females born in the 1860s (fig. 12.3). For males there was some reduction in the rate of increase in age-specific death rates over successive cohorts born after the 1860s, but not a decline. Any cohort-related benefits for males appear to have been offset by adverse influences during adult life, particularly cigarette smoking. Differences between male and female cohort trends were found in an earlier study that reported a decline in age-specific death rates from cancer over successive cohorts of females born between 1871 and 1901, while death rates for males increased.[21] However, for later cohorts born in the mid-20th century, death rates were only increasing for a few sites—kidneys, pharynx, lung, pancreas, male urinary system, and female genital organs.

Trends in Site-specific Cancer Death Rates

The diversity of forms of cancer and multifactorial etiology further complicate explanations of changes in the period death rate from all forms of cancer, which is the only category for considering very long-term trends. Although there are clinical reasons for fragmentation of mortality data into site-specific subcategories, there are advantages to considering trends in death rates for cancer as a whole over the long run. Early studies of cancer death rates suggested that the overall susceptibility to cancer in a population might be relatively constant, such that reductions in incidence of one form could be offset by increased incidence of another. If this were the case, it could account for the widely different incidence of site-specific cancers among populations with similar death rates from cancer as a whole.[22] In considering increasing death rates from cancer among males and females in the 19th century, there are few data on cancer deaths by site, and to some extent it may have been regarded as one disease. Nevertheless, some conclusions can be drawn about the likely contribution of different sites to the overall increase in cancer mortality in the 19th century, based on data for 1911–15 when site was first reported. Lung cancer is unlikely to have contributed

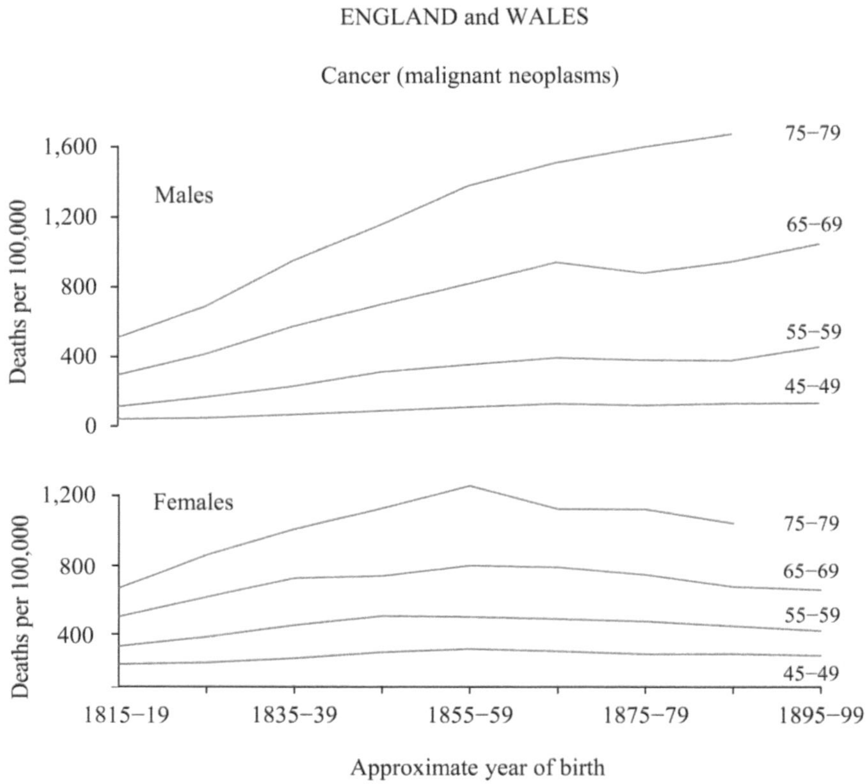

Figure 12.3. Annual average age-specific death rates from cancer in England and Wales for males and females by year of birth from 1815–19 to 1895–99. *Sources:* Registrar General, *Annual Reports*; *Annual Statistical Reviews*; Office of Population Censuses and Surveys, *Mortality Statistics: Cause, Series DH2.*

much to increasing cancer mortality in the 19th century, as only 1.3% of cancer deaths among males and 0.7% among females involved this site in 1911–15. The main contributions to overall cancer mortality were female-specific cancers (36.0%) and cancers of the digestive system among females (36.1%) and among males (50.4%), and these are likely to have contributed most to any genuine increase in cancer mortality in the 19th century.

Cancers of the lung, trachea, and bronchus now account for the largest proportion of total cancer mortality—24% among men and 20% among women in 2008. The increase in death rates for both males and females after World War I is particularly striking (figs. 12.4 and 12.5). The more rapid rate of increase in male lung cancer mortality after World War II underlies the increasing sex differential in the period death rates for all cancer (fig. 12.1). The sex-specific sites of prostate (12.7%) and breast (16.3%) are now the second-largest categories of cancer mortality for males and females, respectively (table 12.1). The period death rate from prostate cancer increased more rapidly in the 20th century than the death rate from breast cancer (figs. 12.4 and 12.5). Other sites contributing to the overall increase in the period death rate from cancer as a whole were bladder, pancreas, and leukemia among males, and bladder, pancreas, leukemia, esophagus, and ovary among females. Meanwhile, death rates from alimentary canal sites, including mouth, stomach, intestine, and rectum, increased in the first three or four decades of the 20th century and then declined.[23]

Risk Factors and Cancer Mortality

Gastrointestinal, epithelial, and breast cancer in particular are associated with nutritional factors. Both experimental and human observations suggest the importance of diet, although evidence has not always been consistent. Doll and Peto found that the evidence suggested control of the components of diet that enhance or inhibit carcinogenesis may be more important for prevention than preventing ingestion of carcinogens.[24] The main role of dietary factors in cancer may be to act as vehicles for carcinogens, or to modify the effect of these. Many aspects of diet, vitamins, trace elements, and other micronutrients could be involved, acting either to enhance carcinogenesis or to inhibit the process through some protective effect.[25] The very high proportion of gastrointestinal cancers in 1911–15, when recording by site began, is likely to reflect the poor hygiene, extremely poor food quality, and nutritional deficiencies experienced by those born in the 19th century. Until the last quarter of that century, there was little control over the quality of food sold, and much of it was adulterated with poisonous chemicals and cheaper foreign substances to increase weight, and contaminated with bacteria, organic, and other matter. The work of pioneering food chemists who published the results of their analyses and campaigned for controls led to Food Adulteration Acts and the appointment of public analysts toward the end of the 19th century. Improved food quality is likely to have reduced the risk of gastrointestinal disorders and cancers of the digestive system, while increased consumption of fresh fruit and vegetables could have had a protective effect.[26] Recent confirmation that *Helicobacter pylori* is a microbial causal agent of stomach cancer suggests that improved hygiene conditions in childhood may also have been particularly important,[27] as discussed below. Reductions in age-specific death rates from cancer of the stomach, intestines, and rectum could all be due in part to protective effects of improved diet and quality of food. However, the contribution of specific dietary factors and carcinogens in food and drink to the increase in the death rate from cancers of the digestive system in the 19th century has not been assessed.

Although cigarette smoking accounts for much of the increase in cancer death rates among men in the 20th century, it cannot explain the increase among men or women in the 19th century. Tobacco was smoked in cigars and

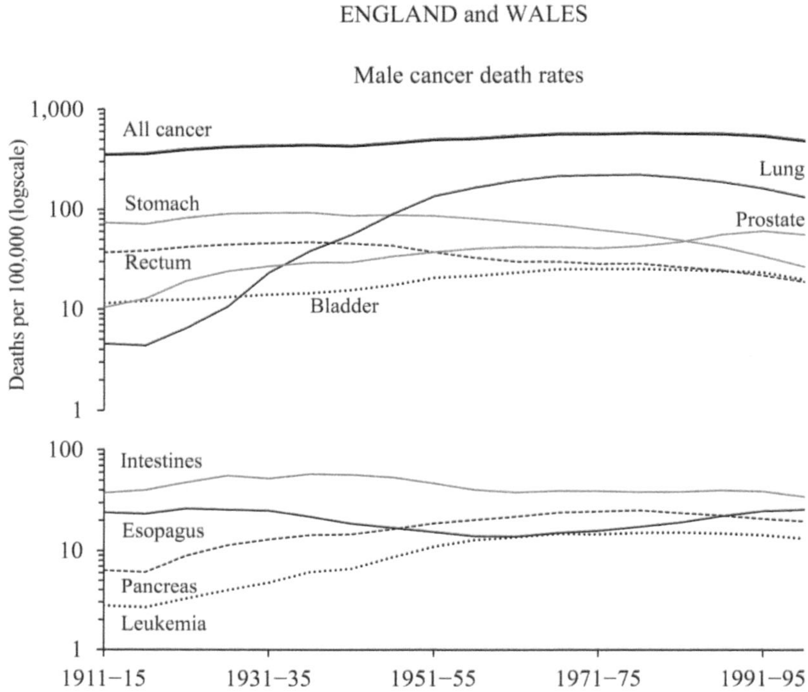

Figure 12.4. Age-standardized death rates for the main sites of cancer among males in England and Wales, for 5-year periods, 1911–15 to 1996–2000. *Source:* Institute of Cancer Research, *Serial Mortality Tables.*

pipes, but the more harmful habit of cigarette smoking did not become common until the 20th century.[28] During World War I, it became much more widespread among young men, and even more common during World War II when cigarettes were issued to soldiers.[29] Trends in consumption for several countries, including England and Wales, indicate rapid increases after the 1930s, particularly among young men.[30] The widening sex differential in cancer mortality reflects the increasing death rate among males from World War I until the 1960s, and the greater increase in cigarette smoking among men. An increase in cigarette smoking among women occurred later, which is reflected in the later increase in the cancer death rate from the 1960s to the 1990s (fig. 12.1). Increasing sex differentials in cancer, bronchitis, and cardiovascular disease mortality in the United States were attributed to differential changes in cigarette smoking.[31] It was estimated that about three-quarters of the increased sex differential in life expectancy at ages over 50 years in the United States between 1910 and 1962 was due to cigarette smoking.[32]

Preston found that mortality varied in the 20th century in the expected manner in relation to daily consumption of cigarettes, age at which smoking began,

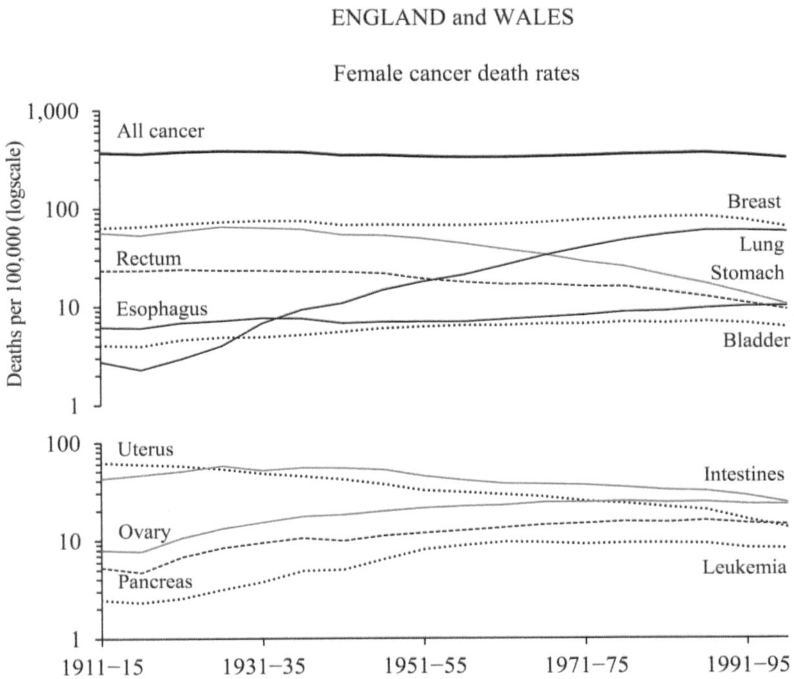

Figure 12.5. Age-standardized death rates for the main sites of cancer among females in England and Wales, for 5-year periods, 1911–15 to 1996–2000. *Source:* Institute of Cancer Research, *Serial Mortality Tables.*

and length of time since discontinuing.[33] Many studies from the 1950s onward had indicated excess mortality associated with cigarette smoking, one-quarter of which was due to lung cancer and chronic lung disease.[34] Doll and Peto estimated that cigarette smoking accounted for about 30% of male deaths from cancer in the United States and 7–8% of female deaths.[35] However, Epstein suggested that the estimate of 5% of cancer deaths linked with exposure to occupational risks was an underestimate, as these can interact with the adverse effects of cigarette smoking to produce an even greater risk of cancer.[36] He also pointed out that 20% of lung cancer deaths in the United States were among nonsmokers, and the risk was similar for smokers and nonsmokers in some occupational groups. The main established environmental risks include asbestos dust, radon daughters, nickel ores, chromium, the products of other industries, and pollution generally. Because of their greater involvement in industrial activities, men may have had greater exposure than women to some of these environmental risks in the 19th century in England and Wales.

Although the etiology of cancer is multifactorial, cigarette smoking is recognized as one of the most important risk factors in several forms of the disease. In 2004 the International Agency for Research on Cancer (IARC) reported that

Table 12.1. Percentage of malignant neoplasm deaths and cases due to cancers at different sites for males and females in England and Wales, 2008

	Percentage of all malignant neoplasms			
	Deaths		Cases	
Site of Malignant Neoplasm	Males	Females	Males	Females
Lung, trachea, and bronchus	23.9	19.9	14.3	11.2
Prostate	12.7	—	24.2	—
Breast	—	16.3	—	31.3
Uterus	—	2.1	—	5.1
Ovary	—	5.3	—	4.2
Urinary system	6.9	4.3	8.3	4.1
Colon	6.4	6.7	8.5	7.8
Esophagus	6.1	3.1	3.5	1.8
Pancreas	4.7	4.9	2.6	2.7
Rectum	4.3	3.4	5.6	3.7
Stomach	3.9	2.6	3.1	1.7
Leukemia	3.1	2.6	2.9	2.1
Non-Hodgkin's lymphoma	3.0	2.8	4.1	3.7
Brain and CNS	2.6	2.0	1.7	1.3
Liver	2.5	1.8	1.5	0.9
Skin, melanoma	1.4	1.3	3.6	4.0
Hodgkin's disease	0.2	0.2	0.6	0.5
Other	18.3	20.7	15.5	13.9
All malignant neoplasms	100.0	100.0	100.0	100.0
Number of deaths and cases	72,095	65,736	137,641	135,248

Source: Office for National Statistics, *Mortality Statistics, Series DR, 2008.*

cigarette smoking contributed in varying degrees to at least 15 types of cancer.[37] Epidemiological studies have provided sufficient evidence to establish a causal association for cancer of the nasal cavities, nasopharynx, stomach, liver, kidney, uterine cervix, adenocarcinoma of the esophagus, and myeloid leukemia. These sites were added to the already established causal association between cigarette smoking and cancer of the lung, oral cavity, pharynx, larynx, esophagus, pancreas, urinary bladder, and renal pelvis. It has been estimated that smoking is responsible for about one-third of cancer deaths in many Western countries, and half of the deaths among smokers can be attributed to tobacco.[38] A meta-analysis also found a consistent and statistically significant association between exposure to environmental tobacco smoke and lung cancer among women who had never smoked.[39]

A review of cancer mortality trends in the 20th century concluded that trends in lung cancer death rates for men and women mostly reflect changes in smoking habits and reduced tar content of cigarettes.[40] Consumption of cigarettes among men in England and Wales reached a peak in 1960 and had almost halved by 1985, while the peak among women was in the mid-1970s. A small part of the declining death rates may also be attributable to a massive reduction in air pollution from the 1950s. As mentioned, the large reduction in stomach cancer mortality also reflects a decline in the prevalence of *H. pylori* as a result of changes in behavior and the domestic environment. Total cancer mortality fell from the 1970s for men under age 70 and for women under 50 as a result of changes in behavior and the prevalence of risk factors, as well as treatment. Improved treatment resulted in a dramatic decline in mortality from testicular cancer and Hodgkin's disease and a reduction in mortality from leukemia. It also contributed to reduced mortality from cancers of the ovary and large bowel, along with a decline in incidence. The continued increase in period death rates at older ages may reflect cohort-related influences such as the age at which smoking became habitual. The cohort of males with the highest lung cancer rates was that born around 1901, who would have been in their late teens during World War I when the prevalence of cigarette smoking among men increased rapidly. For their part, the cohort of females with the highest lung cancer death rates was that born in the mid-1920s, who would have been in their late teens during World War II. These were the first age cohorts in whom the habit was firmly established in early adult life, and only later cohorts appear to have benefited from tar reduction.[41]

An increasing socioeconomic differential in cancer mortality in England and Wales has been attributed mainly to differential changes in cigarette smoking.[42] Death rates from lung cancer increased in the first half of the 20th century for each socioeconomic group (based on men's occupation), although differences in rates of change in smoking led to an increasing differential in mortality. There was no socioeconomic gradient for adult lung cancer mortality in 1931, but by 1961 the death rate was higher among social classes IV–V than among social classes I–II.[43] By 1991 lung cancer mortality for men in social class V was more than four times greater than for social class I.[44] Even for lung cancer, other factors operating throughout life are likely to contribute to socioeconomic differentials as well as cigarette smoking.[45] Socioeconomic differentials in total cancer mortality have been found in studies based on data other than the Registrar General's occupational statistics, including longitudinal studies that suggest they are not due to artifacts such as health selection effects.[46] The Whitehall study of civil servants in London found that lower employment grades (clerical and manual) had a 48% higher risk of cancer than the higher grades (administrators, professionals, and executives), as well as higher overall mortality in a ten year period.[47] Combining employment grade with the socioeconomic indicator car ownership identified even greater differentials in mortality.[48] Higher grades did have higher mortality from 6 of the 13 main sites of cancer, and death rates from prostate and breast cancer in the general population have tended to be higher among higher socioeconomic groups.[49] Even so, the main established risk factors for cancer are likely to contribute to the socioeconomic gradient in total cancer mortality, including cigarette smoking, occupation, alcohol consumption, diet, deprivation, a poor health history, and infections.

Association between Tuberculosis and Cancer

Many different types of study have found associations between infections and cancer. Investigation of a statistical association between death rates from tuberculosis and cancer dates back over a hundred years. In 1902 Coglan observed that the decrease in the period death rate from tuberculosis appeared to be offset by an increase in the period death rate from cancer over the second half of the 19th century in New South Wales, Australia.[50] In an analysis of data from England and Wales, Cherry found that around 20% of deaths among adults aged 25 and over were attributed to cancer or tuberculosis over the period 1851–1920.[51] He also found carcinogenic effects in laboratory tests on animals and suggested there might be a causal link between infection with the tubercle bacillus and development of cancer. When mice were inoculated with minute doses of tubercle bacillus, they developed leukemic conditions, neoplasms, and ulcers.[52] Although no theory of pathogenesis developed linking the two diseases, further evidence of ecological association was reported in studies of period death rates.[53] Later studies focused on analysis of death rates by year of birth, which showed that the risk of dying from cancer or tuberculosis had remained quite constant over successive cohorts in England and Wales.[54]

A comparison of the lifetime probability of dying from tuberculosis or cancer for different populations provided further evidence of association between the diseases. A relatively constant proportion (0.18) died from either disease in decadal cohorts born in England and Wales between 1841–50 and 1891–1900. A slightly higher but constant probability of dying (0.20) was found for cohorts born in Ireland between 1851–60 and 1891–1900, and a lower constant probability of dying (0.16) among cohorts born in Pennsylvania and New Jersey in the United States.[55] The probability of dying from cancer among more recent birth cohorts would be affected by improvements in cancer survival, although the inverse relationship between tuberculosis and cancer mortality risk for those born in the 19th century would more closely reflect morbidity in the absence of effective treatment. Although the association might be coincidental, it could reflect a direct effect of infection contributing to the development of cancer, or some common immunogenetic predisposition that allows either disease to develop.

Further evidence of ecological association between tuberculosis and cancer comes from an analysis of data for counties of England in the 20th century. Tuberculosis death rates in 1901–10 were found to be strongly correlated ($r = +0.71$) with cancer death rates at ages 45 and over in 1971, while death rates in the same period were not significantly correlated ($r = +0.25$).[56] Further analysis using data on tuberculosis cases notified in each county in 1921 indicates that incidence rates were negatively correlated with cancer death rates for males aged 45–64 in 1921 (r = –0.31), but there was an increasingly positive correlation with the cancer death rate 30 years later (r = +0.26) and 60 years later (r = +0.45), with a similar gradient for females.

The evidence of ecological association between tuberculosis and later cancer mortality suggested a relationship that could be tested more rigorously in epidemiological studies. Stronger evidence of association between clinical tuberculosis and subsequent lung cancer has come from several studies, particularly in China, where tuberculosis is still common.[57] A case-control study in Shanghai found a significantly raised risk for lung cancer in those with a self-reported history of tuberculosis in the past. It was suggested that the effects of carcinogenic exposure might be enhanced by the tuberculosis inflammatory process, which could entrap carcinogens in tuberculosis scar tissue leading to a precancerous lesion or abnormal cellular proliferation and growth.[58] A retrospective cohort study in rural China found that the risk of dying from lung cancer was eight times higher among those who reported a history of tuberculosis in the past, compared with people who did not. The risk remained high after controlling for demographic characteristics, other lung diseases, tobacco use, and exposure to indoor smoke from coal.[59]

A recent prospective study in Finland followed up male cigarette smokers and found a fivefold increase in the risk of lung cancer within two years of diagnosed tuberculosis,[60] which is consistent with the findings in China. A systematic review in 2009 of 37 case-control and 4 cohort studies and meta-analysis of risk estimates, found a significantly increased risk of lung cancer in relation to earlier tuberculosis.[61] There was a statistically significant twofold increase in the risk of death from lung cancer among those who had experienced tuberculosis but had never smoked or been exposed to domestic tobacco smoke. There was also a twelvefold increase in the risk of death from lung cancer 1–5 years after diagnosed tuberculosis that was independent of these other risk factors, and a twofold increase 20 years after tuberculosis. The evidence of association after such a long interval between tuberculosis and lung cancer suggests that the increased risk was not due to lung cancer being incorrectly diagnosed as tuberculosis at the earlier stage in life and rules out the possibility of cancer contributing to the development of tuberculosis.

Although the effects of other confounding factors cannot be discounted, these findings are consistent with tubercular infection possibly having a role in the pathogenesis of lung cancer. Pathological studies over many years have found an association between lung cancer and tubercular scars, although the disease is also associated with scars caused by other respiratory diseases.[62] A recent radiographic study found that pulmonary scarring was associated with a higher risk of lung cancer. It was suggested that local inflammatory processes could have promoted carcinogenesis by inducing genetic damage in cells within the lung.[63] Other epidemiological studies have found a significantly raised risk of lung cancer for those who had experienced tuberculosis or other respiratory diseases in the past.[64] Two studies in the United States found an increased risk of lung cancer following respiratory conditions but little association with tuberculosis, although prevalence was low.[65] A recent cohort study among male smokers in Korea found a twofold increased risk of lung cancer in those reporting a history of pulmonary tuberculosis.[66] A pooled analysis of 17 studies mainly conducted in Europe and North America using self-reported data on previous lung disease found that pneumonia, chronic bronchitis, emphysema, and tuberculosis were associated with an increased risk of lung cancer.[67] Elevated risks among nonsmokers who had experienced pneumonia, emphysema, or tuberculosis suggested that previous lung infections affected the risk of lung cancer independently of tobacco use. The effect of previous lung diseases on lung cancer may operate through associated pathogenesis and the inflammatory response, which could be exacerbated in smokers. It was suggested that a biologically plausible mechanism is chronic inflammatory processes in the lung that enhance the effects of other carcinogenic exposures or stimulate cell proliferation and growth. A compromised immune response, which often accompanies chronic inflammatory reactions, might also contribute to the development of cancer.[68]

Most studies have supported a growing body of evidence implicating chronic inflammation and pulmonary scarring in the etiology of lung cancer, and tuberculosis in particular may play a significant role in countries where prevalence is high. Possibly a third of people worldwide have been infected with *M. tuberculosis*,[69] and a primary infection can reactivate in later life to produce clinical tuberculosis. Since the 19th century, people in England were increasingly likely to survive infection with *M. tuberculosis* for the reasons discussed in chapter 9. The declining death rate from tuberculosis among children and young adults before the 1940s, when contact with *M. tuberculosis* was still universal, resulted in the survival to ages at which cancer more often occurs of people who in earlier times would have developed clinical tuberculosis and died. The possibility that people naturally infected with *M. tuberculosis* who have not experienced clinical disease also have a higher risk of lung cancer could be investigated in countries with high prevalence.

The association between tuberculosis and cancer is not confined to lung cancer. Several studies have found that non-Hodgkin's lymphoma is associated with a history of chronic infection, including tuberculosis. For example, a study in Sweden found a raised risk for this form of cancer among individuals who had been diagnosed with tuberculosis before 1953. It was suggested that the association between tuberculosis and non-Hodgkin's lymphoma could involve either a direct causal link with tubercular infection or greater susceptibility to the inflammatory response, which may in part be genetically determined.[70] Further epidemiological studies could assess the relative risk for non-Hodgkin's lymphoma, lung cancer, and any cancer, for those who are tuberculin positive through natural infection (not vaccinated with BCG), as well as those known to have had clinical tuberculosis.

BCG Vaccination and Cancer Prevention

The long history of research into association between tuberculosis and cancer includes many studies since the 1950s into the possible role of BCG vaccine in preventing cancers, particularly leukemia and melanoma. Studies in the early 1970s found evidence of a reduced risk of dying from leukemia among children vaccinated neonatally with BCG in Quebec, Canada,[71] and in Chicago.[72] There were several deficiencies in the methodology, and a review of these and other studies found little evidence that vaccination at older ages had a protective effect.[73] A further review of 14 studies found 3 indicated a high level of protection against cancer, while 3 reported a raised risk of cancer, although methodological deficiencies precluded firm conclusions.[74] The reviewers suggested that a prospective clinical trial was the most appropriate method, but would require a very large sample size and long follow-up, while location would also be problematic. The effectiveness of BCG for prevention of tuberculosis appears to vary considerably between studies, populations, and geographic areas.[75] This may partly depend on the strain of vaccine used, characteristics of the population, and exposure to environmental mycobacteria.[76] It has been suggested that BCG provides some protection against leukemia and other childhood cancers, but only where it protects against tuberculosis.[77] BCG could be a "two-edged sword" because mycobacteria produce two different types of immune response—one protective, the other leading to necrosis of tissues containing mycobacteria. The response depends on prior contact with environmental mycobacteria, and which of two types of T cell has been primed (Th1 or Th2). It may be that BCG tends to boost the response already primed, and that only Th1 reactivity mediates protection against tuberculosis and certain cancers.[78]

In addition to the protective effect of BCG against juvenile leukemia found in several studies, there is evidence of a protective effect against melanoma. A case-control study conducted in seven countries found that those vaccinated against either tuberculosis (with BCG) or smallpox (with vaccinia) in childhood had a reduced risk of melanoma, about 50% lower than those who had neither vaccination.[79] A further cohort study in these countries found an improvement in prognosis for melanoma patients who had previously received vaccinia or BCG, and an even greater improvement for those who had received both.[80] A study in Denmark also reported a 50% lower risk of developing lymphomas among those vaccinated with BCG, but no reduction in relation to smallpox vaccination and no reduction in the risk of leukemia.[81] Despite the variability of results, evidence that BCG has a preventive effect against some cancers as well as tuberculosis in certain locations may add to the case for its continued use, or reintroduction, in view of the resurgence of tuberculosis and emergence of multi drug-resistant strains.

Association between Other Microorganisms and Cancer

BCG and other childhood vaccinations contribute to the maturation of the immune system. Burnet hypothesized that failure of any system of immune surveillance against aberrant cells might allow cancer cells to proliferate,[82] while others suggested that a compromised immune response accompanying chronic inflammatory reactions might predispose to the development of cancer.[83] Burnet suggested that in certain circumstances viruses can enter a cell and cause damage to DNA. The damage can be repaired, but with an increased risk of informational error and the possibility of cancer cells replicating if not checked.[84] There is evidence of excess cancer mortality in cases of immune suppression and immune deficiency, although this involves a few relatively rare types of cancer for which there is evidence of viral etiology.[85] Epstein-Barr virus (EBV) is classified as a causal agent of immune-suppression-related non-Hodgkin's lymphoma. Chronic infection with hepatitis C virus (HCV) can also cause non-Hodgkin's lymphoma. There is evidence of the role of viruses in more common types of cancer, and the infectious agents are classified as carcinogenic to humans. Chronic infection with HCV or hepatitis B virus (HBV) is known to cause hepatocellular carcinoma, and human papillomavirus (HPV) causes cervical, penile, vaginal, and other types of cancer linked with sexual activity.[86] Some cancer-causing viruses are widespread, including EBV, the causal agent in infectious mononucleosis (glandular fever). EBV infects almost everyone and causes several types of cancer, including nasopharyngeal carcinoma, one of the most common cancers in Southeast Asia, and Burkitt's lymphoma in children in Africa, while it may also have a role in gastric carcinomas. Where common viruses have a causal role, other risk factors affecting immunological-cellular processes determine whether exposure leads to cancer in a particular individual.[87]

The involvement of viruses in breast cancer is suspected, with HPV, mouse mammary tumor virus (MMTV), and EBV being the main candidates.[88] MMTV, the cause of breast cancer in mice, has been identified in human breast tumors, although there is still no definitive evidence that it has a causal role rather being an innocuous "bystander." Viral genetic material from each of these types of virus has been identified in breast tumors, and it is rarely found in the normal breast tissue from controls.[89] The involvement of particular viruses in the development of cancer could explain a striking feature of the epidemiology of breast cancer—the large difference in incidence and mortality between some Asian and Western populations. Well-established risk factors for breast cancer relating to estrogens and female growth hormones do not explain this differential or its reduction among second- and third-generation migrants to Western countries. Changes in food consumption could be involved, since diet could affect levels of the sex hormones that promote replication of the hormone-dependent viruses, MMTV and HPV.[90] Unlike most forms of cancer and other chronic diseases, the risk for breast cancer has tended to be higher among higher socioeconomic groups, and other more established risk factors include family history, age at menarche, age at first pregnancy, and parity, with a higher risk for those who have had fewer pregnancies.[91]

Evidence of association between specific microorganisms and specific forms of cancer is particularly important when prognosis is poor, which is the case with stomach cancer. An association between chronic infection with the bacterium *Helicobacter pylori* and gastric cancer was reported in the early 1990s based on clinical, epidemiological, and ecological studies.[92] An international study found a strong association between *H. pylori* prevalence and gastric cancer incidence and mortality.[93] Incidence of gastric cancer is particularly high in certain regions of China, and prevalence of *H. pylori* was found to be associated with gastric cancer mortality.[94] In one region with high gastric cancer mortality, *H. pylori* infection and cigarette smoking were identified as the main risk factors.[95] The IARC concluded on the basis of three prospective epidemiological studies that *H. pylori* is a definite carcinogen in humans causally linked with gastric cancer.[96] In studies in England and Wales, both stomach cancer and *H. pylori* infection in adults were found to be associated with poor housing and socioeconomic circumstances in childhood.[97] Stomach cancer in adulthood may be a delayed consequence of an infection acquired in childhood when the risk of infection was linked with large family size, overcrowded housing, and poor hygiene.[98] There is evidence of a decline in the prevalence of *H. pylori* over cohorts born in the 1970s and 1980s who experienced a decline in the risk of dying from stomach cancer.[99]

Colonization of the stomach with *H. pylori* causes a persistent inflammatory response and chronic gastritis, which predisposes to precancerous changes. Gastric cancer develops in only a minority of those infected, which has been attributed to variations in the interactions between *H. pylori* virulence (strain-specific), pathogenicity, host susceptibility, diet, and environmental factors.[100] Prospective studies testing for *H. pylori* antibodies before cancer had been detected indicated a strong association with noncardial gastric cancer, but not cardial (top of the stomach).[101] The recognition that *H. pylori* has a causal role in gastric cancer has led to progress in treatment using chemotherapy,[102] pointing to the possibility of prevention. The first randomized, placebo-controlled trial of antibiotic treatment for *H. pylori* infection in an area of China at high risk for gastric cancer found that eradicating bacteria from infected people with no precancerous lesions significantly decreased the incidence of gastric cancers. Longer follow-up could assess the effect of eradicating bacteria in people with precancerous lesions already present.[103]

Another widely prevalent bacterium associated with cancer of specific sites and other chronic diseases is *Chlamydia pneumoniae.* Although association with atherosclerosis and other cardiovascular disorders has been investigated in many different types of study, as discussed in chapter 11, research into its association with lung cancer is more recent. The presence of antibodies against *C. pneumoniae* increases with age, and serology can indicate whether a person has an acute infection or was infected in the past. A review of six serological studies found that the evidence was consistent with a causal relationship. Chronic inflammation caused by *C. pneumoniae* infection was considered a plausible mechanism through which bacteria could be involved in the carcinogenic process, as in the case of *H. pylori* and gastric cancer.[104] It was suggested that inflammation can cause damage to DNA, damage to cells that requires repair, and an increased rate of cell division, carrying an increased risk of mutation and cancerous cells that have a selective advantage. In smokers, immune response in the lung may be impaired, allowing *C. pneumoniae* infection and inflammation to persist, with an increased risk of damage to tissue and DNA. A later study found that the risk of lung cancer increased with the level of antibodies and that the risk remained high two to five years after detection of antibodies. A dose-response relationship and evidence that the risk of lung cancer remained high were supportive of the infection having a causal role. It was suggested that a lack of association among those who had never smoked could indicate that *C. pneumoniae* acts synergistically with the carcinogenic effects of tobacco smoke.[105] A later meta-analysis found a slightly raised risk of lung cancer in four prospective studies, and a twofold higher risk in eight retrospective studies, with a higher antibody titer being a better predictor of risk.[106]

The main infections for which a causal role in cancer is established are bacterial infection with *H. pylori* and viral infections with EBV, HPV, HBV, and HCV, as mentioned; and there are already effective vaccines for HPV and HBV. Other microorganisms classified as carcinogenic to humans by the IARC include Kaposi's sarcoma herpes virus, HTLV-1, which causes adult T-cell leukemia and lymphoma, and *Schistosoma haematobium,* which causes urinary bladder cancer.[107] Infectious causation has been accepted for about 15–20% of cancers, and the proportion is higher in less developed countries (23%).[108] Ewald suggested that there is evidence pointing to the possible role of infection in all but 5% of cancers.[109]

Since the 1980s, there has been a dramatic increase in research into the relationship between infections and cancer, which may provide evidence of a causal role of specific pathogens and indicate opportunities for prevention, particularly through immunization. In some cases, association with infections may indicate that they have a more general role in increasing susceptibility to a particular pathogen, which could be the case with colorectal cancer. A review of studies focusing on four pathogens, *Helicobacter pylori, Streptococcus bovis,* JV virus, and human papillomavirus, concluded that there was no strong evidence of a causal role in colorectal cancer for any of the individual pathogens, however, general disruption of the microflora in the gut as a result of infection might increase susceptibility to some highly pathogenic subtypes.[110]

Ongoing research and development of techniques for detection may lead to the identification of other specific microorganisms associated with particular forms of cancer. The association between tuberculosis and cancer is likely to be investigated further, particularly in countries with high prevalence of *M. tuberculosis* infection and high incidence of clinical disease. Clearly, these associations and causal links have implications for any theory of epidemiological transition. Issues relating to the assessment of causality are briefly considered in the final chapter, and evidence of the involvement of microorganisms in other chronic diseases is considered in the next chapter.

Chapter Thirteen

Other Chronic Diseases

The evidence of involvement of microorganisms in the major chronic diseases and in the underlying biophysiological disorders suggests that the infectious disease environment is still a considerable influence on health and mortality risk. The classification of only 3% of deaths in England and Wales as due to infections, including urinary tract infections, is therefore somewhat misleading. External causes (accidents, suicide, and violence) account for 4% of deaths, while other categories include many common chronic diseases that have suspected or confirmed links with infection. About 6% of deaths in 2010 were due to cancers with confirmed infectious etiology, and microbial involvement is suspected in many other forms of cancer that caused a further 22% of deaths. Most of the respiratory diseases that caused 14% of deaths involve infections at some stage, and most forms of cardiovascular disease that caused 32% of deaths have some association with microorganisms, and a causal role is strongly suspected in some disorders. In total, these three major categories of disease—cardiovascular disease, cancer, and respiratory disease—accounted for about 74% of deaths (appendix E). For some of the 15% of deaths attributed to digestive, endocrine, musculoskeletal, nervous, genitourinary, and other diseases, and mental disorders (4%), there is also evidence indicating possible microbial involvement. Some of the associations are referred to at the end of this chapter, while the main focus here is on four of the subcategories of common chronic disease that account for 4% of deaths, as there is strong evidence of microbial involvement or confirmed infectious etiology.

Specific microorganisms and infections are suspected of having some role in the processes underlying cirrhosis of the liver, diabetes mellitus, and nephritis/nephrosis. Peptic ulcer will be considered first as the causal role of a specific microorganism, *Helicobacter pylori*, has already been established. As indicated in chapter 2, criteria for establishing causality are often difficult to apply when a specific pathogen is found to be associated with chronic disease morbidity or mortality. This applies to the other diseases briefly reviewed in the last section of this chapter. The general theme being developed here is that the infectious disease environment continues to be of major significance for morbidity and mortality, despite the decline in mortality attributed directly to acute infectious diseases and tuberculosis and the overwhelming predominance of other chronic diseases. Although the chronic diseases considered here are much less frequently recorded as primary causes of death compared with heart disease or stroke, some cause considerable morbidity and prolonged disability, and contribute to the risk of dying from cardiovascular diseases.

There are complex interrelationships between chronic disorders, and the presence of more than one complicates certification of primary cause of death. For example, a combination of diabetes, chronic kidney disease, and hypertension is now the most common cause of kidney failure. Kidney disease is an independent risk factor for cardiovascular disease, and diabetes and hypertension are established risk factors for chronic kidney disease along with cigarette smoking, obesity, and physical inactivity. Many of the major risk factors for incidence and outcome are common to different forms of chronic disease, and despite major differences in the underlying pathogenic processes, there are similar rates of increase in mortality with age.[1] Atherosclerosis increases with age and consumption of cigarettes,[2] and the pathogenic process may involve tobacco substances enhancing the susceptibility of the blood and arteries to the effects of common microorganisms.[3] Similarly, the excess risk of lung cancer among cigarette smokers may be due to impairment of the capacity to clear the bronchi of bacterial infections.[4] The effects of different lifestyle and environmental factors over the life course, including infections, are likely to be major determinants of the chronic disorders that develop, along with any genetic propensity and influences in early life.

Changes in the prevalence of different risk factors, interrelationships between chronic disorders, and changing practice regarding certification of the primary cause of death need to be borne in mind when considering long-term trends in death rates from chronic diseases. Death rates from peptic ulcer, cirrhosis of the liver, diabetes mellitus, and nephritis/nephrosis increased in the second half of the 19th century. In the 20th century, this group of diseases combined contributed −0.04 to each unit of change in the total death rate (appendix C1). However, the long-term trends in age-and-sex-standardized death rates differed considerably, with a decline beginning toward the end of the 19th century for cirrhosis of the liver, after World War I for nephritis/nephrosis, in the 1940s for diabetes mellitus, and in the 1950s for peptic ulcer (fig. 13.1).

Diseases of the Digestive System

Diseases of the digestive system accounted for 5.2% of deaths in 2010, including liver disease (1.5%), ulcers (0.5%), and intestinal diseases (0.4%). Appendicitis now causes very few deaths (0.03%) compared with 1901 (4%), with the decline in mortality probably reflecting a decline in incidence and improvements in anesthesia and surgery.[5]

Peptic Ulcer

Peptic ulcers (stomach and duodenal) are not in themselves a cause of death, and the risk of fatality is linked with perforation and hemorrhage. Perforation

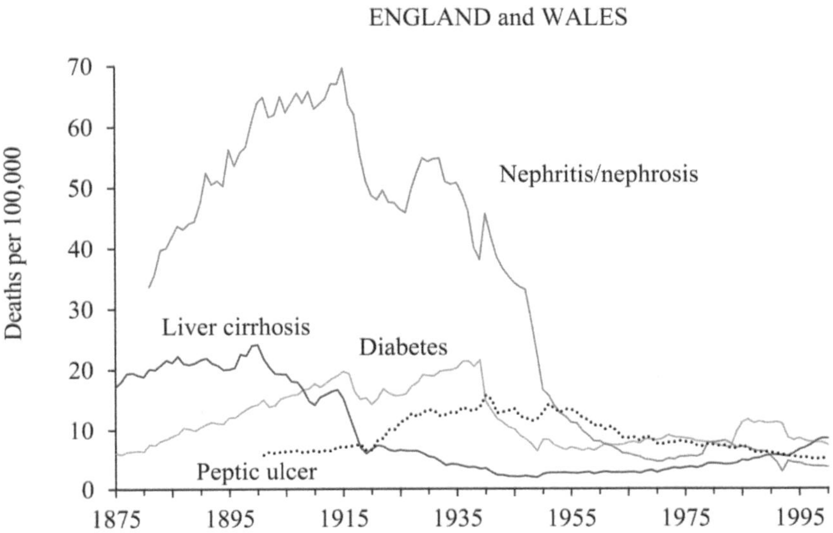

Figure 13.1. Annual age-and-sex-standardized death rates from diabetes mellitus, nephritis/nephrosis, peptic ulcers, and cirrhosis of the liver in England and Wales, 1875–2000. *Sources:* Registrar General, *Annual Reports*; *Annual Statistical Reviews*; Office of Population Censuses and Surveys, *Mortality Statistics: Cause, Series DH2.*

of acute gastric ulcers (stomach) appeared as a new disorder in the 19th century, and became increasingly common, particularly among young women. Toward the end of that century, two other syndromes became more significant: perforation of duodenal ulcers in young and middle-aged men, and perforation of gastric ulcers in older men. Although increasing specificity in recording gastrointestinal diseases may account for some of the increase in peptic ulcer death rates, the increase among males was so great that it seems likely there was a genuine increase.

The sex differential in death rates from peptic ulcer is illustrated by the very large gap between the trends in annual age-standardized death rates for males and females in England and Wales over most of the 20th century (fig. 13.2). As mentioned, cigarette smoking, a major risk factor for peptic ulcer, increased among males between the 1920s and 1960s when peptic ulcer mortality increased sharply. Average consumption was much lower among females and negligible before the 1920s.[6] A strong correlation was found between cigarette smoking and duodenal ulcer mortality in the United States, and similar death rates among men and women with comparable consumption suggested that higher prevalence of cigarette smoking contributed significantly to the sex differential in mortality.[7] The continuing increase in incidence and period death rates from ulcers among males in the first half of the 20th century was initially seen as an indication that ulcer was a "disease of civilisation" linked with industrialization.[8]

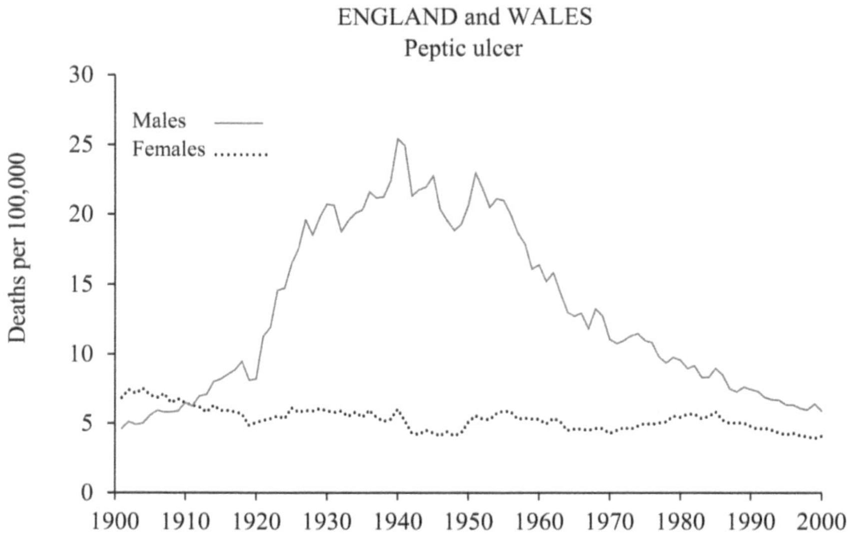

Figure 13.2. Annual age-standardized death rates from peptic ulcer for males and females in England and Wales, 1900–2000. *Sources:* Registrar General, *Annual Reports*; *Annual Statistical Reviews*; Office of Population Censuses and Surveys, *Mortality Statistics: Cause, Series DH2.*

Association of incidence with war, heavy air raids, and work led to a psychosocial hypothesis linking the disease with stress. However, the idea of "executive stress ulcer" was never supported by the evidence. There was no socioeconomic gradient for duodenal ulcer in the early 20th century, and it was common among men in traditional working-class occupations.[9]

Death rates from both gastric and duodenal ulcer among those aged 65 and over continued to increase in the first half of the 20th century when death rates at younger ages had already started to decline. The trends for age-specific death rates from peptic ulcer for adult males and females indicate that the downturn occurred later for older age groups (fig. 13.3). This age differential in period trends suggested a possible cohort-related turning point in mortality linked with influences earlier in life. An analysis of death rates by year of birth by Susser and Stein indicated that males born around 1885 had the highest risk for gastric ulcer and those born around 1890 the highest risk for duodenal ulcer.[10] The trends in death rates from all peptic ulcers at different adult ages by year of birth indicate lower mortality for males born after the 1880s, with a slightly earlier downturn for females (fig. 13.4). Subsequent analysis of age-specific death rates from ulcerative colitis also indicated a peak for cohorts born around 1890 in England and Wales. Data from several industrialized countries revealed similar trends in cohort death rates from ulcer and ulcerative colitis.[11]

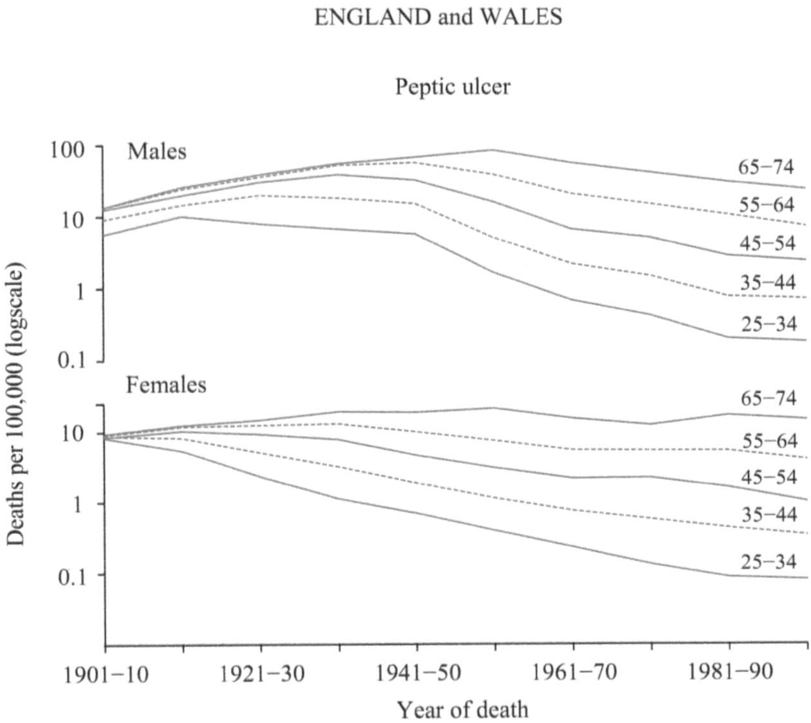

Figure 13.3. Age-specific death rates from peptic ulcer for males and females in England and Wales, 1901–10 to 1991–2000. *Sources:* Registrar General, *Annual Reports*; *Annual Statistical Reviews*; Office of Population Censuses and Surveys, *Mortality Statistics: Cause, Series DH2.*

Changes in the infectious disease environment at the end of the 19th century, particularly changes linked with improved sanitation and domestic hygiene, and with less overcrowding as a result of better housing and smaller families, are possible explanations for long-term changes in the cohort death rates from peptic ulcer. In recent years it has been established that infection of the stomach with the bacillus *Helicobacter pylori* is the main cause of peptic ulcer. The presence of *H. pylori* in association with peptic ulcer was first demonstrated in 1983 by Marshall and Warren, who examined specimens from patients presenting for gastroscopy at a hospital in Perth, Western Australia. They reported that almost all the samples from patients with active chronic gastritis, duodenal ulcer, and gastric ulcer contained a bacillus related to the genus Campylobacter, later named *Helicobacter pylori.*[12] Convincing evidence of the temporal relationship between infection with *H. pylori* and peptic ulcer emerged when Marshall deliberately ingested the pathogen, developed peptic ulcer, and was subsequently treated successfully with antibiotics. Eradication of *H. pylori* from the body

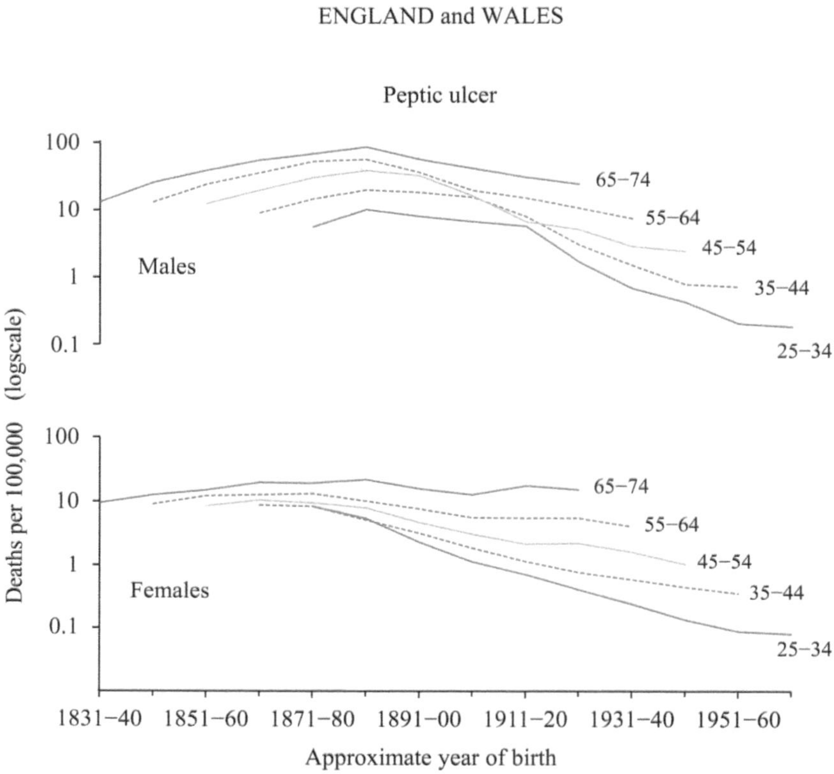

Figure 13.4. Age-specific death rates from peptic ulcer for males and females in England and Wales by year of birth, 1831–40 to 1961–70. *Sources:* Registrar General, *Annual Reports*; *Annual Statistical Reviews*; Office of Population Censuses and Surveys, *Mortality Statistics: Cause, Series DH2.*

results in prolonged and possibly permanent healing of peptic ulcers, suggesting that persistent infection is the critical factor that maintains ulcers.[13]

Helicobacter pylori does not cause ulcers in all those infected, and it has probably been colonizing the digestive system of humans for thousands of years without causing sickness in most people. The pathogen is likely to have been ubiquitous in England and Wales in the 19th century,[14] as indicated by age-related seroepidemiology and evidence from biopsy surveys in recent times.[15] The rapid growth of urban populations and increased contact between people living in rural areas and those in towns and cities may have increased exposure to *H. pylori* at an early, more vulnerable age. Domestic environmental conditions such as fecal contamination of water supplies, poor sanitation, lack of in-house water for washing, poor food storage facilities, large families living in overcrowded conditions, and many children sharing one bed would all have been conducive to rapid transmission.[16] Diet may have contributed, while under-nutrition and weakening of the immune system by intercurrent infections and gastrointestinal diseases may have increased the risk of *H. pylori* infection persisting in the stomach.[17] Toward the end of the 19th century, sociodemographic changes and improvement in the domestic environment of many people may have led to a reduction in the rate of infection in early childhood. Specific factors that could have contributed include improved housing with less overcrowded living conditions,[18] smaller families, and improvements in water supplies, sanitation, and domestic and personal hygiene.

A sharp decline in incidence and prevalence of peptic ulcer in Western countries in recent years has been attributed to a decline in the prevalence of *H. pylori* as well as efforts to eradicate the bacillus from the body of those requiring treatment for peptic ulcer. A systematic review of 93 studies examined evidence of other risk factors associated with incidence and mortality from peptic ulcer.[19] In terms of complications, the most commonly identified risk factor for peptic ulcer hemorrhage is use of nonsteroidal anti-inflammatory drugs (NSAID), and the evidence is strengthened by a dose-dependent increase in risk. Prospective case-control studies in Europe have also found that prior use of acetylsalicylic acid (ASA, "aspirin") increases the risk of hemorrhage from gastric ulcer, although results from different countries provide conflicting evidence regarding the contribution relative to sociodemographic and lifestyle-related factors. The most widely reported risk factor for mortality is older age, particularly in Asia. Other factors associated with mortality following hemorrhage and perforation in Western countries are shock and comorbidity. The review concluded that widespread use of ASA and NSAIDs in these countries was a particular health-care problem that led to peptic ulcer complications, although early-life experience is important as infection by *H. pylori* at an early age is more likely to develop into chronic or atrophic gastritis. Infection is more frequent and more often acquired at an early age in developing countries compared with industrialized countries. As about 80% of the population in developing countries may be infected by age 20 years, this constitutes a large potential burden of disease from peptic ulcer, stomach cancer, and possibly other chronic diseases.[20]

Cirrhosis of the Liver

The age-standardized death rates from cirrhosis of the liver for males and females declined quite rapidly in the first half of the 20th century in England and Wales (fig. 13.5). From 1900 there was a sharp decline until just before World War I. In 1916, alcohol restrictions were introduced and consumption per capita declined dramatically until the 1920s.[21] With alcohol consumption still at a much lower level than before the war, death rates continued to fall, but increased again from the 1950s when alcohol consumption increased again. With alcohol consumption continuing to increase until the 1980s, the

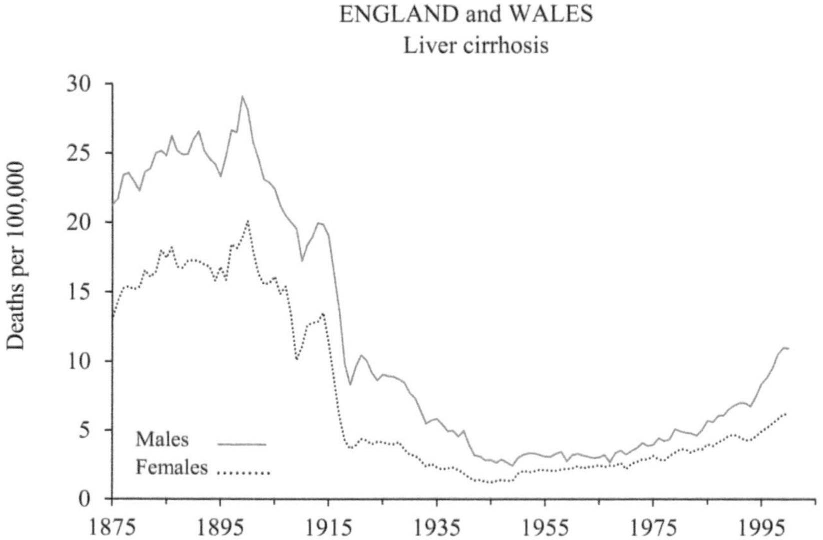

Figure 13.5. Annual age-standardized death rates from cirrhosis of the liver for males and females in England and Wales, 1875–2000. *Sources:* Registrar General, *Annual Reports*; *Annual Statistical Reviews*; Office of Population Censuses and Surveys, *Mortality Statistics: Cause, Series DH2.*

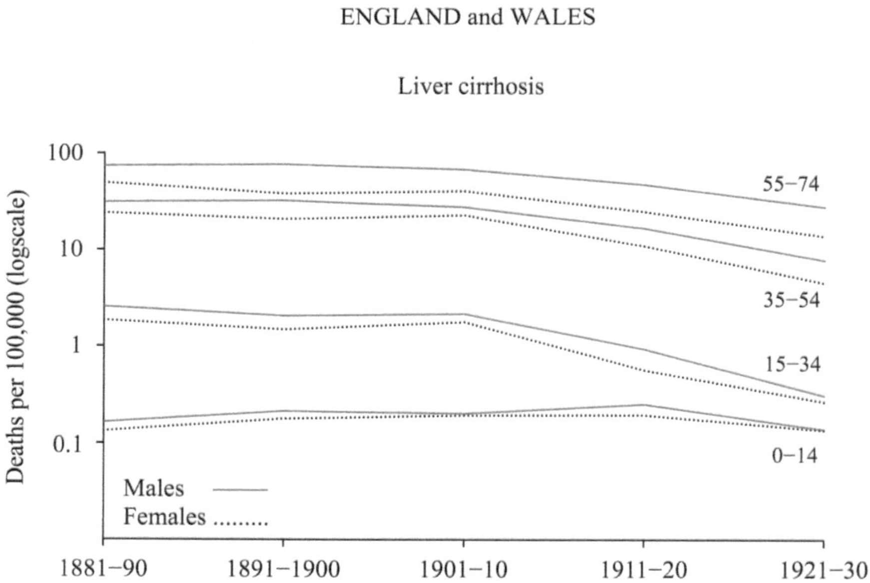

Figure 13.6. Annual average age-specific death rates from cirrhosis of the liver for males and females in England and Wales, 1881–90 to 1921–30. *Sources:* Registrar General, *Annual Reports*; *Annual Statistical Reviews.*

age-standardized death rate for men increased fourfold between 1950–54 and 2000–2002, while that for women increased threefold.[22] The increase occurred at different adult ages, but not among children under 15 years of age (fig. 13.6), which is consistent with an alcohol-related effect among adults. Epidemiological evidence indicates a strong dose-dependent relationship between lifetime alcohol consumption and liver cirrhosis.[23] Alcohol consumption (equivalent liters of 100% alcohol per capita at ages 15 and over) increased considerably in the 1960s and 1970s as in other countries of northern Europe.[24] In view of the evidence of association between per capita alcohol consumption and liver cirrhosis mortality, the increase in death rates and subsequent leveling off in the 1980s is probably linked with the trend in alcohol consumption.[25]

There have also been dramatic changes in the socioeconomic differential in liver cirrhosis mortality in England and Wales. In 1921 liver cirrhosis mortality (standardized mortality ratio) among the professional and managerial occupational groups (social classes I and II) was more than double that for other occupational groups (social classes III–V). By 1991 there was an inverse relationship between liver cirrhosis mortality and socioeconomic status, with mortality being about four times higher for social class V compared with social class I.[26] Although surveys did not reveal evidence of alcohol consumption patterns that might explain socioeconomic differentials and changes since the 1920s,[27] harmful drinking habits and related dietary deficiencies could have contributed to high mortality in socioeconomically deprived areas.[28]

Harmful alcohol consumption, poor diet and nutritional status, exposure to hepatotropic viruses, and access to treatment for alcoholism affect differentials in liver cirrhosis mortality and trends over time. Alcohol and HCV infection are independent risk factors for liver cirrhosis and the major determinants in Western countries. There is evidence of an interactive effect, such that the excess incidence of liver cirrhosis caused by high alcohol intake is even greater among those who have experienced HCV infection (anti-HCV antibodies detected).[29] Trends over the period 1970–89 indicate that alcohol consumption was probably the main cause of liver cirrhosis in many European countries, although the age pattern of mortality suggests that viral infection was also a major contributor in Eastern Europe.[30] The World Health Organization has estimated that about 170 million people are chronically infected with HCV worldwide, with 3–4 million newly infected each year. Chronic cirrhosis develops in about 10–20% of those with chronic HCV infection, and liver cancer in a further 1–5%. In developed countries, chronic infection is mostly due to injecting drugs or receiving transfusion with contaminated blood or blood products. Use of unsterilized injection equipment and unscreened blood transfusion are also the main modes of transmission in developing countries. As there is no vaccine against HCV and treatment is too costly for most people in developing countries, prevention is based on promotion of behavior change, safe injection practices, sterilization of medical equipment, and the screening and testing of blood, plasma-derived products, and organ donors.[31]

Endocrine, Nutritional, and Metabolic Diseases

Endocrine, nutritional, and metabolic diseases accounted for 1.5% of deaths in 2010, with diabetes mellitus being the main cause (1.1%). The number of deaths attributed to diseases in the group declined in the first half of the 20th century and then increased again, with trends in age-specific death rates largely reflecting the trends for diabetes mellitus.

Diabetes mellitus is characterized by raised concentration of glucose in the blood due to a deficiency in the production of the pancreatic hormone insulin. In insulin-dependent diabetes (type-1 diabetes), there is severe deficiency or absence of insulin production and onset is usually in childhood. Non-insulin-dependent diabetes (type-2 diabetes) usually occurs at ages over 40 years, although it is increasingly found to occur at younger ages. These and other forms of diabetes associated with other chronic conditions such as obesity and cirrhosis of the liver are not necessarily fatal, and treatment with insulin since 1922 has probably had considerable impact on death rates at younger ages. However, the overall age-standardized death rates for men and women had already fallen quite dramatically during World War I (fig. 13.7). Data from Ireland indicate a similar long-term trend, with an increase in the age-standardized death rate from the mid-19th century to World War I. Surveys of the diet of laborers indicated an increase in consumption of fat and sugar over this period, which may have increased the risk of diabetes.[32] Reduced availability of these foods and changes in diet during the war probably contributed to reduced mortality attributed to diabetes in Ireland and in England and Wales. In the period of food controls between 1940 and 1954, death rates declined among all age groups (fig. 13.8).[33] As type-1 diabetes is believed to be due to interactions between genetic predisposition, the immune system, and environmental factors, including enteroviruses such as Coxsackie B virus,[34] environmental changes may also have contributed. Most diabetes at younger ages is insulin dependent, and treatment with insulin and antibiotics to control infections from the 1940s onward probably contributed to the decline in death rates at ages under 55. Deaths at older ages have predominated in the overall trend, with the death rate increasing in the 1920s, 1930s, and again from the 1950s.

From about 1950, diabetes death rates among middle-aged and older adult males increased, which could reflect increased prevalence of obesity or being overweight and the consumption of fiber-free energy foods, sugar, and fat, which are considered a risk for those susceptible to diabetes. Studies of diabetes mortality trends have taken into account problems of classification relating to multiple chronic disorders and changes in the rules for certifying the underlying cause, which led to an increase in deaths attributed to diabetes between 1984 and 1992. Multiple-cause coding was introduced as standard practice in England and Wales in 1993, as in many other countries.[35] A study of data from death certificates for the period 1979–98 found that the death rate, based on diabetes coded as the underlying cause, had changed considerably; however, the death rate was almost unchanged for diabetes mentioned anywhere on the record of cause of

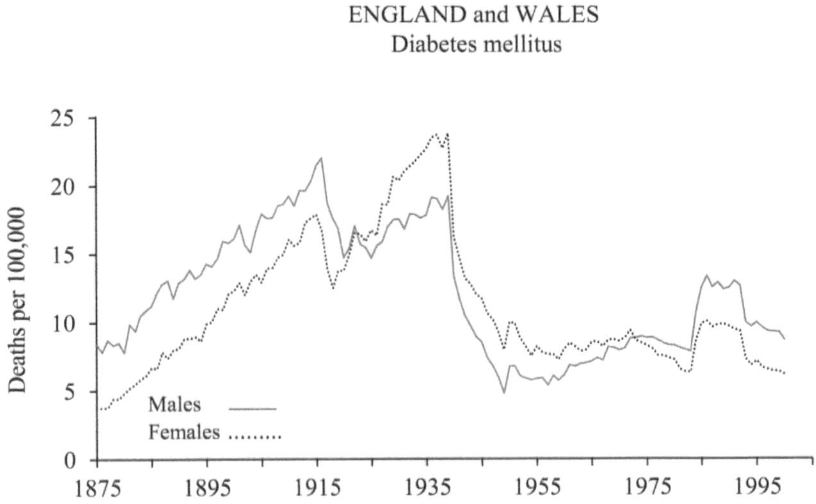

Figure 13.7. Annual age-standardized death rates from diabetes for males and females in England and Wales, 1875–2000. *Sources:* Registrar General, *Annual Reports*; *Annual Statistical Reviews*; Office of Population Censuses and Surveys, *Mortality Statistics: Cause, Series DH2.*

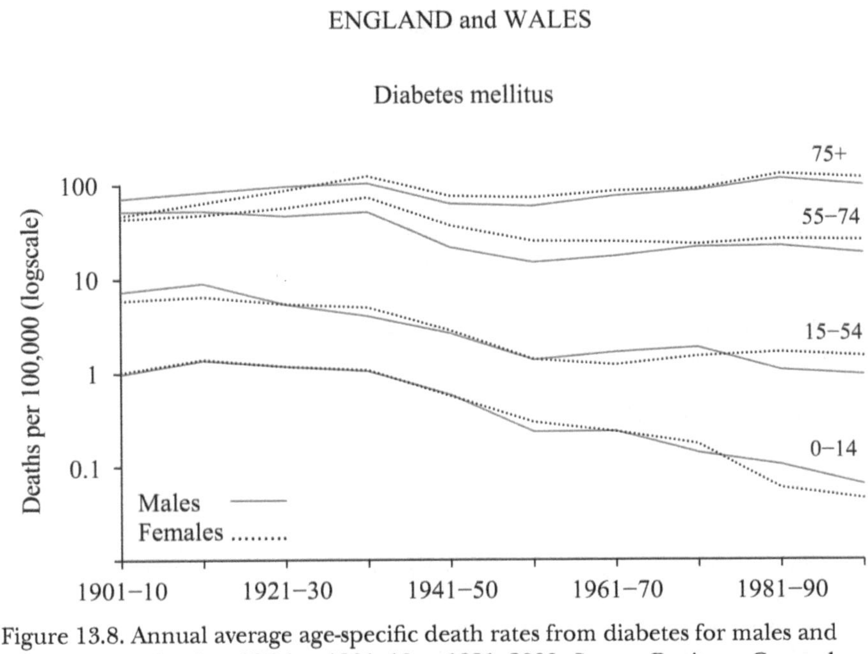

Figure 13.8. Annual average age-specific death rates from diabetes for males and females in England and Wales, 1901–10 to 1991–2000. *Sources:* Registrar General, *Annual Reports*; *Annual Statistical Reviews*; Office of Population Censuses and Surveys, *Mortality Statistics: Cause, Series DH2.*

death. It was concluded that either there had been no improvement in survival for diabetics with other life-threatening conditions such as cardiovascular disorders, or improvement in survival had been offset by increased prevalence of diabetes.[36] Prevalence of type-2 diabetes in the United Kingdom increased from 2.8% in 1996 to 4.3% in 2005.[37]

Studies in the United States cast further light on mortality trends by considering death rates for diabetics. Among self-reported diabetic men in a national health and nutrition survey, the all-cause death rate declined from 42.6 to 24.4 per 1,000 between 1971–86 and 1988–2000, and the cardiovascular disease death rate declined from 26.4 to 12.8 per 1,000. However, the death rates among diabetic women did not decline.[38] A further study analyzed changes in mortality over a longer period (1950–2001) and overcame the limitations of self-reporting by focusing on diabetics identified by routine screening in the Framingham Heart Study. The risk of dying was twice as high for diabetic men and three times as high for diabetic women compared with nondiabetics. However, between 1950–75 and 1976–2001, mortality declined considerably (between 39–60%) for both diabetic and nondiabetic men and women. There was a considerable reduction in cardiovascular mortality among diabetic men (69%) and diabetic women (75%), but no significant decline in mortality from other causes. It was suggested that several factors could explain the decline, including reduced prevalence of the main risk factors for cardiovascular disease, including smoking, total blood cholesterol, and systolic blood pressure, as well as the benefits of other prevention therapies specifically for diabetics.[39]

Diabetics have a much higher risk of dying from cardiovascular disease than nondiabetics, yet diabetes is recorded as the underlying cause in relatively few deaths among them. Heart disease is the most common cause of death recorded among type-2 diabetics in the United States and the United Kingdom.[40] Both diabetes and cardiovascular disease are associated with obesity. This is now commonly defined in Western populations as a weight-for-height, body mass index (BMI) of $> 30 kg/m^2$, although risks for type-2 diabetes in Asian countries increase sharply at BMI levels considered acceptable for white Westerners. Obesity and type-2 diabetes are becoming increasingly common as a consequence of changes in lifestyle toward more sedentary work and leisure, coupled with higher-energy-density diets.[41] Humans evolved for a different active lifestyle of hunting and gathering, with consumption of food to provide sufficient energy. It has been suggested that natural selection may actually have favored those with a genetically related capacity to store dietary glucose as fat when food shortage and starvation were a recurring threat in the premodern era. The increasing reliability of food supplies in Europe may have been accompanied by a slow rise in the prevalence of diabetes over many years.[42] In recent times, an imbalance between diet and physical activity, together with inflammatory processes, could be a common link between obesity, diabetes, and cardiovascular disorders.[43]

The increase in incidence of type-1 diabetes, other autoimmune diseases, and allergies such as asthma has also been linked with recent improvements in the infectious disease environment, in a "hygiene hypothesis."[44] The immune system evolved through exposure to many different microorganisms, some of which were able to survive because they inhibited particular immune responses. Contact with certain types of bacteria and worms (helminths) may have contributed to the development of an immune system capable of a strong anti-inflammatory response. Reduced exposure to nonpathogenic environmental bacteria and helminths commonly encountered during human evolution as a result of relatively recent improvements in hygiene and living conditions may have restricted the development of the immune system's capacity for anti-inflammatory regulation. A deficiency in immunoregulation of inflammation could allow allergies and autoimmune disorders such as diabetes to develop. The infectious disease environment continues to be significant in other ways, as both diabetes and cardiovascular disorders are associated with microorganisms that remain widely prevalent.

A causal role for microorganisms in diabetes has long been suspected. Similarities in the seasonal patterns of incidence suggest that viral infection might be initiating the underlying process,[45] although there is conflicting evidence regarding the effect of specific infections in promoting or protecting against type-1 diabetes.[46] In the 19th century diabetes was thought to follow some cases of mumps and other acute infectious diseases. A study in the 1960s found no evidence of excess antibodies to mumps virus or common respiratory viruses among diabetics, although higher antibody titers to Coxsackie B virus were found among insulin-dependent diabetics within three months of onset of the disease.[47] This association was investigated in several studies, although results from case-control studies lacked consistency.[48] Epidemiological studies provided some support for the hypothesis of an etiological role for enteroviruses, such as higher incidence of type-1 diabetes following an epidemic of Coxsackie B5 virus in the United States.[49] A study of pancreatic tissue from diabetics infected with Coxsackie B4 virus found evidence that the virus can infect beta cells and that infection is associated with inflammation and functional impairment.[50]

A review of epidemiological and serological studies, and genetic analysis of host susceptibility, concluded that beta cell destruction could be linked with infection, and that certain enteroviruses (picornaviruses) were the most likely candidates.[51] Biological plausibility is based on the view that type-1 diabetes is a consequence of selective autoimmune destruction of pancreatic beta cells in genetically predisposed individuals. Enteroviruses may trigger or accelerate the pathogenic process in different ways such as direct destruction of beta cells, an inflammatory reaction, or a pathogenic immune response.[52] A recent review of studies of prevalence found strong evidence of association between enterovirus infection and type-1-diabetes-related autoimmunity.[53] Although it may not be possible to determine causality by randomized controlled trial, prospective international studies could clarify the interactions between infection and environmental, geographic, and genetic factors contributing to the multifactorial etiology of type-1 diabetes.

Evidence of the involvement of viruses in the development of type-2 diabetes has come from studies of hepatitis C virus (HCV). A recent review of evidence concluded that both cross-sectional and longitudinal studies indicate that HCV infection is associated with an increased risk for type-2 diabetes. Longitudinal prospective studies considered whether HCV infection preceded type-2 diabetes. A significantly higher risk of type-2 developing in HCV-infected people compared with controls suggested a possible causal role.[54] Among persons already at risk for diabetes, those with HCV infection were many times more likely to develop diabetes than those without HCV infection.[55] Although the mechanism through which HCV infection increases the risk of diabetes is not clear, evidence suggests that viral proteins affect different cellular processes.[56] A review of studies suggested that HCV interferes with glucose metabolism.[57] Some of the risk factors for development of type-2 diabetes, including HCV infection, coinfection with HCV and hepatitis B virus (HBV), and being overweight or obese, also increase the risk of liver disease. Type-2 diabetes is a common complication of liver disease affecting the rate of progression to cirrhosis, along with age, gender, alcohol consumption, being overweight, immune status, and coinfections.[58]

Musculoskeletal Diseases

Musculoskeletal diseases accounted for less than 1% of deaths in 2010 (0.8%), with rheumatoid arthritis (0.16%) and osteoporosis (0.26%) being the main causes certified. The conditions are often not recorded on the death certificate, making mortality trends difficult to interpret. Although not immediately life threatening, they are a significant cause of disability particularly among older adults, and prevalence has increased dramatically since the 19th century. Possibly half of all adults over 75 years of age have some locomotion disability.[59] Rheumatoid arthritis usually begins in small joints, and an inflammatory process erodes cartilage and underlying bone, eventually causing deformity and disability. Prevalence may have increased in the late 19th and early 20th century, with a peak of about 1% of the adult population in the 1950s. Osteoarthritis (joint failure) is the most common joint disorder, resulting from trauma and gout, as well as rheumatoid arthritis. Prevalence rises with age, and over half of adults aged 65 and over are likely to have some form of osteoarthritis. Osteoporosis (reduction of bone mass) is associated with bone fractures, and is a significant cause of morbidity among older adults.

Diseases of the Nervous System

Diseases of the nervous system accounted for 3.8% of deaths in 2010, including Alzheimer's disease (1.4%), Parkinson's disease (1.0%), motor neuron disease (0.4%), epilepsy (0.2%), and multiple sclerosis (MS) (0.2%). Clearly certification of these diseases as primary cause is not a good indicator of relative prevalence as death can be attributed to other chronic conditions. There has been a considerable increase in the number of people with chronic neurological conditions since the 19th century along with the increase in longevity.

A review of trends in the 20th century reported that Alzheimer's disease has become the most common cause of dementia accounting for more than half of the cases of deteriorating cognitive function at older adult ages, while cerebrovascular disease is also a common cause.[60] Part of the gradual increase in deaths attributed to dementia in the second half of the 20th century may be due to increasing preference for this diagnostic label, while recording of deaths as "senility" has declined. Parkinson's disease was known in the 19th century as *paralysis agitans*. Age-period cohort analysis indicated that the risk of death increased over successive cohorts born in the second half of the 19th century, then declined after a peak at the turn of the century. Such a clear cohort trend is likely to be due to a change in risk-factor exposure rather than changes in certification. Period death rates for age groups under 75 declined consistently from the 1930s, predating the introduction of L-dopa treatment in the 1960s. Motor neuron disease is a syndrome of progressive muscular wasting and weakness due to degeneration of motor neurons in the brain and spinal cord. Death rates increased with age for those born after 1900, and period death rates were increasing rapidly in industrialized countries in the second half of the 20th century. Although this may in part reflect decreasing mortality from competing causes, changes in exposure to risk factors could be involved. Epilepsy is a tendency to recurrent seizures in which cerebrovascular disease, cerebral tumors, alcohol, and trauma have been implicated. It is recorded as primary cause in very few deaths (0.2%), and prevalence does not appear to be changing. Multiple sclerosis is an inflammatory disease affecting the myelin sheaths of neurons in the central nervous system, and there are variations in distribution that suggest environmental influences or the effect of late childhood infections. Infections with measles, mumps, rubella, and Epstein-Barr virus tend to have occurred later in life in those with MS compared with those without.

Genitourinary Diseases

Age-specific death rates from genitourinary diseases generally declined in the 20th century, largely reflecting trends for the group of kidney diseases—nephritis, nephrosis, and nephrotic syndrome. The whole group of genitourinary diseases accounted for 2.5% of all deaths in 2010, with 0.8% of deaths attributed to kidney diseases, which can cause progressive chronic renal failure and ultimately end-stage renal failure.

The main causes of kidney failure are glomerulonephritis in which glomeruli are destroyed by the body's immune response, diabetes mellitus, pyelonephritis caused by infection, polycystic kidney disease, and high blood pressure.[61] The complex relationship between kidney disease and cardiovascular disease illustrates the interrelated nature of chronic disorders that are potentially causes of death, although only one will be certified as the primary cause. Kidney disease is an independent risk factor for cardiovascular disease in both men and women,[62] while hypertension and diabetes are established risk factors for chronic kidney disease, along with lifestyle-related factors such as cigarette smoking, obesity, and physical inactivity.[63] As mentioned, the combination of diabetes, hypertension, and chronic kidney disease is now the most common cause of kidney failure worldwide.[64] The "epidemic" of type-2 diabetes and aging populations are contributing to a global increase in the prevalence of chronic kidney disease.[65] Renal failure is common in developing countries, as are secondary kidney disorders related to infection. In many countries, poststreptococcal glomerulonephritis is still common, contributing to the risk of kidney failure along with other infectious diseases and factors related to adoption of a "Western lifestyle."[66]

Changes in terminology and classification pose considerable problems for assessment of long-term trends in kidney disease mortality in England and Wales. The general term nephritis refers to inflammation of the kidney, and includes acute and chronic forms. The main acute forms are acute pyelonephritis caused by bacterial infection, and acute glomerulonephritis due to an inflammatory response linked with the immune reaction to streptococcal infections such as scarlet fever and sore throat. The main chronic renal conditions are now known as chronic pyelonephritis, which is due to chronic bacterial infection of the kidney, and chronic glomerulonephritis, which can take different forms and is due to immunological problems. In view of these distinctions between types of kidney disease and related classification changes affecting chronic nephritis and subcategories, long-term trends in death rates can be considered for nephritis as a whole.

In England and Wales, there was a sharp decline in the death rate from nephritis from World War I up to 1925, mainly due to a decline among older adults (figs. 13.9 and 13.10). A study of trends in death rates from acute nephritis, chronic nephritis, and kidney infections between 1940 and 1965 reported a sharp decline after World War II, which also occurred in other Western countries.[67] It was suggested that when diabetics with kidney disease died, the primary cause could have been recorded as diabetes in an increasing proportion of cases, which might explain some of the decline in the death rate from chronic nephritis. Growing interest in urinary tract infections may have focused attention on infections of the kidney, leading to an increase in deaths attributed to this cause rather than acute nephritis, for which the death rate declined between 1950 and 1964. The death rate from coronary heart disease also increased, and some deaths that would previously have been attributed to chronic nephritis may have been transferred to this category.

The considerable decline in kidney disease mortality in the first half of the 20th century occurred before effective treatment, with reduced exposure to toxins and hence incidence suggested as a possible contributing factor.[68] Although renal replacement therapy by dialysis or kidney transplantation was in use from the 1950s, it was not until the 1980s that the number of transplants increased significantly when rejection problems had been overcome by immunosuppression.

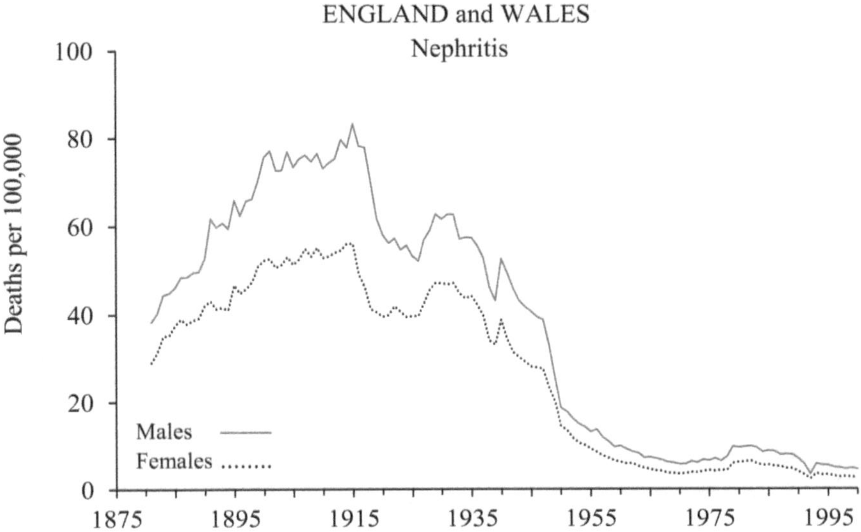

Figure 13.9. Annual age-standardized death rates from nephritis for males and females in England and Wales, 1875–2000. *Sources:* Registrar General, *Annual Reports*; *Annual Statistical Reviews*; Office of Population Censuses and Surveys, *Mortality Statistics: Cause, Series DH2.*

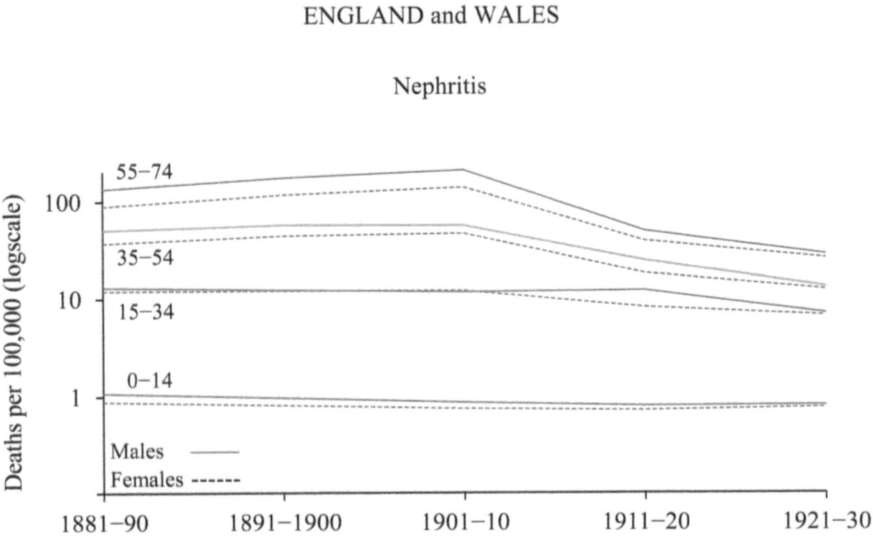

Figure 13.10. Annual average age-specific death rates from nephritis in England and Wales for 10-year periods, 1881–90 to 1921–30. *Sources:* Registrar General, *Annual Reports*; *Annual Statistical Reviews.*

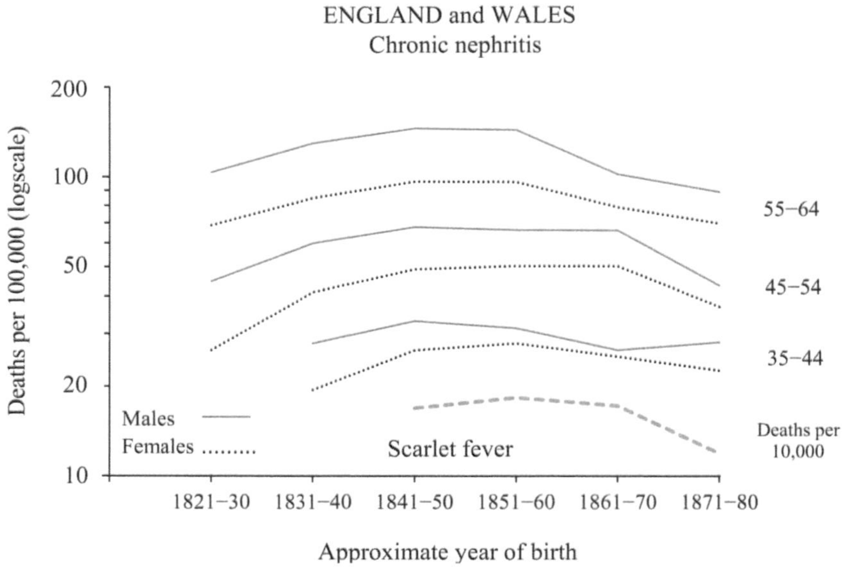

Figure 13.11. Annual average death rates from chronic nephritis and scarlet fever in England and Wales, by year of birth, 1821–30 to 1871–80. *Sources:* Registrar General, *Annual Reports*; *Annual Statistical Reviews*; Office of Population Censuses and Surveys, *Mortality Statistics: Cause, Series DH2.*

A decline in the combined death rate from kidney diseases (nephritis, nephrosis, and kidney infections) between 1949 and 1965 was reported among men at all ages, and among women under 65 years of age but not older women.[69] Hansen and Susser suspected a generation effect on chronic nephritis, which accounted for over 80% of all deaths from kidney disease. Analysis of age-specific death rates by year of birth indicated a peak in chronic nephritis mortality among those born in the mid-19th century.[70] This roughly corresponds with the peak in scarlet fever mortality among children born in the 1850s (fig. 13.11).

Hansen and Susser suggested that streptococcal infection could have been the main cause of chronic nephritis in the past, with successive generations experiencing increasing mortality from scarlet fever and chronic nephritis up to the 1850s and declining mortality from the 1860s.[71] A similar decline in mortality before the antibiotic era was observed for rheumatic fever, which was recognized in the 1940s to be a consequence of infection with *Streptococcus pyogenes*, the causal agent in scarlet fever and other throat infections.[72] The decline in scarlet fever mortality in Western countries appears to reflect a decline in case fatality rather than declining incidence, as discussed in chapter 8. Hansen and Susser concluded that in the past, chronic nephritis was linked with preceding streptococcal infection.[73] Life-threatening scarlet fever could have become less common over successive cohorts if a milder strain of streptococcus began to gain an ecological advantage, or because enteric coinfections that increased the severity of streptococcal infection became less prevalent. As discussed in chapter 8, there is an ecological association between the decline in the death rate from scarlet fever and the decline of typhoid and other enteric fevers that impaired absorption of micronutrients important for resistance to infectious diseases. Whatever the cause, a decline in severity of scarlet fever infections experienced in childhood probably reduced the risk of ill health and kidney disease in later adult life.

Microorganisms and Other Chronic Diseases

When considering links between microorganisms and chronic diseases, two possible pathways should be kept in mind. Some microorganisms may directly trigger or activate a specific pathogenic process, while others trigger an immune response that contributes to the disease process in a susceptible host. Several examples of microbial triggers for chronic disease were reported by the American Academy of Microbiology in 2005.[74] It was suggested that pathogens might activate chronic disease processes in unknown ways, while genetic susceptibility has been recognized in some disorders. Crohn's disease, an inflammatory disease that can occur in any part of the gut, does not result from infection alone, but from the interrelationship between the immune response and genetic susceptibility in particular hosts.[75] A causal role for specific microorganisms, based on epidemiological association, is particularly difficult to establish for chronic gastrointestinal diseases in general. Application of Koch's and Hill's criteria (see chapter 2) in the case of Crohn's disease and Whipple's disease, for example, is complicated by the presence of many microorganisms.[76] Infections may be innocuous, although evidence of association can generate hypotheses about chronic disease processes. Whipple's disease, a rare condition that prevents the small intestines from properly absorbing nutrients, was linked with the bacterium *Tropheryma whipplei* when bacilli were found in diseased tissue.[77] Some studies have implicated measles virus in inflammation of the intestine, and other microorganisms are suspected as well. The exposure of the human colon to high concentrations of bacteria and viruses has also added to the complexity of assessing association between infectious agents and colorectal cancer (see chapter 12). With some disorders, chronic disease can occur after an initial infection has cleared, and if the causal agent is no longer detectable, this will inhibit confirmation of a suspected association. For example, the gastrointestinal or sexually transmitted infection that leads to Reiter's syndrome involving polyarthritis, urethritis, and ocular inflammation is relatively short lived, and the resulting arthritis syndrome occurs weeks or months after infection has cleared.[78] The lack of evidence of a pathogen at the site of a chronic disorder is not evidence against its involvement, and clearly identification of a pathogen is not necessarily an indication of a causal role.

Epidemiological studies can provide supporting evidence regarding a suspected role for a particular pathogen in a specific chronic disorder. Strong evidence in support of causality can come from studies comparing the risk for a chronic disease between people identified as infected with a particular pathogen and those who are not. This type of evidence contributed to the recognition that stomach cancer as well as peptic ulcer is often caused by *H. pylori* bacteria. Epidemiological patterns and concentrations of a chronic disease in particular locations or social groups can suggest infectious etiology. Also, when a similar disease is known to be infectious in origin, microbial involvement is more strongly suspected. This was the case with rheumatoid arthritis, which has many characteristics in common with Lyme disease, an arthritic inflammatory condition caused by a bacterial pathogen.[79] Before *H. pylori* was recognized as a causal agent in gastric cancer, mortality was found to be associated with indicators of overcrowded housing in childhood, such as persons per room and small rooms, and with a lack of proper food storage or sanitary facilities. This suggested that person-to-person transmission of an infection might be involved, particularly as bronchitis and rheumatic heart disease, which have an infectious etiology in childhood, were also associated with indicators of overcrowded housing earlier in life.[80]

Many chronic diseases exhibit one or more of the signs of possible infectious etiology—pathogens are present in diseased tissues; the condition responds to antimicrobial therapy; the onset of the chronic disease occurs after persistent infection; immune-suppressed individuals have increased risk of the disease; the host immune response suggests infection is involved; there is inflammation associated; the disease is multifocal, involving more than one organ; epidemiological patterns are suggestive of infectious origins; or similar diseases are known to have a microbial origin. On the basis of such signs, the American Academy of Microbiology reported in 2004 that many well-known chronic diseases were suspected of having infectious etiology,[81] including multiple sclerosis (EBV), Crohn's disease (*Mycobacterium paratuberculosis* and others), Alzheimer's disease (*Chlamydia pneumoniae*), diabetes (enteroviruses), atherosclerosis (*C. pneumoniae,* cytomegalovirus), Bell's palsy (herpes simplex virus), schizophrenia (intrauterine exposure to influenza), chronic fatigue (HTLV-1, EBV), and prostate cancer (BK virus). Infectious etiology is suspected for other well-known chronic diseases, including pelvic inflammatory disease (*Chlamydia trachomatis*), poststreptococcal glomerulonephritis (group A streptococcus), and arthritis (parvovirus B19 and rubella).[82] At least some of these associations are likely to be added to the growing number of chronic diseases with confirmed infectious etiology. In 2004, Ewald listed 15 chronic diseases for which an infectious cause (virus, bacteria, or protozoan) had been accepted since the 1980s, including AIDS (HIV), cervical cancer (HPV), subacute sclerosing panencephalitis (measles virus), Kaposi's sarcoma (human herpes virus 8), liver cancer (HBV, HBC), stomach cancer and peptic ulcers (*H. pylori*), and rheumatoid arthritis (*Streptococcus pyogenes*).[83]

Infectious etiology is suspected in many chronic debilitating conditions, although causality and biophysiological mechanisms are often difficult to establish. Evidence of involvement is of varying strength from different types of investigation. For example, measles virus has been identified in diseased tissue of patients with rheumatoid arthritis, a chronic inflammatory disease.[84] Rheumatic fever, which appears to involve an autoimmune response, and its sequel rheumatic heart disease continue to be significant causes of morbidity and mortality globally, and epidemiological evidence suggests an association with group A streptococcus infection. However, the pathogenic mechanisms whereby the microbial agent might be triggering an autoimmune disease have proved difficult to establish.[85] Multiple sclerosis, a disease of the brain and spinal cord in which symptoms of tremors and paralysis develop slowly, has been linked with infection. Some epidemiological evidence points specifically to influenza virus as a possible microbial trigger, although MS patients have high levels of antibody against many viruses. A study in Poland found a strong correlation between incidence of influenza and incidence of MS five years later.[86] Other associations with common infectious diseases such as measles and infectious mononucleosis suggest that MS may be more likely to develop among those who acquired infection relatively late in life.[87] This would be similar to the increase in incidence of poliomyelitis paralysis when age at first exposure to poliovirus increased as a result of improvements in hygiene. Evidence concerning a possible causal role of poliovirus in motor neuron disease could come from studies of the impact on incidence of the disease resulting from immunization against poliomyelitis.[88] Parkinson's disease, which is also characterized by neuronal degeneration, could be due to a combination of genetic and toxic environmental factors, although epidemiological evidence suggests that *Bordetella pertussis* may be a microbial trigger operating through the effects of pertussis toxin. Incidence of Parkinson's disease was more common among cohorts born after major whooping cough epidemics in Iceland, for example.[89] Secular trends in several countries were also consistent with an increase following the pandemic of encephalitis lethargica between 1919 and 1926.[90]

A combination of infection and genetic propensity may be involved in other chronic debilitating conditions affecting the nervous system, through the immune response triggered in susceptible hosts.[91] Schizophrenia, like Parkinson's disease and Alzheimer's disease, is now regarded by many as a disease of the brain. Family studies and epidemiological evidence suggested that schizophrenia might be caused by a virus transmitted from existing sufferers to genetically predisposed individuals.[92] Research in the 1980s and 1990s suggested that influenza infection in pregnancy, particularly in the second trimester, can cause damage to the fetal brain, which might increase the risk of schizophrenia in later life for the genetically vulnerable.[93] Although infectious causation of schizophrenia may have been less well demonstrated than a genetic component, it has been suggested that evidence that seems to indicate genetic influences might actually be explained by infectious causation.[94] The evolutionary perspective of Cochran, Ewald, and Cochran has raised doubts about the role of genetic factors in schizophrenia as the illness drastically reduces reproductive fitness. It might be expected that any genetic propensity to the disease would have been selected out over time.[95] There may be different routes to schizophrenia, with different infections or multiple infectious agents having a role. Ewald pointed out that evidence of the possible role of different microorganisms such as Borna disease virus, *Toxoplasma gondii*, and influenza is no reason to doubt the role played by any one of the pathogens.[96]

In the case of other types of brain disorder, it has long been known that atrophy and amyloidosis (deposits of protein) can be caused by chronic bacterial infections. In Alzheimer's disease, the most frequent cause of dementia, inflammation contributes to neurodegeneration, and association with the bacterium *Chlamydia pneumoniae* has been demonstrated using different techniques for detection.[97] A high frequency of *C. pneumoniae* has been found in areas of neuropathology in the brains of Alzheimer's patients.[98] This common bacterial agent in acute respiratory tract infections such as pneumonia, sinusitis, and bronchitis is also suspected of involvement in multiple sclerosis,[99] as well as atherosclerosis, as discussed in chapter 11. A possible mechanism is that monocytes and macrophages scavenging bacteria during an acute or chronic infection may spread them through the bloodstream to susceptible areas of the body including the brain. Microorganisms such as *C. pneumoniae* can establish subclinical and apparently asymptomatic infections that could have long-term, irreversible, and eventually life-threatening effects manifesting as chronic disease.

Considerable research is now focused on the development and application of experimental methods for investigating associations between infection and many chronic disorders. The findings of microbiological and other research on the role of infection in chronic diseases complement those concerning lifestyle-related, social, economic, and environmental determinants of disease. Evolutionary and historical perspectives also contribute to an understanding of how changes in the environment and human activities influence the characteristics of infectious disease agents and their role in chronic diseases. Whether the growing body of empirical evidence linking microorganisms with chronic disorders suggests the possibility of a more unified theory of acute infectious disease and chronic disease will be considered in the final chapter.

Chapter Fourteen

Epidemiological Transition

A New Perspective

Changes in Disease, Mortality, and Life Expectancy

Human beings have been adapting to invasive microorganisms contracted in different environments throughout their history, and long before the existence of microbes was known. The recent epidemiological transition has occurred very late in human history, along with urbanization and industrialization in the last three hundred years. Earlier changes in the predominant way of life exposed humans to new infectious diseases that challenged the immune system and people's ingenuity as they sought to avoid or prevent them. A transition in disease patterns occurred when microorganisms transferred to humans as a result of following herds of animals for food. Later, during the long period of the "Neolithic Revolution," the development of crop cultivation enabled people to live in more settled communities alongside domesticated animals, thus increasing exposure to new infections. Living in villages and eventually towns led to infection with airborne, waterborne, and food-borne microorganisms that were able to adapt to humans as suitable hosts. Human settlement also resulted in new microbial hazards due to living in close proximity to animal and human waste, which could be more easily avoided in a nomadic way of life. Fecal contamination of water and food led to new waterborne and gastrointestinal infections. The increase in size of centers of population brought further changes in the infectious disease environment, with airborne viruses such as measles and smallpox causing regular epidemics among those with no immunity, or becoming endemic where populations were sufficiently large and concentrated. Infectious diseases spread as a result of migration from areas of high prevalence, via rural-urban migration, as a result of increasing contact between people in rural areas and towns, and through trade. Human beings had evolved for a very different way of life of hunting and gathering, and adaptation to a "modern" way of life is still far from complete.

This study of changes in disease and mortality in England since the 17th century indicates the continuing importance of the infectious disease environment despite the dramatic decline in death rates from acute infectious diseases and tuberculosis, as many of the chronic diseases that have replaced them as the predominant causes of death have confirmed or suspected infectious etiology.

Some of the common microorganisms associated with particular chronic disorders may not have caused many deaths from infectious disease in the past. Other microorganisms that did cause high mortality in England in the 19th century are still ubiquitous, although the infectious diseases they cause are usually only fatal in developing countries. Some major epidemic killers in the past such as smallpox, typhus, cholera, and typhoid no longer occur in England, and smallpox has been eradicated globally. However, these diseases could cause high mortality if prevalent today as there is no evidence that the microorganisms became less virulent. Deaths from these highly destructive diseases were almost eliminated from England by the end of the 19th century, and death rates from many other acute infectious diseases and tuberculosis had started to decline. The range of severity of infectious diseases and the diversity of trends in death rates indicate that explanations of mortality decline need to be disease specific, although important generalizations are possible.

Evidence of changes in the economic standard of living and diet does not suggest that these can explain the increase in life expectancy before the end of the 19th century. Improvement in human physiology is not necessarily an indication of increased dietary intake, and it does not provide a satisfactory explanation for declining death rates from infectious diseases, which themselves affect physical development and nutritional status. Indicators of economic standard of living such as real wages and food prices do not suggest any consistent association with turning points and trends in mortality or death rates from specific infectious diseases. Poor nutrition most likely continued to contribute to high infectious disease mortality up to World War I. Although rates of malnutrition declined dramatically in the 20th century along with increased food consumption per capita, it is not clear how much this contributed to the decline in infectious disease mortality, while many components of diet have been detrimental to health in later life. A further problem with the "standard of living/nutrition hypothesis" is that the decline in mortality among the aristocracy is very unlikely to have been due to changes in their economic circumstances or access to food. In general terms, the increase in life expectancy between the 1740s and 1940s when antibiotics became available was largely due to human intervention and changes in behavior that reduced the risk of severe infections. Threatened by devastating epidemics, people had long sought ways to protect themselves and their children. Measures were developed through experimentation, at both the individual and the community level, based on observation of how diseases spread, who was affected, and the association with particular environmental conditions. Preventive measures and public health interventions to control infectious diseases contributed most to the decline in mortality before the end of the 19th century. The extension of these interventions and beneficial changes in behavior in the 20th century led to further reductions in infectious disease mortality, while changes in lifestyle and health-related behavior based on knowledge about risk factors began to have an impact on chronic disease mortality from the 1960s.

Measures to prevent plague, including monitoring epidemics, screening travelers, isolating infected households, and enforcing quarantine of ships, could be a sufficient explanation for the absence of plague in England after the last epidemic in the 1660s. Government famine-relief measures from the mid-18th century helped to prevent local food shortages that fostered typhus epidemics. Recognition that ships and jails were foci of infection led to measures to prevent outbreaks. Improvements in cleanliness and personal hygiene, washable cotton clothes, washing of bedding, and in the second half of the 19th century public health measures to clear slums probably contributed to the decline in typhus mortality. Provision of safer water and sewerage prevented cholera epidemics occurring after the 1860s, and these public health measures most likely reduced mortality from gastrointestinal diseases, dysentery and diarrheal diseases, typhoid, and other enteric infections. Smallpox vaccination after 1800, later supported by revaccination and isolation of the infected, ensured the virtual elimination of the disease from England by the end of the 19th century. This not only prevented deaths from smallpox but many deaths from its sequelae and intercurrent infectious diseases. Smallpox vaccination may explain the decline in tuberculosis mortality in the 19th century as a severe attack of smallpox could "trigger" clinical tuberculosis from a latent or new infection. Isolation of tuberculosis patients in sanatoriums; use of pasteurized milk; vaccination with BCG from the 1920s; health education; preventive behavior with regard to sneezing, coughing, and spitting; and chemotherapy from the 1940s probably account for most of the decline in incidence of clinical tuberculosis in the 20th century.

A decline in maternal and infant mortality between the mid-17th and mid-19th centuries among both the aristocracy and lower socioeconomic groups could reflect reduced exposure to infectious diseases in the late stages of pregnancy. Diarrheal diseases and domestic conditions in the growing towns of England contributed to the lack of further decline in the second half of the 19th century. After this, improvements in domestic hygiene, food hygiene, milk quality, and child care were probably the main contributors to the more rapid decline in infant mortality, with pasteurized milk preventing child deaths from gastrointestinal infections, nonrespiratory bovine tuberculosis, and scarlet fever. Children would have benefited from reduced exposure to dysentery, typhoid, and other enteric fevers as a result of the provision of safer water. As these infectious diseases cause micronutrient deficiency, which would increase the risk of dying from other infectious diseases, provision of uncontaminated water could also have reduced the severity of scarlet fever infections, the most common cause of child deaths. The germ theory and new knowledge about the microbial causes and transmission of infectious diseases led to preventive measures being promoted that parents could adopt, including boiling milk, sterilizing feeding bottles, washing hands, protecting food from flies, and isolating sick family members. Voluntary health visitors provided advice about mother and child health, and school education also increased women's access to information. With the dissemination of information about birth control methods, women gained knowledge about how to prevent pregnancy, extend birth intervals, and limit family size. Reduction in the size of families affects transmission of airborne infectious diseases and is likely to have reduced the severity of measles, whooping cough, and respiratory infections, as severity increases with the number of children in a household. In the 20th century, further extension of these benefits to lower socioeconomic groups, together with improved housing, sanitation, and domestic hygiene, led to a more rapid and sustainable improvement in child survival and life expectancy. Improved domestic, personal, and food hygiene; better care of children and the sick; isolation of cases of severe infectious disease; measures to prevent pregnancy; smaller families and other sociodemographic changes that reduced the severity of infections; and immunization to prevent disease—were probably the main contributors to the decline in mortality from infectious diseases in the 20th century.

The rise to prominence of chronic diseases and the subsequent decline in death rates in the 20th century can be better understood in the historical context of a changing infectious disease environment, particularly as microorganisms are now known to play a significant part in their multifactorial etiology. The increase in death rates from chronic diseases in the second half of the 19th century was not simply due to an increasing proportion of children surviving infectious diseases and reaching ages at which the underlying disorders develop. Health hazards associated with industrial occupations, heavily polluted environments, poor diet, and contaminated food, together with the deleterious effects of infectious diseases in childhood and adult life, contributed to increasing death rates from chronic diseases. Given the air pollution and squalid, damp, crowded living conditions in industrial towns, it is not surprising that death rates from chronic respiratory conditions did not decline before the 1890s. High prevalence and rapid transmission of respiratory infections may also have contributed to cardiovascular deaths, in view of the evidence of association with specific microorganisms.

The increase in chronic nephritis mortality among those born before the 1860s coincided with the increase in scarlet fever severity. Adult death rates from liver cirrhosis increased until the 1890s, reflecting high alcohol consumption and possibly lifetime exposure to chronic infections associated with the disease. Adult death rates from peptic ulcer increased among those born before the 1870s, almost certainly linked with *Helicobacter pylori* infection in childhood in the overcrowded and insanitary domestic conditions. In view of its causal role in gastric cancer, it seems likely that mortality from that disease also increased. Cancers of the digestive system contributed most to total cancer mortality up to World War I, also reflecting extremely poor diet and contaminated food. The high proportion of female-specific cancers may reflect poor sexual hygiene and exposure to infections associated with these cancers. In the 20th century, the adoption of cigarette smoking; increasingly sedentary occupations; lack of exercise; unhealthy diet; and other behavioral, social, and economic factors contributed to higher morbidity and mortality from many chronic diseases. The delayed effects of acute infectious diseases in childhood and contact with microorganisms throughout life also contributed to the disorders that underlie chronic disease and "premature" death.

For the most part, the decline in death rates from major chronic diseases began at different times, and the relative influence of cohort-related factors and risk factors over the life course also differed. Studies in the 1920s and 1930s found that the risk of "premature" death was different for different cohorts, and long-term effects of childhood infections were suspected.[1] Recent studies of morbidity data in the United States found that infectious disease in young adulthood was associated with higher incidence of chronic conditions at older adult ages, including cardiovascular, respiratory, and musculoskeletal disorders.[2] Trends in death rates in England for some of the chronic diseases discussed in chapters 10–13 also suggest influences early in life. The decline in cancer death rates over successive cohorts of women born after the mid-19th century could reflect changes in the experience of infectious disease in childhood. The decline in death rates from peptic ulcer over cohorts of females and males born after the 1870s probably reflects changes in exposure to *H. pylori* in childhood as domestic conditions improved with respect to overcrowding, family size, water quality, sanitation, and hygiene. The decline in adult death rates from chronic nephritis over successive cohorts born after the mid-19th century may be due to reduced exposure to severe streptococcal infections as a result of the improvements in the domestic environment.

Despite evidence of early-life influences on the risk for cardiovascular disease later in life,[3] period-related influences have predominated in the trends in age-specific death rates and overall mortality. The period death rate from all cardiovascular disease peaked in 1891 and again in 1951, a quite distinct long-term trend. However, the common peak in cardiovascular and respiratory disease mortality in 1891, similar trends between 1875 and 1915, and correspondence of short-term fluctuations with influenza epidemics are consistent with other evidence of association. Reduced exposure to severe respiratory infections as a result of sociodemographic changes may explain the early phase of cardiovascular disease mortality decline between 1891 and 1910. This reflected the decline in cerebrovascular disease death rates for men and women, which continued in the first half of the 20th century long before anticoagulant and antihypertension treatments were introduced in the 1950s. The later decline in the death rate from heart disease from the 1970s reflects the development of prevention strategies, changes in health-related behavior, and treatment. Epidemiological studies have estimated that over half the decline in heart disease mortality in the 1980s and 1990s was due to beneficial lifestyle changes with respect to diet, exercise, and particularly cigarette smoking. Treatment with aspirin, drugs for reducing hypertension and cholesterol, thrombolysis, and coronary bypass surgery are likely to have improved survival times for many of those with cardiovascular disorders.

Age-specific death rates from respiratory disease declined fairly consistently from the 1890s, reflecting less severe infections in childhood; improved housing; and in the second half of the 20th century, reduced air pollution and the decline in cigarette smoking. Reduced prevalence of cigarette smoking has contributed to the decline in death rates from many other chronic diseases and cancers,[4] while treatment measures have increased survival rates for most types of cancer in recent decades.[5] Improved food quality with regard to adulteration with chemicals and other substances[6] together with the protective effects of an improved diet are likely to have contributed to the decline in death rates from some cancers of the digestive system. The rapid decline in the death rate from liver cirrhosis in the first half of the 20th century probably reflects changes in alcohol and dietary intake, and possibly reduced exposure to infections. Cirrhosis was the main component of the decline in the death rate from all diseases of the digestive system, and in the upturn in the 1980s and 1990s, most likely linked with alcohol consumption. The decline in mortality from diseases of the genitourinary system was more rapid and consistent, reflecting the trends for chronic nephritis and infections of the urinary system.[7] The lack of any consistent decline in the death rate from diseases of the endocrine system reflected the trend for diabetes mellitus at older adult ages. The decline in the death rate from diabetes mellitus during and just after the two world wars probably reflects changes in diet, with insulin treatment and control of infections with antibiotics having an impact on death rates at younger ages from the 1940s.

Despite reductions in death rates from chronic diseases at different times in the 20th century, they have accounted for an increasing proportion of total deaths as death rates from acute infectious diseases and tuberculosis declined consistently and more rapidly. During this epidemiological transition, there was a major shift in the age pattern of mortality, with an increasingly high proportion of deaths among older adults rather than children and young adults. Survival chances for children (1–4 years) improved fairly consistently from the 1860s. The decline in death rates at ages 1–4, 5–19, and 20–34 years each accounted for about one-quarter of the overall decline in mortality in the second half of the 19th century. While infants benefited from improved hygiene and weaning practices from the end of the 19th century, children and adults had benefited more from the improvements in water supplies and sewerage from the 1860s, and adolescents and young adults experienced lower death rates from respiratory tuberculosis. There were further improvements from the end of the 19th century when death rates from measles and respiratory diseases declined, death rates among older adults (age 45 and older) began to decline, and infant mortality declined rapidly.

Changes in disease patterns and mortality decline, mostly due to human interventions and changes in behavior to protect lives and health, have contributed to increased life expectancy since the early 18th century.[8] Average life expectancy at birth increased steadily from about 30 years in the first half of the 18th century to 40 years in 1851 and 46 years in 1901. It increased much more rapidly in the 20th century to reach 66 years by 1951 and 76 years in 2001. By 2010 life expectancy at birth in England had reached 78 for males and 82 for females. The increase in life expectancy at age 1 and at age 5 between 1851 and 2001 contrasts with the lack of improvement at adult ages between 1851 and 1951. Life expectancy at age 25 increased very little before the 20th century. Adults aged 65 in 1851, in 1901, and in 1951, could expect to reach 76, but an

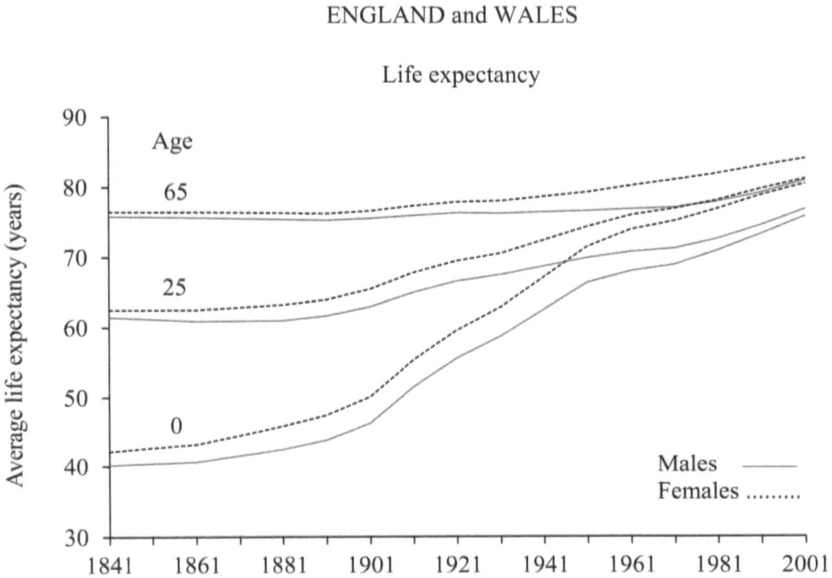

Figure 14.1. Changes over time in average life expectancy at different ages in England and Wales, 1841–2001. *Sources:* Preston, Keyfitz, and Schoen, *Life Tables for National Populations*, 224–66; Office for National Statistics, "English life tables, nos. 1–16"; "Report: Decennial life tables," 110.

increase to 81 came only in the second half of the 20th century (appendix F; trends for males and females in fig. 14.1). In that period, declining death rates from major chronic diseases contributed to a more rapid improvement in life expectancy among adults, with a decline in death rates from cardiovascular disease, cancer, and respiratory diseases contributing the most.

Epidemiological Paradigms and Research

When more children survived to adulthood as a result of the decline in mortality from infectious diseases, medical attention began to focus in the 1920s and 1930s on the chronic diseases that were seen to cause "premature" adult mortality. After World War II, a new epidemiological paradigm emerged focusing research on risk factors associated with chronic disease. Some epidemiologists suggest that the ensuing era of "chronic disease risk factor" epidemiology has come to an end because further investigation of risks at the individual level will not lead to a comprehensive understanding of contemporary disease patterns and variations.[9] In focusing on identification of risk factors for chronic disease, epidemiologists generally paid less attention to intervening biophysiological mechanisms and pathways, or the broader sociocultural and economic context in which individuals become exposed to risks.

Epidemiology has faced the challenge of developing new approaches in the past, with paradigm shifts occurring in response to empirical findings about infectious disease patterns and new hypotheses about causation. "Miasma" was the prevailing paradigm or theory of disease in the 19th century, and individuals were thought to be poisoned by foul emanations from the soil, water, and air. The theory was based on observation of an association between diseases and slum conditions. In the mid-19th century, Chadwick proposed remedial measures to "reduce miasma" and hence mortality, such as closed drainage, new sewage systems, public baths, and new housing, and Engels identified poverty as a major cause of ill health among people living in appalling conditions in industrial Manchester. Evidence presented here (see chapters 5 and 6) suggests that preventive measures, particularly smallpox vaccination, environmental hygiene, and public health interventions to improve water and sewage systems, contributed most to the reduction in mortality in the 19th century, despite being based on inadequate understanding of the causes of disease and transmission. An equivalent contemporary strategy might be expansion of immunization programs to prevent infections suspected of having a role in chronic disease, before causality is confirmed.

Long before the era of "miasma theory" ended, scientific approaches to the study of disease were developing that laid the foundations for a new phase in epidemiological investigation. A better understanding of infectious disease transmission started to develop before bacteriological research provided a sound empirical basis for the germ theory.[10] Farr had a strong influence on the operation of the national registration system and identified clusters of morbidity and mortality in England by analyzing statistics. Snow's work between 1849 and 1854 linking cholera with water sources led to appropriate preventive measures, long before specific microbial agents of disease were detected or even widely suspected. Although Henle hypothesized as early as 1841 that infection by minute organisms was a major cause of disease, it was not until 1865 that Pasteur became the first to identify a specific living microorganism linked with infection in his study of silkworms. Koch's discovery in 1882 that a mycobacterium was the cause of tuberculosis led to a search for microbial causal agents of other diseases.

A new paradigm was founded on the principle that particular infectious diseases were each linked with a specific microorganism, and causality could be demonstrated by applying Koch's criteria (see chapter 2). This microbiological emphasis on identifying single causal agents of disease diverted epidemiological investigation away from an earlier focus on association between disease, the environment, and social conditions.[11] Koch's causal criteria may have promoted an oversimplified view of infectious disease etiology, although it was later broadened to include characteristics of the microbial causal agent, the host, the environment, and the population.[12] Despite the inadequacies of earlier theories of disease, severe and highly destructive acute infectious diseases such as plague, smallpox, cholera, and typhus were virtually eliminated from England and other parts of Europe through organized interventions aimed at protecting people from these diseases, long before the germ theory provided a scientific explanation of their cause and transmission.

As the risk of dying from acute infectious diseases or tuberculosis declined, concern grew in the first half of the 20th century over the chronic diseases that were causing an increasing number of deaths. After World War II, epidemiology once again began to focus on social and environmental determinants of disease, when associations with chronic disorders were observed. The "risk factor paradigm" evolved, with epidemiological research focused on peptic ulcer, heart disease, and lung cancer among middle-aged men, in observational and distribution studies.[13] Methods for case-control and cohort studies were developed, which enabled risk ratios or odds ratios to be calculated that linked exposure to risk factors with outcomes. These studies provided strong statistical evidence of association that suggested causality, particularly when a "dose-response" relationship was observed. Such a relationship helped to establish cigarette smoking as a cause of lung cancer through the studies of Doll and Peto and many others from the 1950s onward. Supporting biological evidence of possible mechanisms for observed associations was often lacking, although tar was found to have a carcinogenic effect when applied to the skin of mice. Mainstream epidemiology was less concerned with the process of pathogenesis in chronic diseases and departed from a "single specific cause" model of disease. The emphasis was on developing "multicausal" models of chronic disease under a new paradigm that linked a "black box" of risk factors to outcome.[14] The objective was to establish the statistical probabilities of risk for morbidity and mortality relating to intermediate determinants of disease, while researchers in other disciplines investigated mechanisms of pathogenesis.

Risk factors have usually been conceptualized in terms of individuals, although public health issues have arisen over broader aspects of social responsibility. A primary focus on individual lifestyle and the exercise of choice carries implications of individual responsibility, although behaviors and lifestyles are partly determined by sociocultural and economic circumstances, and commercial activities can be highly exploitative and deleterious to health. The report of a British government working group on health in the 1970s (the Black Report) concluded that smoking behavior is a secondary symptom of underlying social and economic determinants, and it recommended that policy makers consider how these could be addressed in addition to provision of health education and counseling for individuals.[15] Tobacco companies sell products that are known to be addictive and kill many consumers "prematurely." This fact has raised legal as well as ethical issues about culpability for individual deaths, although governments still allow tobacco companies to conduct their business and some do little to restrict the promotion of extremely harmful tobacco products.[16]

Cigarettes are likely to have killed many more people prematurely than HIV/AIDS, which galvanized international efforts to implement awareness-raising and behavior-change prevention programs in the 1980s. The pandemic of human immunodeficiency virus (HIV) challenged the prevailing chronic disease "risk factor paradigm" as it exposed the limitations of aiming for control through focusing on changing the behavior of individuals.[17] The pandemic of acquired immune deficiency syndrome (AIDS) led to chronic disorders that were clearly linked with the immune response to a specific virus that had been identified. Infectious causation was accepted on the basis of many different types of scientific evidence, despite being questioned on the grounds that not all Koch's criteria had been fulfilled. In fact, the criteria were not fulfilled for most of the chronic diseases for which infectious causation was accepted in the 1980s and 1990s, including cervical cancer, liver cancers, and adult T-cell leukemia, as well as AIDS.[18]

Links between infections and chronic disorders were suspected as early as the 1890s. A hypothesis was proposed that the skin disorder shingles is a delayed manifestation of chickenpox, although the causal connection was only accepted much later, in the 1940s.[19] Ewald suggested that the lack of progress in investigating hypotheses of links between microbial agents and chronic diseases such as peptic ulcer, cardiovascular disease, and cancer, between the 1940s and the 1980s, was due to rigid adherence to Koch's criteria as the only basis for assessing infectious causation.[20] As mentioned, fulfillment of the requirements of Koch's criteria can be particularly difficult for chronic diseases, as they can manifest many years after an infection. Ewald pointed out that a hypothesis of infectious etiology does not exclude other possible influences on the disease process, and microbial agents operate in the context of environmental, lifestyle-related, and genetic determinants.[21] Infectious etiology has recently been accepted over a relatively short period of time for cancers that account for between 15–20% of all cancers, and microorganisms are suspected of a possible causal role in most other types of cancer.[22]

Evidence of microbial involvement in chronic diseases is of varying strength, based on the results of different types of scientific investigation. The focus here has been on diseases responsible for a relatively high number of deaths, and the strongest empirical evidence for microbial causation relates to gastric cancer and peptic ulcer (*H. pylori*), hepatocellular carcinoma (HBV and HCV), and AIDS (HIV). Infectious etiology is also accepted for adult T-cell leukemia (HTLV-1); cervical, penile, and anal cancer (HPV); nasopharyngeal carcinoma and Hodgkin's disease (EBV); rheumatic fever, and poststreptococcal glomerulonephritis (group A streptococcus). There is considerable evidence indicating a causal role of microorganisms in atherosclerosis (*H. pylori* and *C. pneumoniae*), cerebrovascular disease, and coronary heart disease (*H. pylori, C. pneumoniae,* and influenza viruses).[23] Several other disorders under investigation for possible infectious etiology were mentioned in chapters 12 and 13. Future research and improvements in technologies for microbial detection could lead to confirmation of a causal role of infection in many of these chronic diseases and possibly others. The relationship between *M. tuberculosis* infection and cancer discussed in chapter 12 is likely to be investigated further in different types of study, including assessment of the impact on incidence of tuberculosis and cancer of a range of preventive measures, including BCG vaccination in populations where it provides protection against tuberculosis.

Further research into associations between microorganisms and chronic diseases would be consistent with a new paradigm for investigation of multifactorial chronic diseases encompassing pathogenesis and the underlying biophysiological processes as well as risk factors and the sociocultural, economic, and environmental determinants. A proposed "eco-epidemiology paradigm" would explicitly recognize multilevel causation and the link between epidemiology and public health.[24] A more integrated approach to the investigation of health and disease based on multilevel causality would encompass risk-factor analysis, a life-course perspective, and analysis of historical trends. The aim would be explanation of disease in terms of pathogenesis as well as risk factors and an understanding of causal pathways at cellular-genetic, individual, societal, and population levels. Further research into the role of microorganisms in chronic disease is likely to make a significant contribution to the understanding of pathogenesis.

Research on the development and application of experimental methods for investigating association between infections and chronic disorders is likely to continue. Advances in microbiological techniques can contribute to a better understanding of pathogenesis and the underlying causes of chronic disease, including infection, immune responses, and inflammatory processes. New molecular techniques could enhance the scope for empirical research guided by an "eco-epidemiology paradigm" that encompasses unexplained pathogenesis.[25] Techniques such as genetic recombination and imaging may also contribute to a more complete understanding of diseases, as genetic factors may be involved in some of the differences in people's susceptibility. Advances in DNA-sequencing technology and genomewide association studies have revealed a vast number of common DNA variations linked with the risk of developing common chronic diseases, such as diabetes, heart disease, cancer, and autoimmunity, although most variations identified so far confer only a relatively small incremental risk.[26] Cochran, Ewald, and Cochran suggested that the possibility of infectious causation has tended to be dismissed when genetic or environmental influences are established empirically.[27] Evidence interpreted as indicating genetic causation might in some cases be explained by infectious etiology.[28] Their evolutionary perspective on associations between microorganisms and chronic diseases is consistent with an "eco-epidemiology paradigm" that might be characterized by a blurred distinction between infectious disease and chronic disease.[29]

With new microbiological techniques and resources for research, more of the suspected links between microorganisms and chronic disease may be confirmed as causal. Reconciliation of the biological and social determinants will be required to achieve a more unified understanding of disease and ill health. A more comprehensive understanding of current disease patterns requires determinants and outcomes to be understood at different levels, including microbiological systems of molecules, cells and tissues, physiological systems, single individuals, social groups, societies, populations, and the physical environment. Even considering just the confirmed links between infections and chronic disease, any theory of epidemiological transition will need to encompass microbial, biophysiological, immunological, and genetic processes, as well as environmental, lifestyle, behavioral, sociocultural, and economic factors. Research on the role of microorganisms, infections, immune responses, and inflammatory processes is likely to further enhance understanding of pathogenesis, leading to a more comprehensive understanding of the multifactorial etiology of chronic diseases.

Whether or not an "eco-epidemiology paradigm" supersedes the chronic disease "risk factor paradigm," contemporary disease patterns can be better understood in historical context. This study has considered the emergence of chronic diseases as the predominant causes of death in the context of dramatic long-term changes in the infectious disease environment. The review of changes in disease and mortality has highlighted a new perspective on the epidemiological transition by focusing on the relationship between microorganisms and different forms of acute and chronic disease. The many established and suspected causal links between microorganisms and chronic diseases referred to have implications for any theory of epidemiological transition aimed at understanding, rather than just describing, the process of change in disease and mortality. In the past, both individual-level and public health measures were adopted to prevent acute infectious diseases such as plague, typhus, smallpox, and cholera, long before their causes were understood. The risk of dying from other acute infectious diseases and tuberculosis was reduced through targeted preventive interventions and changes in health-related behavior at the individual and household level. Knowledge about risk factors from recent scientific research has offered opportunities for individuals to reduce the risk of chronic disorders or delay their effects by adopting healthier behaviors and lifestyles. In the future, much research is likely to focus on the role of microorganisms in chronic diseases, which could expand the knowledge base for more effective prevention strategies at the population level.

Challenges for Public Health and Prevention

One of the main conclusions of this review of historical change in disease and mortality is that people have experienced fewer severe infections since the 17th century, and health-related human intervention and behavior change have been the most important factors contributing to the decline in mortality and increased life expectancy. The infectious diseases that killed most people from the 17th century through the 19th century in England were controlled through preventive measures, public health interventions, social organization, and changes in health-related behaviors. Without preventive measures, plague, smallpox, typhus, typhoid, and cholera are unlikely to have become less destructive of life. Although average life expectancy at birth increased more rapidly in the 20th century, it was the virtual elimination of the severest acute infectious diseases that prepared the way for more dramatic improvements in the length and quality of life. From the end of the 19th century, sociodemographic changes, particularly families having fewer children, are likely to have reduced the severity of other airborne infectious diseases such as measles and respiratory infections. New knowledge about the microbial causes of acute infectious diseases and tuberculosis contributed to the development of further measures to restrict rapid transmission and control them. Improvements in personal, domestic, and food hygiene; smaller families; better care of children and the sick; isolation of infectious disease cases; and immunization are likely to have been the main contributors to declining mortality in the first half of the 20th century before the introduction of antibiotics in the 1940s. In the second half of the 20th century, the decline in overall mortality was largely due to reductions in cardiovascular disease, cancer, and respiratory disease mortality, to which preventive strategies, changes in lifestyle, and especially reduced cigarette smoking are likely to have contributed more than treatment measures.

The influences that contributed to mortality decline in England after the last plague epidemic in the 17th century affected all socioeconomic groups, regardless of their economic standard of living and diet, albeit with differences in the timing and the rate of decline. This explanation of mortality decline in terms of health-related interventions and changes in behavior is consistent with the explanation of mortality decline in other industrialized and developing countries in the 20th century (see chapter 1). Preston identified preventive measures in the home as the main cause of improved child survival in the United States in the first few decades of the 20th century, with public health interventions contributing most to reductions in mortality at older ages.[30] Costa concluded that improvements in adult health in the second half of the 20th century could partly reflect reduced exposure to infectious diseases among cohorts who had benefited from improved public health measures and preventative interventions earlier in the century.[31] Increases in life expectancy at birth in developing countries in the 20th century were due mainly to health interventions that had proved successful in Western countries, including safer water, environmental sanitation, health education, basic mother and child health care, and use of antibiotics.[32]

Acute infectious diseases and tuberculosis are still a major problem in many low-income and middle-income countries, and they accounted for 59% of deaths and disability among the world's poorest 20% in 1990.[33] Much of the increasing burden of chronic disease in these countries can be explained by increased cigarette smoking, consumption of unhealthy quantities of saturated fats and sugars, and reduced levels of physical activity when people move to the towns.[34] Low-income countries will not have sufficient resources to provide the costly treatments for chronic diseases, and only a small minority are likely to gain access to such treatments, either in their own country or abroad. The educationally and economically better-off, like their counterparts in industrialized countries, also gain access more quickly to information about prevention and ways of modifying lifestyle and behavior in the interests of health.[35] Governments in all countries face issues of equity in allocating resources to health facilities in urban and rural areas, and the cultural context has to be taken into account in developing locally appropriate health strategies.[36] An increasing burden of chronic disease is affecting all subgroups of the population in countries at different stages of economic development. For example, about 80% of all cardiovascular deaths in 2001 occurred in countries with an annual per capita income of less than US$9,000,[37] and 80% of all chronic diseases usually assumed to be noncommunicable occur in low-income and middle-income countries.[38]

Chronic diseases usually classified as "noncommunicable" now account for about 60% of all deaths worldwide. In England, a relatively high-income country, these diseases account for most deaths from disease, and they place an increasing burden on health-care services and financial resources. In high-income countries in the 20th century, medical interventions and resources were focused more on treatment than on prevention, although many chronic diseases are largely preventable.[39] In the 1970s McKeown challenged the orthodoxy of focusing on curative medicine, pointing out that it had not contributed significantly to the considerable improvement in life expectancy before the 1940s.[40] However, some of his main conclusions about the causes of mortality decline were not evidence based, and he greatly underestimated the role of preventive measures—particularly immunization, changes in health-related behavior, and sociodemographic changes. In the future, treatment costs are likely to be unsustainable given increases in the cost of technological inputs and medicines. A particular concern is the declining proportion of economically active adults to generate resources with which to meet the growing demand for treatment and health care for growing numbers of older people in "aging populations." Based on past experience, strategies to reduce the burden and cost of health care would give more priority to prevention. In high-income countries preventive strategies can focus on health education; promotion of healthier lifestyles; control of pollution; much stronger regulation of the tobacco and food industries in the interests of public health; and measures to reduce poverty, income inequality, and the lack of control many people have in their work situation and life generally. The challenge for health policy makers and responsible agencies is to promote lifestyles, economic activity, and environmental conditions that are conducive to people spending more of their longer lives in good health.

In low-income countries with much more limited resources, most people will not gain access in the foreseeable future to costly treatments for heart disease, cancer, and other chronic diseases currently available to many in high-income countries, making locally appropriate prevention programs a particularly high priority. Reducing the prevalence of major risk factors may be more complex than prevention of the infectious diseases that are still a major challenge in low-income countries. However, the main lifestyle-related risk factors are well established, many are common to different forms of chronic disease, and risks for individuals are similar in all countries.[41] These risks include cigarette smoking and other tobacco use; foods high in saturated fats, trans fats, salt, and sugar (especially sweetened drinks); physical inactivity; and harmful alcohol consumption.[42] Part of the challenge for prevention relates to the difficulty of encouraging people to change behaviors and unhealthy aspects of lifestyle upheld by their local culture and socioeconomic circumstances. Choices over tobacco and alcohol use, diet, and physical activity can be influenced by pressures that are difficult for many individuals to overcome, particularly children and adolescents.[43] While responsibility ultimately lies with adults to adopt healthier lifestyles, it is for governments to invest in education, public health, and prevention programs to enable people to protect their health and that of their children. Governments and international agencies can support the development of healthy lifestyles through training for health professionals, targeted public health programs, and regulation of large-scale commercial activities at the national and international levels in the interests of public health.

Many large-scale commercial organizations fail to take sufficient responsibility for the social consequences of their activities, which poses a threat to public health and people's lives through environmental degradation, the marketing of harmful products, and generation of enormous inequalities in income and wealth that are socially divisive. Evidence suggests that wide income inequality within a country is itself associated with worse health and social indicators.[44] Great disparity in wealth and the social forces that give rise to it can be detrimental to social cohesion, and the adverse effects appear to be greatest among young adults.[45] Together with high unemployment among young adults, this constitutes a threat to social stability as well as to the health and well-being of individuals. A vast amount of research has contributed to knowledge about social and economic determinants of disease and mortality, leading to evidence-based recommendations for achieving greater equity in health.[46] Much of the action required is outside the scope of traditional public health policy.[47] However, public health professionals in collaboration with nongovernmental and international agencies can act to influence broader policies that affect health at the individual and population level. Collaborative action of this kind can be seen as complementing targeted public health interventions.[48] The concept of public health action has broadened to encompass human activities of all kinds that have important health consequences.[49]

The globalized marketing of products that are known to be harmful to the health of consumers poses a particular challenge because of powerful commercial interests. Tobacco and food companies pursue their economic interest in "new susceptibles" becoming dependent on, or addicted to, their products, which kill far more people "prematurely" than do illegal drugs. Many of the cigarette marketing strategies particularly targeting women and young people in developing countries have already been banned in some industrialized countries.[50] Although individual governments can seek to regulate the activities of tobacco companies in their own country, only internationally coordinated action is likely to achieve a proposed target for global prevalence of cigarette smoking of below 5% by 2040.[51] An international treaty, the Framework Convention on Tobacco Control, supports demand reduction and supply-side action by individual countries on advertising, labeling, and other control priorities. Demand can be reduced through taxes on tobacco products, health warnings, mass media antismoking campaigns,[52] smoke-free public places and work environments, and a complete ban on any form of tobacco promotion. Individual governments can take even stronger measures to control currently legal and illicit supply-side activities, depending on the level of political commitment and public support.

In 2008 the World Health Organization published an action plan for prevention and control of chronic diseases conventionally assumed to be noncommunicable diseases (NCD). In addition to tobacco control, four other preventive interventions were prioritized by the Lancet NCD Action Group and the NCD Alliance—salt reduction, improved diets, physical activity, and reduction of hazardous alcohol intake. Beaglehole and colleagues suggested that interventions directed at whole populations, such as tobacco control and reduction of salt in foods, are likely to be pro-poor, reduce inequalities, and bring the greatest benefits.[53] Increases in child and adult obesity in industrialized and developing countries have been linked with the shift to sedentary urban lifestyles and consumption of more processed foods, fat, and sugar.[54] Improvements in food industry practices could have a beneficial impact on future health, and some multinational food corporations have begun to make changes to their product and marketing strategies in the interests of public health and public relations.[55] Governments have an important role in regulation and promotion of fruit and vegetable consumption, foods low in salt, saturated and trans fats, and sugar. Promotion of physical activity, inclusion of obesity prevention in maternal and child health programs, and measures to reduce alcohol-related harm all require commitment by governments to reduce the future burden of chronic disease and associated health-care costs.

Much costly ill health, disability, and "premature death" among adults in industrialized and developing countries is a consequence of conditions in early childhood. Considerable evidence links low birth weight with chronic respiratory and cardiovascular disorders in adulthood; birth injury and asphyxia with neurological, mental, and physical disabilities; and congenital, perinatal, and childhood infections with long-term chronic conditions.[56] Child health interventions such as immunization and preventive measures that could reduce the risk of more than one type of chronic condition will have benefits for adult health. Interventions in developing countries can aim to improve hygiene and sanitation and prevent childhood infections linked with chronic disease in adult life, such as *Helicobacter pylori*, a cause of gastritis, peptic ulcer, and gastric cancer; and Epstein-Barr virus, a causal agent in Burkitt's lymphoma and nasopharyngeal carcinoma. Early detection and treatment of pharyngitis can prevent rheumatic fever, an inflammatory manifestation of group A streptococcal infection, which can lead to rheumatic heart disease, a common cause of cardiovascular deaths among young adults in developing countries. Treatment of syphilis and gonorrhea prevents maternal transmission to infants, thus also avoiding serious disabilities in adult life. Maternal-infant transmission of hepatitis B virus, a cause of liver cancer, is largely preventable through immunization, and effective vaccines against human papillomavirus are available for prevention of cervical cancer.[57]

Immunization has been a highly successful population-level strategy for control of infectious disease worldwide, bringing dramatic reductions in morbidity and mortality from smallpox, measles, whooping cough, diphtheria, poliomyelitis, and other infectious diseases affecting children in particular.[58] A life-course perspective indicates the importance of preventing infections in childhood that can have lifelong effects, as well as other infections contracted in adult life that can contribute to the development of chronic disorders. Many of the major public health advances in the second half of the 20th century were the result of immunization and other measures to prevent acute infections that cause liver cancer, cervical cancer, ulcers, and hepatitis, as well as the childhood epidemic diseases.[59] If the causal role of specific microorganisms in more chronic diseases is established, immunization could become a cost-effective strategy for prevention of chronic diseases and "premature" adult deaths in low-income countries, complementing health education and health promotion to address lifestyle-related risks.

Microorganisms and Epidemiological Transition

Studies of immunization in low-income countries as well as industrialized countries could provide further evidence concerning the role in cardiovascular disease of common respiratory pathogens, including *C. pneumoniae* and *H. influenzae.* So far, there is only limited evidence regarding any protective effect against cardiovascular accidents of vaccination against pneumonia and influenza.[60] However, research has already established that the relationship between influenza and coronary heart disease meets several of Hill's criteria for causality.[61] Clinical trials in different parts of the world could determine whether influenza vaccination provides protection against cardiovascular accidents in those most at risk. Because children are frequently the source of respiratory infections affecting adults, preliminary evidence that vaccinating children against influenza can decrease incidence and mortality from cardiovascular disease among older people warrants further investigation.[62] Vaccination against seasonal and pandemic influenza continues to be important for older adults, particularly those at risk of heart attack and stroke because of underlying cardiovascular disorders.[63] International immunization programs can be expanded to include prevention of influenza, pneumonia, and other respiratory infections linked with chronic disease among adults. BCG vaccination in early childhood may be cost-effective for prevention of some childhood cancers in populations where it is effective in preventing tuberculosis. Vaccines, antimicrobials, and hygiene improvements could become the most effective measures for the control of some chronic diseases. Ewald suggested that programs would need to take into account the evolutionary ecology of causative microorganisms and problems of resistance, directing the evolution of pathogens toward milder forms rather than seeking to decimate harmful ones that are difficult to eradicate.[64]

The infectious disease environment continues to have a hugely detrimental and costly effect on human health globally. Some infectious diseases have resisted control, in some cases due to antibiotic resistance, and many new ones such as Lyme disease, Ebola fever, and severe acute respiratory syndrome (SARS) have emerged.[65] Antibiotic use, effectiveness, and resistance will be an important consideration in developing appropriate treatment and prevention strategies.[66] This study has emphasized that common microorganisms, infections, related immune responses, and inflammatory processes contribute significantly to the development of many chronic diseases. The evidence relates to various cancers, heart disease, cerebrovascular disease, peptic ulcer, diabetes, diseases of the liver and kidneys, and many other chronic diseases. Other well-established risk factors for morbidity and mortality are common to the different forms of chronic disease that are replacing acute infectious diseases as the main causes of death worldwide. Behavioral and lifestyle-related risk factors contribute to the development of the underlying biophysiological disorders along with environmental agents, including microorganisms.

The original concept of "epidemiologic transition" oversimplified the changing pattern of disease and cause of death, by viewing it as a replacement of one category of predominant diseases (infectious) by another category of supposedly unconnected diseases ("degenerative"). Later characterizations of the transition in terms of a shift from communicable diseases to diseases assumed to be noncommunicable, or from infectious diseases to chronic diseases, have also assumed the categories were distinct. This does not take into account the many interrelationships between infectious diseases, between infections and chronic diseases, and between the chronic disorders themselves. In the light of many established and suspected links between microbial infection and chronic diseases, Omran's "theory of epidemiologic transition" appears simplistic and descriptive, although he focused attention on an extremely important global phenomenon. The evidence presented here confirms the basic components of the transition—a shift in age at death from children and young adults to older adults, increased average life expectancy, "aging populations," and acute infectious diseases being superseded by chronic diseases as the main causes of death. However, this study has highlighted another dimension of epidemiological transition based on evidence of ecological and statistical associations between diseases and the findings of many clinical, observational, and epidemiological studies linking specific microorganisms, immune responses, and inflammatory processes with chronic diseases. Any theory of epidemiological transition needs to encompass the role of microorganisms in the pathogenic processes underlying chronic disease, as well as other environmental, lifestyle-related, behavioral, sociocultural, and economic factors. Without this perspective, the concept of epidemiological transition can be a misleading descriptive framework for assessing change in disease and mortality that does not reflect the interrelated nature of disease.

In the long-term historical context in which human beings are adapting to an urban way of life and a changing infectious disease environment, with old infections reemerging and new ones emerging,[67] the potential for rapid global transmission and the emergence of chronic diseases have brought new challenges for public health, prevention, and health care. With the growing proportion of older people due to longer lives and "population aging," and an increasing burden of chronic disease, the majority of people in low-income countries will not gain access in the foreseeable future to costly treatments provided in industrialized countries. Even in relatively high-income countries, the increasing burden of chronic disease is likely to make equitable provision unattainable. Past experience and future projections indicate the need to focus more on public health and prevention strategies. The science of epidemiology, which generates the knowledge base for public health, can inform both the general public and policy makers about the effects on the health of individuals and populations of changing social, economic, environmental, and ecological circumstances. Collaboration between different disciplines and coordination of epidemiological and microbiological research will be required to achieve a more complete understanding of the pathogenesis and the multifactorial etiology of chronic diseases. In particular, the many suspected links between infection and the underlying chronic disorders require further investigation. Depending on any specific microorganisms confirmed as causal agents in chronic disease, and the significance of infection relative to other environmental, economic, occupational, social, cultural, behavioral, and lifestyle-related determinants of disease, appropriate population-level prevention strategies can be developed. Whatever new findings emerge, the infectious disease environment will continue to be a significant ecological determinant of health, disease, and mortality in industrialized countries and in developing countries undergoing the epidemiological transition from acute infectious disease to chronic disease.

Appendix A

Disease Classification Codes

Data for 1901–2000 were extracted from the CD-ROM dataset *Twentieth Century Mortality* produced by the Office for National Statistics (ONS) of the UK Statistics Authority. The codes of the International Classification of Diseases (ICD) included in different categories of disease are shown below using the numbering system from the CD-ROM. The ICD is the standard diagnostic tool for epidemiology, health management, and clinical purposes. The first classification (ICD-1) was introduced in 1900, and the 10th revision (ICD-10) was endorsed by the World Health Assembly in May 1990 and came into use in World Health Organization (WHO) member states in 1994. The WHO periodically updates a manual for using the classification system (see bibliography for the latest edition.

ICD codes included in the cardiovascular category were those specified for examining trends in the ONS publication *Health Statistics Quarterly* 18 (Summer 2003). Hemiplegia/other paralysis was also included under cerebrovascular disease, which is consistent with its inclusion under stroke in a study of comparability over time published by the Centers for Disease Control and Prevention in the United States (www.cdc.gov/nchs/data/statab/comp2.pdf). The codes included in the cancer category were those for malignant neoplasms (including neoplasms of the lymphatic and hematopoietic tissues) under ICD-6 and later ICD revisions (see www.wolfbane.com/icd/index.html). The codes used for the respiratory disease category were those recommended in the above ONS publication. Data prior to 1901 were extracted from the Registrar General's *Annual Report for England and Wales* using the disease categories listed below.

All cardiovascular disease:

1881–1900		Circulatory diseases, chorea, apoplexy, hemiplegia, softening of the brain
1901–1910	ICD-1	63, 64, 87, 99–113
1911–1920	ICD-2	47, 64–66, 72, 77–85, 189A
1921–1930	ICD-3	51, 74, 75, 81, 83, 87–96, 205 (1)
1931–1939	ICD-4	56, 82, 87a, 90–97, 99–103, 200 (1)
1940–1949	ICD-5	58, 83, 87a, 90–97, 99–103, 200a (1)
1950–1957	ICD-6	330–34, 400–454, 456–68, 782
1958–1967	ICD-7	330–34, 400–454, 456–68, 782

1968–1978	ICD-8	390–438, 440–44.1, 444.4–458, 782
1979–2000	ICD-9	390–438, 440–59

Cerebrovascular disease:

1881–1900		Apoplexy, hemiplegia, softening of the brain
1901–1910	ICD-1	84, 106, 107
1911–1920	ICD-2	64–66, 82a
1921–1930	ICD-3	74, 75, 83, 91b(1)
1931–1939	ICD-4	82, 97(1), 97(2)
1940–1949	ICD-5	83
1950–1957	ICD-6	330–34
1958–1967	ICD-7	330–34
1968–1978	ICD-8	430–38
1979–2000	ICD-9	430–38

Cancer (malignant neoplasms):

1848–1880		Cancer
1881–1900		Cancer
1901–1910	ICD-1	68–70
1911–1920	ICD-2	39–45, 53
1921–1930	ICD-3	43–49, 65
1931–1939	ICD-4	45–53, 72
1940–1949	ICD-5	44b, 45–55, 74
1950–1957	ICD-6	140–205
1958–1967	ICD-7	140–205
1968–1978	ICD-8	140–209
1979–2000	ICD-9	140–208

Respiratory disease:

1848–1880		Diseases of the respiratory organs, influenza
1881–1900		Diseases of the respiratory system, influenza
1901–1910	ICD-1	12, 36–39, 118–22
1911–1920	ICD-2	10, 86–87, 89–98, 100
1921–1930	ICD-3	11, 97–107, 109
1931–1939	ICD-4	11, 104–14, 115(3)
1940–1949	ICD-5	33, 104–14, 115b–d
1950–1957	ICD-6	240, 241, 470–527
1958–1967	ICD-7	240, 241, 470–527
1968–1978	ICD-8	460–519
1979–2000	ICD-9	460–519

Respiratory tuberculosis:

1848–1880		Phthisis
1881–1900		Phthisis
1901–1910	ICD-1	46–47
1911–1920	ICD-2	28–29
1921–1930	ICD-3	31
1931–1939	ICD-4	23
1940–1949	ICD-5	13a, b
1950–1957	ICD-6	1–8
1958–1967	ICD-7	1–8
1968–1978	ICD-8	10–12
1979–2000	ICD-9	10–12

Nonrespiratory tuberculosis:

1848–1880		Tabes mesenterica, hydrocephalus, scrofula
1881–1900		Tubercular meningitis, tabes mesenterica, other TB
1901–1910	ICD-1	48–54
1911–1920	ICD-2	30–35
1921–1930	ICD-3	32–37
1931–1939	ICD-4	24–32
1940–1949	ICD-5	13c, 14–22
1950–1957	ICD-6	10–19
1958–1967	ICD-7	10–19
1968–1978	ICD-8	13–19
1979–2000	ICD-9	13–18

Nephritis:

1875–1880		Nephritis, nephria (Bright's disease)
1881–1900		Acute nephritis, Bright's disease
1901–1910	ICD-1	143–44
1911–1920	ICD-2	119–20
1921–1930	ICD-3	128–29
1931–1939	ICD-4	130–32
1940–1949	ICD-5	130–32
1950–1957	ICD-6	590–94
1958–1967	ICD-7	590–94
1968–1978	ICD-8	580–84
1979–2000	ICD-9	580–89

Cirrhosis of the liver:

1875–1880		Cirrhosis of the liver
1881–1900		Cirrhosis of the liver
1901–1910	ICD-1	136
1911–1920	ICD-2	113a, b
1921–1930	ICD-3	122
1931–1939	ICD-4	124
1940–1949	ICD-5	124
1950–1957	ICD-6	581
1958–1967	ICD-7	581
1968–1978	ICD-8	571
1979–2000	ICD-9	571

Diabetes mellitus:

1875–1880		Diabetes
1881–1900		Diabetes mellitus
1901–1910	ICD-1	75
1911–1920	ICD-2	50
1921–1930	ICD-3	57
1931–1939	ICD-4	59
1940–1949	ICD-5	61
1950–1957	ICD-6	260
1958–1967	ICD-7	260
1968–1978	ICD-8	250
1979–2000	ICD-9	250

Peptic ulcer:

1901–1910	ICD-1	125
1911–1920	ICD-2	102
1921–1930	ICD-3	111
1931–1939	ICD-4	117
1940–1949	ICD-5	117
1950–1957	ICD-6	540–41
1958–1967	ICD-7	540–41
1968–1978	ICD-8	431–533
1979–2000	ICD-9	531–533

Appendix B

Number of Deaths in Carlisle by Recorded Cause and Age in 1779–87

	Age in years					
Cause of death	0–4	5–19	20–49	50+	All	%
Infant causes	217	—	—	—	217	13.5
Measles	28	3	—	—	31	1.9
Whooping cough	18	1	—	—	19	1.2
Scarlet fever	31	7	1	—	39	2.4
Thrush	63	2	—	—	65	4.0
Smallpox	225	10	3	—	238	14.7
Fevers	29	23	49	33	134	8.3
Jail fever (typhus)	4	5	5	—	14	0.9
Jaundice	3	—	6	4	13	0.8
Venereal disease	—	—	2	—	2	0.1
Consumption	34	40	110	30	214	13.3
Dropsy	3	9	13	29	54	3.3
Pleurisy	3	4	3	9	19	1.2
Asthma	1	—	2	24	27	1.7
Looseness	7	3	4	5	19	1.2
Indigestion	—	—	7	14	21	1.3
Stones	—	—	2	7	9	0.6
Cancer	—	—	—	5	5	0.3
Rheumatism	—	—	—	6	6	0.4
Gout	—	—	1	3	4	0.2
Apoplexy	—	1	7	24	32	2.0
Palsy	—	—	1	13	14	0.9
Fainting	—	1	3	2	6	0.4
Epilepsy	—	1	2	1	4	0.2

(continued)

	Age in years					
Cause of death	0–4	5–19	20–49	50+	All	%
Difficult delivery	—	—	9	—	9	0.6
Accidents	7	11	9	2	29	1.8
Old age	—	—	—	226	226	14.0
Other/unknown	36	21	29	59	145	9.0
Total	709	142	268	496	1,615	100.0
% of total	43.9	8.8	16.6	30.7	100.0	

Source: Lonsdale, *Life of John Heysham MD.*
Note: Lonsdale found data for 1780 were missing.

Appendix C1

Contribution of Changes in Cause-Specific Death Rates to Change in Total Death Rate, 1751–2000

	Contribution to unit change in death rate from all causes			
	London	England and Wales		
Cause of death	1751–1800	1851–1900	1901–50	1951–2000
Measles		–0.013	–0.026	–0.002
Whooping cough		–0.023	–0.029	–0.001
Scarlet fever and diphtheria		–0.124	–0.038	–0.001
Cholera, diarrhea, dysentery		–0.120	–0.092	–0.058
Nonrespiratory tuberculosis		–0.043	–0.047	–0.009
Diabetes mellitus		0.014	–0.005	–0.005
Peptic ulcers		N/A	0.003	–0.014
Liver cirrhosis		–0.004	–0.019	0.000
Nephritis		0.071	–0.028	–0.018
Other kidney/urinary		–0.010	–0.006	–0.006
Nervous diseases		–0.002	–0.021	–0.008
Respiratory disease		0.104	–0.174	–0.146
Cerebrovascular diseases		–0.018	–0.009	–0.121
Heart and other circulatory diseases		0.199	0.040	–0.356
Cancer (malignant neoplasms)		0.110	0.023	–0.152

(continued)

	Contribution to unit change in death rate from all causes			
	London	England and Wales		
Cause of death	1751–1800	1851–1900	1901–50	1951–2000
Congenital/immature/ perinatal		0.026	–0.124	–0.008
Fevers (typhoid/typhus)	–0.250	–0.170	–0.015	0.000
Consumption	–0.091	–0.333	–0.099	–0.049
Smallpox	–0.084	–0.052	–0.001	0.000
Convulsions/ teething	–0.399	–0.139	–0.061	0.000
Childbirth/ pregnancy	–0.005	–0.012	–0.005	–0.003
Old age, senility	–0.090	–0.106	–0.080	–0.011
Accidents/ violence	–0.006	–0.025	–0.028	–0.061
Other causes	–0.077	–0.330	–0.160	0.028
All causes	1.0	1.0	1.0	1.0

Sources: London Bills of Mortality data from Marshall, *Mortality in the Metropolis*; Registrar General, *Annual Reports, Annual Statistical Reviews*; Office of Population Censuses and Surveys, *Mortality Statistics, Series DH2*, 2001.
Note: Death rates for England and Wales standardized for age and sex to population in 1901 (actual death rates shown in appendixes C2 and C3).

Appendix C2

Annual Average Cause-Specific Death Rates in London and Percentage Contribution to Overall Mortality, 1746–55 and 1796–1805

	1746–55		1796–1805	
Category of deaths	Death rate per million	% of total	Death rate per million	% of total
Fevers/typhoid/typhus	570	15.2	266	10.5
Consumption	700	18.7	590	23.3
Smallpox	322	8.6	220	8.7
Convulsions/"infancy"	978	26.1	493	19.4
Childbirth/pregnancy	31	0.8	26	1.0
Old age/senility	298	7.9	189	7.4
Accidents/violence	42	1.1	35	1.4
Other causes	811	21.6	717	28.3
All causes	3,752	100.0	2,536	100.0

Sources: London Bills of Mortality data from Marshall, *Mortality in the Metropolis*.

Appendix C3

Age-and-Sex-Standardized Death Rates for England and Wales, 1848–54, 1901, 1951, and 2001

	Deaths per million			
Cause of death	1848–54	1901	1951	2001
Measles	342	278	7	0
Whooping cough	423	312	7	0.5
Scarlet fever and diphtheria	1,016	407	2	0
Cholera, diarrhea, dysentery	1,819	1,232	259	2
Nonrespiratory tuberculosis	753	544	42	0.2
Diabetes mellitus	24	91	42	19
Peptic ulcers	N/A	47	75	12
Liver disease	239	220	18	15
Kidney/urinary disease	184	482	118	7
Nervous diseases	316	305	87	51
Respiratory disease	2,239	2,747	906	259
Cerebrovascular diseases	890	803	710	174
Heart and other circulatory	698	1,673	2,098	517
Cancer (malignant neoplasms)	307	844	1,083	406
Congenital/premature/perinatal	1,249	1,375	64	28
Typhoid/typhus (Fevers)	990	155	0	0
Respiratory TB (Consumption)	2,901	1,268	218	1
Smallpox	263	10	0	0
Convulsions/teething	1,322	643	0	0
Childbirth/pregnancy	130	71	13	0
Old age, senility	1,447	930	83	32

(continued)

	Deaths per million			
Cause of death	1848–54	1901	1951	2001
Accidents/violence	761	640	341	69
Other causes	3,543	1,881	187	321
All causes	21,856	16,958	6,360	1,914

Sources: Registrar General, *Annual Reports*; *Statistical Reviews*; Office of Population Censuses and Surveys, *Mortality Statistics, Series DH2,* 2001.
N/A= not available.
* Age-and-sex-specific death rates applied to the age structure of the England and Wales population (persons) in 1901.

Appendix C4

Death Rates in England and Wales, and Cause-Specific Death Rates as Percentage of Total Death Rate, 1848–54, 1901, 1951, and 2001

	1848–54		1901		1951		2001	
Cause of death	Death rate	% of total	Death rate	% of total	Death rate	% of total	Death rate	% of total
Measles	389	1.7	278	1.6	7	0.0	0	0.0
Whooping cough	487	2.1	312	1.8	13	0.1	0	0.0
Scarlet fever and diphtheria	902	3.9	407	2.4	2	0.0	0	0.0
Cholera, diarrhea, dysentery	897	3.9	1,232	7.3	64	0.5	0	0.0
Nonrespiratory tuberculosis	837	3.7	544	3.2	40	0.3	2	0.0
Diabetes mellitus	23	0.1	91	0.5	85	0.7	117	1.2
Peptic ulcers	N/A	N/A	47	0.3	128	1.0	73	0.7
Liver disease	211	0.9	220	1.3	30	0.2	116	1.1
Kidney/urinary disease	195	0.8	482	2.8	200	1.6	147	1.4
Nervous diseases	971	4.2	305	1.8	136	1.1	273	2.7
Respiratory disease	2,833	12.4	2,747	16.2	1,839	14.6	1,285	12.7
Cerebrovascular diseases	448	1.9	803	4.7	1,562	12.4	1,116	11.0
Heart and other circulatory	665	2.9	1,673	9.9	4,493	35.6	2,924	28.9
Cancer (malignant neoplasms)	293	1.3	844	5.0	1,965	15.6	2,654	26.2
Congenital/ premature/ perinatal	1,063	4.6	1,375	8.1	412	3.3	28	0.3

(continued)

Cause of death	1848–54 Death rate	1848–54 % of total	1901 Death rate	1901 % of total	1951 Death rate	1951 % of total	2001 Death rate	2001 % of total
Typhoid/typhus (fevers)	995	4.4	155	0.9	0	0.0	0	0.0
Respiratory TB (consumption)	2,825	12.4	1,268	7.5	275	2.2	5	0.0
Smallpox	291	1.3	10	0.1	0	0.0	0	0.0
Convulsions/ teething	1,339	5.9	643	3.8	1	0.0	0	0.0
Childbirth/ pregnancy	122	0.5	71	0.4	13	0.1	1	0.0
Old age/senility	1,486	6.5	930	5.5	217	1.7	227	2.2
Accidents/violence	788	3.4	640	3.8	458	3.6	316	3.1
Other causes	4,809	21.0	1,881	11.1	693	5.5	831	8.2
All causes	22,869	100.0	16,958	100.0	12,633	100.0	10,115	100.0

Sources: Registrar General, *Annual Reports*; *Statistical Reviews*; Office of Population Censuses and Surveys, *Mortality Statistics, Series DH2,* 2001.
N/A = not available.

Appendix C5

Infant Mortality Rates for Main Causes in England and Wales, 1851, 1901, and 1951, and Contributions to Change in Overall Infant Mortality, 1901–51

	Infant deaths per 1,000 births			Contribution to unit of change
Cause of death	1851*	1901	1951	1901–51
Smallpox	2.2	0.0	0.0	0.00
Scarlet fever	1.8	0.2	0.0	–0.00
Whooping cough	5.9	5.2	0.4	–0.04
Diphtheria	0.0	0.5	0.0	–0.00
Measles	2.1	2.2	0.1	–0.02
Syphilis	0.6	1.2	0.0	–0.01
Nonrespiratory TB	7.6	10.2	0.1	–0.08
Respiratory TB	2.7	0.4	0.0	–0.00
Respiratory disease	20.0	23.7	4.7	–0.16
Convulsions/teething	36.6	18.9	0.0	–0.16
Gastroenteritis and diarrheal diseases	15.1	21.3	1.3	–0.16
Prematurity/debility, atrophy/ congenital	38.8	43.9	0.8	–0.35
Accidents/violence	9.9	2.5	2.3	–0.00
All causes	155.3	151.3	29.8	–1.00

Source: Registrar General, *Annual Reports; Statistical Reviews.*
* An average of the years 1848–54 to allow for epidemic fluctuations.

Appendix DI

Contribution of Age-Specific Death Rates to Overall Age-and-Sex-Standardized Death Rate in England and Wales between 1846–50 and 1996–2000

	Age-and-sex-standardized death rates per 1,000			
Ages (years)	1846–50	1896–1900	1946–50	1996–2000
<1	4.54	4.41	0.88	0.13
1–4	3.34	2.12	0.16	0.02
5–9	1.00	0.44	0.08	0.01
10–14	0.57	0.24	0.06	0.02
15–19	0.77	0.34	0.11	0.05
20–24	0.94	0.43	0.16	0.05
25–34	1.76	0.97	0.30	0.11
35–44	1.68	1.24	0.36	0.15
45–54	1.62	1.45	0.62	0.29
55–64	1.88	1.83	1.02	0.54
65–74	2.19	2.09	1.39	0.85
75+	2.03	1.80	1.44	1.09
All ages	22.31	17.37	6.59	3.30

Sources: Registrar General, *Annual Reports*; *Statistical Reviews*; Office of Population Censuses and Surveys, *Mortality Statistics, Series DH2*, 2001.

Appendix D2

Contribution of Age-Specific Death Rates to Changes in Overall Age-and-Sex-Standardized Death Rate in England and Wales, 1850–99, 1900–1949, and 1950–99

	Contribution to change in death rate			% contribution to decline in death rate		
Ages in Years	1850–99	1900–1949	1950–99	1850–99	1900–1949	1950–99
<1	–0.13	–3.53	–0.75	2.7	32.7	22.9
1–4	–1.22	–1.96	–0.14	24.7	18.2	4.1
5–9	–0.56	–0.36	–0.07	11.3	3.4	2.1
10–14	–0.33	–0.18	–0.05	6.6	1.7	1.4
15–19	–0.42	–0.23	–0.07	8.6	2.1	2.1
20–24	–0.51	–0.27	–0.10	10.3	2.5	3.2
25–34	–0.78	–0.68	–0.19	15.8	6.3	5.9
35–44	–0.44	–0.88	–0.20	8.9	8.2	6.2
45–54	–0.17	–0.83	–0.33	3.3	7.7	10.1
55–64	–0.05	–0.80	–0.49	1.0	7.4	14.9
65–74	–0.10	–0.70	–0.54	2.1	6.5	16.5
75+	–0.23	–0.36	–0.36	4.7	3.3	10.9
Total change	–4.94	–10.78	–3.28	100	100	100

Sources: Registrar General, *Annual Reports*; *Statistical Reviews*; Office of Population Censuses and Surveys, *Mortality Statistics, Series DH2*, 2001.

Appendix E

Main Causes of Death in England and Wales in 2010 and Percentage Contribution to Overall Death Rate

Main causes of death	Male deaths	% of all deaths	Female deaths	% of all deaths
Infectious and parasitic diseases	2,284	1.0	2,753	1.1
Malignant neoplasms	72,734	30.6	65,530	25.7
Other neoplasms	1,533	0.6	1,649	0.6
Diabetes mellitus	2,393	1.0	2,830	1.1
Mental and behavioral disorders	6,299	2.6	13,617	5.3
Diseases of the nervous system	8,551	3.6	9,932	3.9
Cardiovascular diseases	77,260	32.5	80.824	31.7
Respiratory diseases	31,563	13.3	35,713	14.0
Gastric and duodenal ulcer	1,230	0.5	1,286	0.5
Chronic liver disease and cirrhosis	4,724	2.0	2,779	1.1
Other diseases of the digestive system	6,210	2.6	9,433	3.7
Kidney disease	1,608	0.7	2,041	0.8
Urinary tract infection (site not specified)	3,285	1.4	5,472	2.1
External causes (accidents, suicide, violence)	10,545	4.4	6,656	2.6
Other causes	7,697	3.2	14,811	5.8
All causes	237,916	100	255,326	100

Source: Office for National Statistics, UK Statistics Authority, *Mortality Statistics, Series DR, 2010.*

Appendix F

Life Expectancy in England and Wales at 50-Year Intervals between 1851 and 2001

	Life expectancy in years at different ages			
Age	1851	1901	1951	2001
0	40.4	46.3	66.4	76.0
1	48.0	55.0	68.7	76.4
5	55.0	59.7	69.0	76.5
10	57.2	60.7	69.2	76.5
25	61.2	62.9	70.0	77.0
45	67.9	67.7	71.5	78.0
65	75.8	75.6	76.7	81.1

Sources: Office for National Statistics, "Report: Decennial Life Tables," 110.

Notes

Introduction

1. Omran, "The epidemiologic transition." Omran first outlined his "theory" of transition in this paper in 1971.

2. Barrett et al., "Emerging and re-emerging infectious diseases"; Harper and Armelagos, "Changing disease-scape."

3. Caldwell, "Population health in transition"; Omran, "Epidemiologic transition."

4. Derrick, "Changes in generation mortality"; Kermack, McKendrick, and McKinlay, "Death rates in Great Britain and Sweden"; Jones, "Aging, disease and life expectancy."

5. See Lynch and Smith, "Life course approach to chronic disease epidemiology."

6. Barrett et al., "Emerging and re-emerging infectious diseases."

7. Ewald, *Plague Time.*

8. Susser and Susser, "Choosing a future for epidemiology," pts. 1–2.

9. Kirk, "Demographic transition theory"; Lee, "Demographic transition."

10. Kirk, "Demographic transition theory," 384.

11. Caldwell and Caldwell, "What have we learnt?," 3; Caldwell, "Health transition," 125.

12. Fogel, "Disparities in chronic disease." The percentages have been calculated using data in his table 1, which shows the percentage of the eligible cohorts in five-year age groups (16–39) examined and the percentage of examinees rejected.

13. Costa, "Understanding the twentieth-century decline."

14. Fogel and Costa, "A theory of technophysio evolution."

15. Fogel, "Disparities in chronic disease."

16. Riley, *Sickness, Recovery and Death*, 188–89.

17. Riley, *Sick, Not Dead*, 11–12.

18. Riley analyzed data from friendly societies, which were nonprofit organizations providing sickness benefits for working people funded by collection of premiums. In the period 1896–1919, respiratory diseases accounted for 22% of sickness episodes among men in three friendly societies, compared with 17% of deaths in England and Wales. Tuberculosis, the cause of about 14% of deaths, was not recoded as a cause of sickness, which may reflect stigma and possible loss of employment if the diagnosis were divulged. Accidents accounted for a much higher proportion of sickness (16%) than deaths (5%), while rheumatism and lumbago were significant causes of sickness (7%) but not causes of death. Riley, *Sick, Not Dead*, 192.

19. Schofield and Reher, "Decline of mortality in Europe," 3–4; Caselli, "Health transition and cause-specific mortality."

20. Szreter and Mooney, "Urbanization, mortality and standard of living," 88.

21. Wrigley and Schofield, *Population History of England*, 531–35.

22. Brownlee, "History of birth and death rates"; Griffith, *Population Problems*; Loschky, "Urbanisation and England's eighteenth-century crude birth and death rates."

23. Jacob et al., "Acute forms of tuberculosis."

24. Morens et al, "Emerging and re-emerging infectious diseases," 242.

25. Up to the end of 2011, there had been 20,458 deaths among HIV-infected persons in the United Kingdom, with an average of 561 per year between 2001 and 2010. It is likely that there were other deaths among people who were not known to be HIV-infected. A total of 122,228 people had been diagnosed as HIV-infected up to the end of 2011, with 27,548 diagnosed as having AIDS. Health Protection Agency, *HIV in the United Kingdom*, 25.

26. Schofield and Reher, "Decline of mortality in Europe," 2–4.

Chapter One

1. Ütterström, "Population problems in pre-industrial Sweden"; Chambers, "The Vale of Trent, 1670–1800."

2. McNeill, *Plagues and Peoples*. 40–81.

3. McKeown and Record, "Reasons for the decline in mortality"; McKeown, *Modern Rise of Population*, 138, 142, 153–54, 159.

4. Omran, "The epidemiologic transition."

5. Fogel, *Long-Term Trends in Health and Longevity*, 42, 67–68, 82.

6. McKeown, *Modern Rise of Population*, 138, 142, 153–54, 159. McKeown acknowledged the lack of evidence of an improvement in diet, in "Fertility, mortality and causes of death."

7. Szreter, "Population health approach in historical perspective," 428.

8. McKeown, *Modern Rise of Population*, 134–42.

9. Anonymous, "Pathogenesis of measles."

10. Newberne and Williams, "Nutritional influences on infections"; Keusch, "History of nutrition."

11. Lunn, "Nutrition, immunity and infection"; Floud, "Medicine and the decline of mortality."

12. An early study by Krause, "English fertility and mortality," suggested that the standard of living may have deteriorated between 1720 and 1821. See also Woods and Woodward, "Mortality, poverty and the environment," 31–32; Szreter, "Urbanization, mortality, and standard of living," 110.

13. Riley, *Sick, Not Dead*, 262.

14. Szreter, "Economic growth, disruption, deprivation, disease and death."

15. Szreter, "Population health approach in historical perspective," 423–24.

16. Ibid., 427–28; Szreter, "Rethinking McKeown."

17. Easterlin, "How beneficent is the market?," 15–16, 45–46.

18. Fogel, "Trends in life expectation and chronic diseases"; *Escape from Hunger and Premature Death*, 21; Fogel and Costa, "A theory of technophysio evolution," 49.

19. Fogel, *Escape from Hunger and Premature Death*, 18.

20. Fogel, *Long-Term Trends in Health and Longevity*, 80–82.

21. Ibid., 9, 67.

22. Ibid., 67–68, 107; Fogel, *Escape from Hunger and Premature Death*, 46.

23. Caldwell, "Mortality in relation to economic development."

24. Preston, "Mortality and level of economic development," 486. See also, for example, Wyon and Gordon, *Khanna Study*.

25. Caldwell, Reddy, and Caldwell, "Social component of mortality decline."

26. Langford, "Reasons for the decline in mortality in Sri Lanka."

27. Arriaga and Davis, "Pattern of mortality change in Latin America."

28. Mandle, "Decline in mortality in British Guyana."

29. Preston, "Causes and consequences of mortality declines," 297–98.

30. Cook and Borah, *Mexico and the Caribbean*, 409–35.

31. Diaz-Briquets, "Determinants of mortality transition in developing countries."

32. Caldwell, "Health transition," 126.

33. Ratcliffe, "Social justice and the demographic transition."

34. Caldwell, "Routes to low mortality in poor countries"; Caldwell, "Health transition," 126.

35. Caldwell, "Routes to low mortality in poor countries"; Caldwell, "Health transition"; Cleland and van Ginneken, "Maternal education and child survival"; Caldwell and Caldwell, "What have we learnt?," 5.

36. Caldwell, "Health transition," 126.

37. Gwatkin, "Poverty and inequalities in health."

38. Ibid., 219. See also Gwatkin and Guillot, *Burden of Disease*; Gwatkin, Guillot, and Heuveline, "Burden of disease"; Murray and Lopez, *Global Burden of Disease*.

39. Gwatkin, "Poverty and inequalities in health," 228.

40. Ibid., 230.

41. World Health Organization, *World Health Report 1999*, 19, 114. Poverty was defined as income per capita of less than or equal to one dollar per day, expressed in dollars adjusted for purchasing power.

42. Gwatkin, "Poverty and inequalities in health," 223–24.

43. Leon, "Common threads," 59; Preston, *Mortality Patterns in National Populations*.

44. Caldwell, "Health transition," 131–32; Mensch, Lentzner, and Preston, *Socioeconomic Differentials in Child Mortality*, 19–56, 290.

45. Orubuloye and Caldwell, "Impact of public health services"; Caldwell, "Education as a factor in mortality decline."

46. Cleland and van Ginneken, "Maternal education and child survival," 1363.

47. Caldwell, "Major new evidence on health transition," 227.

48. Pritchett and Summers, "Wealthier is healthier."

49. Preston, *Mortality Patterns in National Populations*.

50. Riley reached a similar conclusion in *Rising Life Expectancy*, suggesting that maternal education and basic public health and medical services, including safe water, immunization, and medications, had played a major role in reducing child death rates in developing countries in the second half of the twentieth century.

51. Preston, "Mortality and level of economic development."

52. Ibid.; Preston, *Mortality Patterns in National Populations*; Szreter, "Importance of social intervention," 3–4.

53. Preston, "Mortality and level of economic development"; Preston and Haines, *Fatal Years*.

54. Caldwell, "Health transition," 131.

55. Preston and Haines, *Fatal Years*, 177–87.
56. Ewbank and Preston, "Personal health behaviour."
57. Riley, *Eighteenth-Century Campaign to Avoid Disease*, 29, 55.
58. Ibid.
59. Razzell, "Modern rise of population in Europe."
60. Riley, *Eighteenth-Century Campaign to Avoid Disease*, 133.
61. Woodward, "Medicine and the city," 72.
62. Cherry, "Hospitals and population growth," pt. 2, 252, 265.
63. Woodward, "Medicine and the city."
64. McKeown and Brown, "Medical evidence related to English population changes"; McKeown and Record, "Reasons for the decline in mortality"; McKeown, Record, and Turner, "Interpretation of the decline in mortality"; McKeown, *Modern Rise of Population*, 91–109, 149–50; *Role of Medicine*.
65. Only about 0.3% of deaths were recorded as due to syphilis in the Registrar General's *Annual Report* (1851–1920) and *Statistical Review* (1921–51). The number of annual deaths reached a peak of 2,313 in 1883, when 1,912 (82.7%) deaths were at ages under 2 years and 290 (12.5%) at ages 25–64. An unknown proportion of adult deaths involving syphilis may have been recorded in ill-defined or other categories.
66. Mercer, "Smallpox and epidemiological-demographic change."
67. McKeown, *Modern Rise of Population*, 107–8, 153.
68. Ibid., 72.
69. Great Britain, Royal Commission on Vaccination, *Report of the Royal Commission on Vaccination: 1889*.
70. Cartwright, *Social History of Medicine*, 138–39.
71. Ibid., 140.
72. Riley, *Sickness, Recovery and Death*, 161–71.
73. Howe, *Man, Environment and Disease in Britain*.
74. See Anderson and May, "Population biology of infectious diseases"; Anderson, "Transmission dynamics and control" and other chapters in Anderson and May, *Population Biology of Infectious Diseases*.
75. For a discussion of the double burden of infectious and chronic disease in developing countries see Boutayeb, "Communicable and non-communicable diseases."

Chapter Two

1. Omran, "The epidemiologic transition." Omran's paper was reprinted in 2005 as "The epidemiologic transition: A theory of the epidemiology of population change."
2. McKeown, "Epidemiologic transition," 7.
3. Omran, "The epidemiologic transition."
4. Omran, "Epidemiologic transition theory"; Weisz and Olszynko-Gryn, "Theory of epidemiologic transition," 308, 313–14.
5. Caldwell, "Population health in transition"; McKeown, "Epidemiologic transition," 8.

6. Mackenbach, "Epidemiologic transition theory," 330.

7. Pearson, "Education and income," S2-158–S2-160.

8. Mackenbach, "Epidemiologic transition theory."

9. See Townsend and Davidson, *Inequalities in Health*; Great Britain, Department of Health and Social Security, *Inequalities in Health.*

10. Mackenbach, "Epidemiologic transition theory," 330.

11. Gaylin and Kates, "Refocusing the lens," 615–16; Barrett et al., "Emerging and re-emerging infectious diseases"; Caldwell, "Population health in transition."

12. Vallin, "Commentary," 385.

13. Garrett, *Coming Plague*, 415; Gaylin and Kates, "Refocusing the lens," 615.

14. Olshansky and Ault, "Fourth stage of the epidemiologic transition," 356.

15. Ibid.

16. Gaziano, "Fifth phase of epidemiologic transition."

17. McMichael, "Population, environment, disease, and survival."

18. Vallin and Meslé, "Convergences and divergences in mortality"; Sanders et al., "Epidemiological transition"; Harper and Armelagos, "Changing disease-scape."

19. Kunitz, "Value of particularism."

20. Omran, "Epidemiologic transition in the United States"; Gaylin and Kates, "Refocusing the lens"; Rogers and Nelson, "Epidemiologic transition revisited."

21. Lerner, "Modernization and health."

22. Mosley and Chen, "Analytical framework for the study of child survival."

23. Frenk et al., "Elements for a theory of the health transition," 24–31.

24. Ibid.

25. Omran, "Epidemiologic transition theory."

26. Lorber, "Infectious causes of chronic illness."

27. O'Connor, Taylor, and Hughes, "Emerging infectious determinants of chronic diseases."

28. Carbonne, Luftig, and Buckley, *Microbial Triggers of Chronic Human Illness.*

29. Ibid., 1; Ewald, *Plague Time*, 50.

30. Hill, "Environment and disease"; Carbonne, Luftig, and Buckley, *Microbial Triggers of Chronic Human Illness*, 10.

31. Susser and Susser, "Choosing a future for epidemiology," pts. 1–2; Susser, "Eco-epidemiology"; Pearce, "Traditional epidemiology, modern epidemiology, and public health"; Ewald, *Plague Time.*

32. Riley, "From a high mortality regime to a high morbidity regime," 74.

33. McKeown, *Modern Rise of Population*, 8–10.

34. Black, *Mortality of the Human Species*; Heberden, *Increase and Decline of Different Diseases.*

35. A copy of a London Bill of Mortality (1665) and a comparison of the main causes with registration data is shown in Glass, *Numbering the People*, 22, 190–91. Data from the London bills for 1629–1831 used in the current study are from Marshall, *Mortality in the Metropolis;* other data for 1832–35 were extracted from the original bills in the Guildhall Library in London.

36. Eyler, *Victorian Social Medicine*, 42–53.

37. Ibid., 53; Farr, *Vital Statistics.*

38. Glass, *Numbering the People*, 188.

39. McKeown, *Modern Rise of Population*, 53.

40. Mooney, "Public health versus private practice"; Noymer and Jarosz, "Causes of death"; Condrau and Worboys, "Epidemics and infections."

41. Ackland et al., "Non-communicable disease and chronic disease"; Unwin et al., "Non-communicable disease and chronic disease."

42. Choi et al., "Bringing chronic disease epidemiology and infectious disease epidemiology together."

43. O'Connor et al., "Infectious etiologies of chronic diseases"; Knobler et al., *Infectious Etiology of Chronic Diseases.*

44. Choi et al., "Bringing chronic disease epidemiology and infectious disease epidemiology together"; Unwin et al., "Non-communicable disease and chronic disease."

45. Waldron and Vickerstaff, *Intimations of Quality*, 14–21; Office for National Statistics, *Death Certification Reform.*

Chapter Three

1. Burnet, *Cellular Immunology*, 21–29.

2. Burnet and White, *Natural History of Infectious Diseases*; Cockburn, *Evolution and Eradication of Infectious Diseases*; Cockburn, *Infectious Diseases*; Cockburn, "Infectious disease in ancient populations"; McNeill, *Plagues and Peoples.*

3. Cockburn, *Evolution and Eradication of Infectious Diseases*, 222–23.

4. Merle, Cunha, and Rodrigues, "BCG vaccination and leprosy protection."

5. Greenwood, Topley, and Wilson, *Experimental Epidemiology*; Magill, "Immunologist and the evil spirits."

6. McNeill, *Plagues and Peoples*, 38, 23–77.

7. Caldwell, *Demographic Transition Theory*, 51–63.

8. Sandbach, "History of schistosomiasis research," 261.

9. Cockburn, *Evolution and Eradication of Infectious Diseases*; Cockburn, *Infectious Diseases*; Cockburn, "Infectious disease in ancient populations."

10. Cohen, *Health and the Rise of Civilization*, 32–47.

11. Ibid.

12. McNeill, *Plagues and Peoples*, 54–55.

13. Bartlett, "Measles periodicity and community size."

14. Burnet and White, *Natural History of Infectious Diseases*, 16.

15. Kunitz, "Mortality change in America."

16. Ibid.

17. Omran, "Century of epidemiologic transition."

18. Kunitz, "Mortality change in America."

19. Ibid.

20. Flinn, *European Demographic System*, 95–101.

21. McNeill, *Plagues and Peoples*, 227.

22. Chambers, *Population, Economy and Society*, 98.

23. Goubert, *Malades et Médecins en Bretagne.* See other records from north Europe in Bruneel, *La Mortalité dans les Campagnes*, 452; Lee, *Population Growth, Economic Development and Social Change*, 100.

24. Kunitz, "Speculations on the European mortality decline."

25. Ibid.

26. Sogner, *Folkevekst og Flytting.*

27. Hatcher, *Plague, Population and the English Economy*, 70–73.

28. Flinn, *European Demographic System*, 56–57; Karlen, *Plague's Progress*, 76–77; McNeill, *Plagues and Peoples*, 120.

29. Burnet and White, *Natural History of Infectious Diseases*, 225. See also McNeill, *Plagues and Peoples*, 120–21, 150–56.

30. Burnet and White, *Natural History of Infectious Diseases*, 227.

31. Hatcher, *Plague, Population and the English Economy*, 21–25.

32. Slack, *Plague*, 75.

33. Flinn, *European Demographic System*, 58–61.

34. Slack, *Plague*, 74–84.

35. Ibid., 79.

36. In 1665 there were 97,306 burials in London (the City, out-parishes, and distant parishes), of which 68,596 (60%) were attributed to plague. Graunt showed that a significant number of deaths from plague were recorded in other categories. Glass suggested that total deaths were almost certainly under-recorded. He estimated that the total population of London before this plague epidemic was 500,000–600,000, in which case up to one in five of the population died in that plague year. Glass, *Numbering the People*, 9.

37. Slack, *Impact of Plague*, 313.

38. Cartwright, *Social History of Medicine*, 71.

39. Slack, *Plague*, 83–84.

40. Cartwright, *Social History of Medicine*, 71.

41. Hardy, "Smallpox in London," 125–27.

42. Burnet and White, *Natural History of Infectious Diseases*, 227.

43. Pollitzer, *Plague*, 282–89; Appleby, "Famine, mortality and epidemic disease."

44. Post, "Famine, mortality and epidemic disease."

45. Biraben, "Current medical and epidemiological views on plague."

46. Tranter, *Population and Society*, 66; Flinn, *European Demographic System*, 56–61.

47. Slack, *Plague*, 74.

48. McNeill, *Plagues and Peoples*, 221.

49. Razzell, *Conquest of Smallpox*, 133.

50. Perrenoud, "La mortalité à Genève"; *La Population de Genève*, 458–79.

51. Widen, "Mortality and causes of death in Sweden."

52. Lindskos, "Mortalitaetsdiagnosen in Suedschweden."

53. Turpeinen, "Les causes des fluctuations annuelles du taux de mortalité finlandaise."

54. Creighton, *History of Epidemics in Britain*, 775.

55. Heysham, *Bills of Mortality for Carlisle.*

Chapter Four

1. Wrigley and Schofield, *Population History of England*, 244, 332.

2. Flinn, *European Demographic System*, 80.

3. Schofield, "Impact of scarcity and plenty"; Wrigley and Schofield, *Population History of England*.

4. Fogel, *Long-Term Trends in Health and Longevity*, 67.

5. Ibid., 80–82.

6. Ibid., 67–68. Fogel, *Escape from Hunger and Premature Death*, 8–12.

7. Fogel, *Long-Term Trends in Health and Longevity*, 80–82.

8. McKeown, Record, and Brown, "Modern rise of population in Europe"; McKeown, *Modern Rise of Population*, 128–29, 142, 153–54.

9. Razzell, "Modern rise of population in Europe," 5.

10. See, for example, Taylor, *Standard of Living in Britain*; Hobsbawm, "British standard of living"; Lindert and Williamson, "English workers' living standards."

11. Newberne and Williams, "Nutritional influences on the course of infections," 93.

12. Ütterström, "Population problems in pre-industrial Sweden."

13. Tranter, *Population and Society*, 84.

14. Flinn, *British Population Growth*, 50–51.

15. Galloway, "Variations in fertility, nuptiality, mortality and prices."

16. Chambers, "Vale of Trent."

17. Flinn, *European Demographic System*, 72, 96.

18. Fridlizius, "Mortality decline in the demographic transition."

19. Perrenoud, "Mortality decline in its secular setting."

20. Flinn, *European Demographic System*, 96.

21. Razzell, "Modern rise of population in Europe," 8; Hobsbawm, "British standard of living."

22. Wrigley and Schofield, *Population History of England*, 403–12.

23. Fogel, *Escape from Hunger and Premature Death*, 9; Charlton and Quaife, "Trends in diet 1841–1994," 98–102.

24. Fogel, "Trends in life expectation and chronic diseases," 14. Thomas Malthus in *An Essay on the Principle of Population* suggested that food prices would increase with the pressure of population growth.

25. Fogel, "Trends in life expectation and chronic diseases," 9.

26. Fogel, *Long-Term Trends in Health and Longevity*, 54–56, 61–66.

27. Flinn, *European Demographic System*, 97.

28. Wrigley and Schofield, *Population History of England*, 416–17.

29. Appleby, "Nutrition and disease."

30. Flinn, *European Demographic System*, 97.

31. Fogel, *Long-Term Trends in Health and Longevity*, 66.

32. See the brief review of studies by Floud and Harris, "Health, height and welfare"; Floud, Wachter, and Gregory, *Height, Health and History*; and Floud, "Heights of Europeans since 1750."

33. See Goldstein, "Factors influencing the height of seven year-old children"; Muthayya, "Maternal nutrition"; Lawn, Cousens, and Zupan, "4 million neonatal deaths."

34. Steckel, "Industrialization and health in historical perspective."

35. See the section "Industrialisation and stature" in Floud and Harris, "Health, height and welfare," 18–27.

36. Floud and Wachter, "Poverty and physical stature"; Floud, Wachter, and Gregory, *Height, Health and History.*

37. Floud and Harris, "Health, height and welfare"; Harris, "Health height and history," 311.

38. Floud, Wachter, and Gregory, *Height, Health and History,* 165–71.

39. Ibid.; Floud and Harris, "Health, height and welfare," 19–20.

40. Floud and Harris, "Health, height and welfare," 29–32.

41. Ibid., 26–27; Floud, Wachter, and Gregory, *Height, Health and History,* 206–7.

42. Voth and Leunig, "Did smallpox reduce height?"

43. Floud, Wachter, and Gregory, *Height, Health and History,* 196–200.

44. Morris, *Uses of Epidemiology,* 162. Data are presented from Clay, *Report of the Commission for Enquiry,* appendix, 81.

45. Engels, *Conditions of the Working Class,* 137–40.

46. See, for example, the "real wages debate" in Floud and Harris, "Health, height and welfare"; see also Razzell, "Modern rise of population in Europe," 7; Taylor, *Standard of Living in Britain,* 11–13; and Lindert and Williamson, "English workers' living standards," 12–13.

47. Wrigley and Schofield, *Population History of England,* 528–29.

48. See the graph of trends for bricklayers and blue-/white-collar workers in Floud and Harris, "Health, height and welfare"; see also Lindert and Williamson, "English workers' living standards," 12–13; Tucker, "Real wages of artisans in London"; Flinn, "Trends in real wages"; Von Tunzelmann, "Trends in real wages, revisited."

49. Taylor, *Standard of Living in Britain,* 1–20.

50. Burnett, *Plenty and Want,* 134, 144, 173, 178.

51. Ibid., 107–8; Feinstein, "New look at the cost of living."

52. Burnett, *Plenty and Want*; Rowntree, *Poverty*; Booth, *Life and Labour.*

53. Oddy, "Health of the people"; Charlton and Quaife, "Trends in diet 1841–1994," 101–3.

54. Hollingsworth, "Demographic study of British ducal families"; "Demography of the British peerage."

55. Wrigley and Schofield, *Population History of England,* 231, 243.

56. Census data from Mitchell, *European Historical Statistics*; estimates for England in the 18th century from Wrigley and Schofield, *Population History of England.*

57. Schofield, "Population growth after 1750."

58. Wrigley and Schofield, *Population History of England,* 453.

59. Flinn, *British Population Growth,* 124–25.

60. Wrigley and Schofield, *Population History of England,* 350–55, 403–29.

61. Goldstone, "Demographic revolution in England."

62. Wrigley and Schofield, *Population History of England,* 363.

63. Data from ibid., 324.

64. Flinn, *European Demographic System,* 94.

65. Schofield, "Population growth after 1850."

66. Razzell, *Conquest of Smallpox,* 108–10.

67. Phadke, Samant, and Dewal, "Smallpox as an etiologic factor in male sterility."

68. Hollingsworth, "Demographic study of British ducal families," 29–31.

Chapter Five

1. Razzell, *Conquest of Smallpox*, 133.

2. Hedrich showed that epidemics of measles corresponded with peaks in the proportion of nonimmune "new susceptibles" in the population. Hedrich, "Corrected average attack rate for measles."

3. Creighton, *History of the Epidemics in Britain*, 518–19.

4. Razzell, "Smallpox controversy."

5. Bradley, "Reply to a review."

6. Creighton, *History of the Epidemics in Britain*, 554.

7. Razzell, *Conquest of Smallpox*, 105.

8. Creighton, *History of Epidemics in Britain*, 513, 525–26.

9. Ibid., 539.

10. Landers, "Mortality and metropolis," 66, 73; "Historical epidemiology," 61, 63.

11. Duncan, Scott, and Duncan, "Dynamics of smallpox epidemics in Britain," 419.

12. Wong and Wu, *History of Chinese Medicine*, 140.

13. Silverstein, *History of Immunology*, 254–57.

14. Zwanenberg, "Suttons and the business of inoculation," 75–77.

15. Razzell, *Conquest of Smallpox*; "Population change in eighteenth-century England"; *Population and Disease*, 193.

16. Great Britain, Royal Commission on Vaccination, *First Report*. See also Haygarth, "Population and disease of Chester," in which he reported opposition to use of inoculation in his medical practice.

17. Creighton, *History of Epidemics in Britain*, 513.

18. McNeill, *Population and Disease*, 230; "Migration patterns and infection in traditional societies."

19. Zwanenberg, "Suttons and the business of inoculation," 80; Razzell, *Conquest of Smallpox*; "Population change in eighteenth-century England."

20. Razzell, *Population and Disease*, 188.

21. Brunton, "Smallpox inoculation and demographic trends."

22. Mercer, "Smallpox and epidemiological-demographic change."

23. Dobson, *Disease*, 128.

24. Great Britain, Royal Commission on Vaccination, *Final Report*, 2–3. See also Cartwright, *Social History of Medicine*, 84.

25. Skold, "Offer and request," 78.

26. Cartwright, *Social History of Medicine*, 88; Razzell, *Edward Jenner's Cowpox Vaccine*; *Conquest of Smallpox*; Luckin, "Decline of smallpox and the demographic revolution."

27. Cartwright, *Social History of Medicine*, 85–86; Dobson, *Disease*, 128.

28. Fenner et al., *Smallpox and Its Eradication*.

29. Mercer, "Smallpox and epidemiological-demographic change."

30. Gregory King estimated the population of London in 1695 at about 528,000. Jones and Judges were critical of King's method, which was based on a national average household size and may have led to underestimation. Wrigley suggested that the population in 1700 may have been closer to 575,000. Although the London Bills indicate no natural increase in the 18th century (usually more burials than baptisms in a year), population increased due to in-migration, reaching about 880,000 by

the census of 1801. Glass, "Socioeconomic status and occupation"; Wrigley, "Simple model of London's importance"; Landers, "Historical epidemiology."

31. About 85% of the population of London lived in the parishes included in the Bills of Mortality in 1801. For the purpose of illustrating trends in cause-specific death rates (fig. 4.1), it was assumed that the population of that area increased from roughly 500,000 in 1700 to 750,000 in 1801. In view of the uncertainty about the population in 1700, trends were also calculated using a low estimate of 450,000 and a high estimate of 550,000, but neither assumption affected the conclusion that the crude death rate declined from the 1740s.

32. Watt, *History, Nature and Treatment of Chincough*; Guy, "250 years of smallpox."

33. Holy Trinity Parish, Whitehaven, parish registers for 1752–80.

34. Percival, *Essays on Smallpox and Measles.*

35. Cherry, "Hospitals and population growth," pt. 1. Although the figures for the early decades of the 19th century might reflect a low point for accuracy of recording in the parish registers, a similar change in several towns suggested a more genuine common influence.

36. Great Britain, Royal Commission on Vaccination, *Final Report*, appendix 5.

37. Lonsdale, *Life of John Heysham MD.*

38. Armstrong, "Trend of mortality in Carlisle."

39. Edwardes, *Concise History of Smallpox and Vaccination.* See also Hardy, *Epidemic Streets*, 125.

40. Huck, "Shifts in seasonality of infant deaths."

41. Szreter and Mooney, "Urbanization, mortality, and standard of living," 88.

42. Hardy, *Epidemic Streets*, 124.

43. Parish, *Victory with Vaccines*, 57–58.

44. Fraser, "Leicester and the smallpox."

45. Hardy, *Epidemic Streets*, 124.

46. Ibid., 130–31, 147.

47. Fridlizius, "Mortality decline in the demographic transition"; Fridlizius and Ohlsson, "Mortality patterns in Sweden." Interest in the possibility of genetically determined resistance to smallpox has renewed recently in view of the suggestion that natural selection of those with the relevant genes might explain the prevalence of a gene mutation that conveys resistance to HIV infection in European populations. Galvani and Slatkin, "Evaluating plague and smallpox." HIV and *Variola major* both infect leukocytes resulting in dysfunction of the immune system, which might indicate the biological plausibility of a hypothesis that absence of the CCR5 receptor confers resistance to both smallpox and HIV. The receptor protein CCR5 is fundamental for HIV-1 to gain entry into cells of the immune system and establish an infection. Individuals who carry a mutation in the gene encoding CCR5 (delta 32) are resistant to HIV-1 infection. An estimated 10% of the European population carries the CCR5-delta 32 deletion, although it is very rare in African, Asian, Middle Eastern, and American Indian populations. Some evidence suggests that the smallpox virus, *Variola major*, could have been responsible for the high prevalence of CCR5-delta 32 deletion among Europeans as a result of natural selection, as the virus infected the majority of Europeans before the age of 10 years until the end of the 19th century and case fatality was high. It has been suggested that regular epidemics and high mortality from smallpox could have provided sufficient

selective pressure to result in 10% of the population having resistance to infection, despite case fatality remaining high.

48. Razzell, "Modern rise of population—a critique," 143.

49. Ütterström, "Population problems in pre-industrial Sweden."

50. McNeill, *Plagues and Peoples*, 231–36; Miller, *Adoption of Inoculation for Smallpox.*

51. Henry and Blayo, "La population de la France."

52. Great Britain, Royal Commission on Vaccination, *First Report*, appendix, 107–8.

53. Skold, "From inoculation to vaccination," 253.

54. Great Britain, Royal Commission on Vaccination, *First Report*, appendix, 112–13.

55. Skold, "From inoculation to vaccination," 255.

56. Mitchell. *European Historical Statistics*, 23.

57. Ütterström, "Population problems in pre-industrial Sweden."

58. Nelson and Rogers, "The right to die?"; Rogers and Nelson, "Epidemiologic transition revisited," 251.

59. Skold, "From inoculation to vaccination," 255.

60. Hofsten and Lundström, *Swedish Population History.*

61. Widen, "Mortality and causes of death." For England, Lettsom estimated that there may have been twice as many deaths linked with smallpox than the number recorded. See Razzell, *Conquest of Smallpox*, 107–9.

62. Turpeinen, "Finnish death rates"; "Fertility and mortality in Finland"; "Les causes des fluctuations annuelles du taux de mortalité finlandaise."

63. Pitkanen, Mielke, and Jorde, "Smallpox and its eradication,"98–101.

64. Mielke et al., "Historical epidemiology of smallpox," 275, 280–81.

65. Pitkanen, Mielke, and Jorde, "Smallpox and its eradication."

66. Great Britain, Royal Commission on Vaccination, *First Report*, appendix, 109–10.

67. Mitchell, *European Historical Statistics*, 19–24.

68. Edwardes, *Concise History of Smallpox and Vaccination.*

69. Ibid.

70. Registrar General, *Statistical Review* (1962), pt. 1, "Medical," 14, 351.

71. Great Britain, Royal Commission on Vaccination, *First Report*, 74; *Final Report*, 12–14.

Chapter Six

1. Heysham, *Bills of Mortality in Carlisle*; Creighton, *History of Epidemics in Britain.*

2. Creighton, *History of Epidemics in Britain*, 775.

3. Considering the contribution of different categories of "cause" of death to a unit of change in the total death rate over a period is more meaningful than referring to percentage contributions as some are arithmetically negative and some positive. Clearly, a contribution of a disease to x% of mortality decline when death rates for all cause groups are declining is very different from a contribution of x% to decline when death rates for some diseases increased. The contribution to a unit of change in the death rate over a period is the change in the death rate from a cause category divided

by the change in the total death rate, so it can be either arithmetically negative or positive, and the contributions of all the categories add up to one.

4. Differentiation of the specific infectious diseases involved in "fevers" would have been difficult in many cases. Typhus was referred to as "purples and spotted fever" in 1629, but was included in the general category of "fevers" from 1729. Zinsser, *Rats, Lice and History*, 217; Appleby, "Nutrition and disease."

5. Creighton, *History of Epidemics in Britain*, 82–84, 133.

6. Zinsser, *Rats, Lice and History*, 217; Appleby, "Nutrition and disease."

7. Burnet and White, *Natural History of Infectious Diseases*, 146–47; Zinsser, *Rats, Lice and History*, 218–28.

8. Dobson, *Disease*, 37, 41.

9. Appleby, "Nutrition and disease."

10. Ibid.

11. Razzell, "Modern rise of population—a critique."

12. Creighton, *History of Epidemics in Britain*, 82.

13. Riley, *Eighteenth-Century Campaign to Avoid Disease*, 99.

14. Ibid., 89–98.

15. Porter, "Cleaning up the Great Wen," 67–68; Razzell, *Population and Disease*, 168–71.

16. Razzell, *Population and Disease*, 171.

17. Riley, *Eighteenth-Century Campaign to Avoid Disease*, 102–3, 120.

18. Porter, *Disease, Medicine and Society*, 53–56; Riley, *Eighteenth-Century Campaign to Avoid Disease*, 132–37; Szreter, "Economic growth, disruption, deprivation, disease and death," 709; "Importance of social intervention," 23–24.

19. Razzell, *Population and Disease*, 173.

20. Porter, *Disease, Medicine and Society*, 37.

21. Razzell, "Modern rise of population in Europe."

22. Hardy, *Epidemic Streets*, 199, 203.

23. Ibid., 200–203.

24. Ibid., 207.

25. Luckin, "Evaluating the sanitary revolution," 114.

26. Bourdelais, "Cholera: A victory for medicine?," 122.

27. Parry, *Infectious Diseases*, 166.

28. Bourdelais, "Cholera: A victory for medicine?," 120.

29. Cartwright, *Social History of Medicine*, 103.

30. Szreter, "Health, economy, state and society," 208–11.

31. Chadwick, *Report on Sanitary Conditions.*

32. Cartwright, *Social History of Medicine*, 105; McNeill, *Plagues and Peoples*, 249–52.

33. McNeill, *Plagues and Peoples*, 250; Wohl, *Endangered Lives*, 102–6.

34. Snow, *Mode of Communication of Cholera*, 39–40, 51.

35. Ibid., 68–69.

36. Ibid., 80, 109.

37. Wohl, *Endangered Lives*, 110–12.

38. Rosen, "Disease, debility and death."

39. Szreter, "Importance of social intervention," 24.

40. Cartwright, *Social History of Medicine*, 106; Porter, *Disease, Medicine and Society*, 57.

41. Hardy, "Smallpox in London," 125.

42. Szreter, "Importance of social intervention," 24; "Economic growth, disruption, deprivation, disease and death," 708–9.

43. Van Poppel and van der Heijden, "The effects of water supply on infant and childhood mortality."

44. Longmate, *King Cholera*, 228; Bourdelais, "Cholera: A victory for medicine?," 122.

45. Woods and Woodward, *Urban Disease and Mortality*; Woods, *Demography of Victorian England and Wales.*

46. Engels, *Condition of the Working Class*, 60–61, 69–77, 83–88; Dickens, *Hard Times.*

47. Peters, "Observations upon the natural history of epidemic diarrhoea."

48. Hardy, *Epidemic Streets*, 151, 177–81.

49. Luckin, "Evaluating the sanitary revolution," 108–9.

50. Ibid., 116–17.

51. Hardy, *Epidemic Streets*, 172–81.

52. Woods, "Mortality and sanitary conditions," 200–201.

53. Thompson, "Infant mortality in Bradford," 131–32.

54. Ibid.

55. Luckin, "Evaluating the sanitary revolution," 116–18.

56. Ibid., 117.

57. Woods, *Demography of Victorian England and Wales*, 318, 334.

58. Guha, "Importance of social intervention," 109.

59. The Registrar General's annual reports for the 1890s discussed the relationship between hot summers and diarrheal disease mortality. Registration data indicate summer peaks in deaths from diarrhea and dysentery, as reported by Landers. Gale also presented graphs of temperature and diarrheal disease deaths. Gale, *Epidemic Diseases*, 85; Landers, "Historical epidemiology."

60. Hardy, *Epidemic Streets*, 190.

61. Guha, "Importance of social intervention," 111. This source shows data on cases of diarrhea from a report to the Local Government Board published in 1889.

62. Ewald, *Plague Time*, 203.

63. Preston and Van de Walle, "Urban French mortality."

64. Ewald, *Plague Time*, 203, 242.

65. Ibid., 204–5.

66. Condran and Cheney, "Mortality trends in Philadelphia."

67. Cutler and Miller, "Role of public health improvements."

68. Smith, The decline of infectious diseases."

69. Omran, "Century of epidemiologic transition."

70. Szreter, "Population health approach," 424.

71. Longmate, *King Cholera*, 222–32.

Chapter Seven

1. Hardy, "Diagnosis, death and diet," 390.

2. Fildes, *Breasts, Bottles and Babies*, 253, 390.

3. Hardy, "Diagnosis, death and diet," 390.

4. Fildes, *Breasts, Bottles and Babies*, 390.

5. Razzell, *Conquest of Smallpox*, 105.

6. Pearsons product-moment correlation coefficients based on detrended series of quinquennial data for the period after the plague, 1671–75 to 1831–35, were smallpox with infancy +0.59 ($p < 0.0005$), smallpox with fevers +0.64 ($p < 0.0005$), smallpox with total burials +0.49 ($p < 0.0005$). The use of quinquennial rates removes short-term epidemic fluctuations, which may be less strongly correlated. See Landers, "Mortality and metropolis," 73.

7. Smith, *People's Health*, 87.

8. Wrigley and Schofield, "English population history," 157.

9. See for example Wrigley, "Births and baptisms"; Jones, "decline in infant mortality."

10. Wrigley and Schofield, "English population history," 157.

11. Landers, "Mortality and metropolis."

12. Hollingsworth, "Demographic study of British ducal families."

13. Guha, "Importance of social intervention," 110.

14. Woods, *Demography of Victorian England and Wales*, 258–59.

15. Woods, "Infant mortality in Britain," 79; Woods, Watterson, and Woodward, "Causes of rapid infant mortality decline."

16. Woods, Watterson, and Woodward, "Causes of rapid infant mortality decline"; Woods, *Demography of Victorian England and Wales*, 283.

17. Woods, "Infant mortality in Britain," 82–83; Woods, Williams, and Galley, "Differential mortality patterns," 64.

18. Chalmers, "Infant mortality."

19. Woods, "Infant mortality in Britain," 83.

20. Registrar General, *Annual Report* (1890–99); Gale, *Epidemic Diseases*, 85.

21. Mosley and Chen divided socioeconomic determinants into individual parental factors (productivity, traditions, norms, and attitudes); household variables (income and wealth); and community-level variables (ecological, political, economic, and health systems). These operate through proximate determinants of morbidity and mortality risk, including maternal characteristics (health status, age, parity, and birth intervals); environmental contamination (air, water, food, hands, other objects, and insect vectors); nutrient deficiency; injury; and personal illness control (preventive measures and treatment). Mosley and Chen, "Child mortality in developing countries."

22. Hobcraft, McDonald, and Rutstein, "Determinants of infant and early child mortality"; Preston, "Mortality in childhood"; Preston, *The Effects of Infant and Child Mortality on Fertility*; Woods, "Fertility transition in Victorian England"; Woods, Watterson, and Woodward, "Causes of rapid infant mortality decline."

23. Winter, "Impact of the First World War."

24. Watterson, "Infant mortality by father's occupation," 295.

25. Woods, Watterson, and Woodward, "Causes of rapid infant mortality decline"; Winter, "Decline of mortality in Britain."

26. Wrigley et al., *English Population History*, 313; Woods, "Medical and demographic history," 495.

27. Loudon, "Maternal mortality in the past," 245S.

28. Dobson, *Disease*, 76–79.

29. Ewald, *Plague Time*, 17–19.

30. Loudon, "Maternal mortality in the past."

31. Woods, *Demography of Victorian England and Wales,* 332.

32. Preston, *Mortality Patterns in National Populations,* 44.

33. Watterson, "Environmental factors in mortality decline."

34. Thompson, "Infant mortality in Bradford," 126, 142–44.

35. Woods, "Infant mortality in Britain," 83; Thompson, "Infant mortality in Bradford," 129–30.

36. Thompson, "Infant mortality in Bradford," 143.

37. Fildes, *Breasts, Bottles and Babies,* 81, 88.

38. A period of natural infertility allows a mother to regain her physical and emotional strength between pregnancies and confers advantages on her children in terms of better health and development. The Medical Research Council Unit of Reproductive Biology found that the main variables involved in postpartum infertility were suckling frequency and suckling duration. Howie et al., "Effect of supplementary food." The mechanism may be neural with increased hypothalmic sensitivity to the negative feedback effect of ovarian steroids leading to inadequate production of the gonadotrophin required for ovulation. McNeilly, "Effects of lactation on fertility." Abandonment of prolonged breastfeeding contributes to resumption of ovulation at an earlier stage. Konner and Worthman, "Nursing frequency, gonadal function and birth spacing"; Howie and McNeilly, "Effect of breast-feeding patterns." Although breastfeeding is not a reliable way of avoiding pregnancy, the aggregate effect in a population can be important for controlling fertility if contraception is not commonly used.

39. Fildes, *Breasts, Bottles and Babies,* 81, 88.

40. Woods, *Demography of Victorian England and Wales,* 284–87.

41. Ibid., 286; Woods, "Infant mortality in Britain," 83.

42. Caldwell and Caldwell, "What have we learnt?," 7.

43. Dwork, "*War is Good for Babies*"; Woods, *Demography of Victorian England and Wales,* 284.

44. Smith, *People's Health,* 113–35.

45. Ewbank and Preston, "Personal health behaviour."

46. Ibid.; Preston and Haines, *Fatal Years.*

47. Caldwell, "Major new evidence on health transition"; Hobcraft, McDonald, and Rutstein, "Determinants of infant and early child mortality"; Caldwell, "Education as a factor in mortality decline"; Cleland, "Maternal education and child survival"; Cleland and van Ginneken, "Maternal education and child survival."

48. Preston and Haines, *Fatal Years,* 206; Caldwell, "Old and new factors," 212.

49. Draper, *Birth Control in the Modern World,* 317.

50. Woods, *Demography of Victorian England and Wales,* 303, 305.

51. Ibid., 304.

52. Watterson, "Environmental factors in mortality decline."

Chapter Eight

1. Scrimshaw, Taylor, and Gordon, "Interactions of nutrition and infection"; Behar, "Deadly combination"; Fogel, *Escape from Hunger and Premature Death,* 46.

2. Hedrich, "Corrected average attack rate for measles."

3. Age-specific data on childhood infectious diseases at the national level were first recorded toward the end of the 19th century in the Registrar General's annual reports. Heysham's data for Carlisle in the 18th century suggest that most deaths from scarlet fever at that time were also under the age of five years (Heysham, *Bills of Mortality in Carlisle*; see also appendix B).

4. Swedland and Donta, "Scarlet fever epidemics," 159.

5. Burnet and White, *Natural History of Infectious Diseases*, 200.

6. Gale, *Epidemic Diseases*, 89–92; Rosen, *History of Public Health*, 65–66.

7. Gale, *Epidemic Diseases*, 90–91; Creighton, *History of Epidemics in Britain*, 706, 719–20.

8. Rosen, "Disease, debility and death."

9. Gale, *Epidemic Diseases*, 90.

10. Ibid., 90.

11. Pooley and Pooley, "Health, society and environment," 165–67.

12. Woods, *Demography of Victorian England and Wales*, 323–24.

13. Duncan, Duncan, and Scott, "Dynamics of scarlet fever epidemics."

14. Hardy, *Epidemic Streets*, 70–73.

15. Ibid., 56–59.

16. Creighton, *History of Epidemics in Britain*, 727.

17. Gale, *Epidemic Diseases*, 92.

18. McKeown, *Modern Rise of Population*, 85–86.

19. Hardy, *Epidemic Streets*, 66, 79; Woods, Williams, and Galley, "Differential mortality patterns."

20. Katz and Morens, "Severe streptococcal infection."

21. Gale, *Epidemic Diseases*, 90.

22. Burnet and White, *Natural History of Infectious Diseases*, 198–201.

23. Katz and Morens, "Severe streptococcal infections"; Krause, "Evolving microbes."

24. Swedland and Donta, "Scarlet fever epidemics."

25. Smith, *People's Health*, 226–27; Burnett, "Housing and decline in mortality," 175.

26. Woods, "Mortality and sanitary conditions," 179, 189.

27. Burnet and White, *Natural History of Infectious Diseases*, 108.

28. Gale, *Epidemic Diseases*, 89.

29. Ibid., 93. When diphtheria was first recorded in the Registrar General's *Annual Report* in 1855, it was noted that deaths before this may have been recorded as "cynanche maligna" or "putrid throat." There was some confusion with scarlet fever, while croup was a general term for obstructed breathing. Burnet and White, *Natural History of Infectious Diseases*, 193.

30. Burnet and White, *Natural History of Infectious Diseases*, 193.

31. Gale, *Epidemic Diseases*, 94.

32. Burnet and White, *Natural History of Infectious Diseases*, 193.

33. Hardy, *Epidemic Streets*, 82, 90–104.

34. Gale, *Epidemic Diseases*, 94.

35. Hardy, *Epidemic Streets*, 96–104.

36. Magill, "Immunologist and the evil spirits." Magill pointed out that a decline in the death rate occurred before the 1890s in the United States, although epidemic variation might account for lower rates just before the long-term decline.

37. Condran and Cheney, "Mortality trends in Philadelphia."

38. Hardy, *Epidemic Streets*, 104.

39. Burnet and White, *Natural History of Infectious Diseases*, 198; Gale, *Epidemic Diseases*, 95.

40. Burnet and White, *Natural History of Infectious Diseases*, 198.

41. Ewald, *Plague Time*, 214–15.

42. Middleton and Weitzman, *Place for Everyone.*

43. Preston and Van de Walle, "Urban French mortality."

44. Hardy, *Epidemic Streets*, 50–51.

45. Fine and Clarkson, "Measles in England and Wales."

46. Bartlett, "Measles periodicity and community size."

47. Woods, *Demography of Victorian England and Wales*, 323–25.

48. Woods, "Mortality and sanitary conditions," 200.

49. Reves, "Declining fertility in England and Wales."

50. Halsey, Eddins, and Henman, "Measles mortality in the United States"; US Census Bureau, *Historical Statistics of the United States, Colonial Times to 1970.*

51. Aaby et al., "Overcrowding and intensive exposure"; "Severe measles in Sunderland, 1885."

52. Mercer, "Relative trends in mortality."

53. Aaby et al., "Severe measles in Sunderland, 1885."

54. Reves, "Declining fertility in England and Wales."

55. Aaby et al., "Overcrowding and intensive exposure"; Aaby et al., "Determinants of measles mortality."

56. Anderson and May, "Population biology of infectious diseases"; Fine et al, "Control of infectious disease"; Smith, "Practical problems."

57. McNeilly, "Effects of lactation on fertility"; Howie and McNeilly, "Effect of breast-feeding patterns."

58. Hardy, *Epidemic Streets*, 24–25.

59. Preston and Haines, *Fatal Years*, 200.

60. Ewbank and Preston, "Personal health behaviour."

61. Davey Smith, Gunnell, and Ben-Schlomo, "Life course approaches to socioeconomic differentials," 113–14.

Chapter Nine

1. Dubos and Dubos, *White Plague.*

2. Black, *Mortality of the Human Species.*

3. Hardy, "Diagnosis, death and diet."

4. Puranen, "Tuberculosis and decline of mortality," 99.

5. Hardy, "Diagnosis, death and diet."

6. Guha, "Importance of social intervention," 98–100.

7. There are few data on mortality by cause of death in the second half of the 19th century for other countries, so it is difficult to assess how typical the disease profile of England and Wales was. Even for the twentieth century, different proportions of ill-defined and unknown causes make comparison between countries difficult. An analysis of international data indicated that respiratory tuberculosis contributed −0.10 toward each unit of change in the overall death rate for females, and −0.12 for

males, much the same as for England and Wales. Preston and Nelson, "Structure and change in cause of death."

8. McKeown, Record, and Turner, "Decline in mortality in England and Wales"; McKeown, *Modern Rise of Population*, 142, 153–54.

9. Cockburn, *Evolution and Eradication of Infectious Diseases*, 221.

10. Schofield, Review of *The Modern Rise of Population.*

11. Dubos and Dubos, *White Plague*, 199–207, 232–33.

12. Increases in tuberculosis death rates in some southern states were recorded in the censuses: US Bureau of the Census, *Census of the United States, 1860–*. Increases in New York were mentioned by Van de Walle; see "Accounting for population growth," 653. Data from Massachusetts indicate that tuberculosis mortality was declining from at least 1863. US Bureau of the Census, *Historical Statistics of the United States, Colonial Times to 1970*, pt. 1.

13. Dubos and Dubos, *White Plague*, 233, appendix B, chart 4.

14. Grange and Collins, "Bovine tubercle bacilli and disease in animals and man," 228.

15. Dubos and Dubos, *White Plague*, 116; Burnet and White, *Natural History of Infectious Diseases*, 213–24.

16. Burnet and White, *Natural History of Infectious Diseases*, 215.

17. Stead, "Pathogenesis of chronic pulmonary tuberculosis."

18. Dubos and Dubos, *White Plague*, 115–18.

19. Bentzon, "Effect of certain infectious diseases"; Starr and Berkovich, "Effects of measles on the tuberculin test"; Flick, "Does measles really predispose to tuberculosis?"

20. Nemir, "Pertussis pneumonia," 737.

21. Lettsom estimated that there could have been twice as many deaths from smallpox as the number recorded, as well as deaths from diseases whose effects were exacerbated by smallpox. See Razzell, *Conquest of Smallpox*, 107–9.

22. Black, *Mortality of the Human Species*, 102.

23. Great Britain, Royal Commission on Vaccination, *First Report*, appendix, 90.

24. Dixon, *Smallpox.*

25. Sundbärg, *Dodligheiten af Lungtuberculos i Sverige.*

26. Puranen, "Tuberculosis and decline of mortality," 101.

27. Preston and Van de Walle, "Accounting for population growth."

28. Dubos and Dubos *White Plague*, appendix C.

29. Beaver, "Population, infant mortality and milk."

30. Cronje, "Tuberculosis and mortality decline," 91–93, 97.

31. Ibid., 91.

32. Woods, *Demography of Victorian England and Wales*, 336, 354.

33. Cronje, "Tuberculosis and mortality decline," 95.

34. Guha, "Importance of social intervention," 100.

35. Rosen, in "Disease, debility and death," suggested it was well-known in the early 19th century that tuberculosis was associated with poor working conditions. Riley considered the places in which ventilation might have improved, in *Eighteenth-Century Campaign to Avoid Disease*, 29, 132.

36. Engels, *Conditions of the Working Class*, 129, 191.

37. Ibid.; Dubos and Dubos, *White Plague*, 200–206.

38. Dickens, *Hard Times*, 102. Other descriptions of living and working conditions can be found in Dickens's *Bleak House* and *Oliver Twist* and in Engels's *Conditions of the Working Class*, 60–61.

39. Burnett, "Housing and decline in mortality," 162.

40. Ibid., 173.

41. Guha, "Importance of social intervention," 101; Wohl, "Housing of Artisans and Labourers," 458.

42. Burnett, "Housing and decline in mortality," 174.

43. Yelling, *Slums and Slum Clearance,* 9–30.

44. Pooley and Pooley, "Health, society and environment," 173.

45. Szreter, "Importance of social intervention," 29; Burnett, "Housing and decline in mortality," 173.

46. Burnett *Plenty and Want,* 107–8; Feinstein, "Cost of living"; Davies et al., "Historical declines in tuberculosis"; Hardy, "Diagnosis, death and diet," 399.

47. Burnett, *Plenty and Want,* 158–91; Charlton and Quaife, "Trends in diet 1841–1994."

48. Oddy, "Health of the people."

49. Floud, Wachter, and Gregory, *Height, Health and History.*

50. Oddy, "Health of the people."

51. Morley, *Paediatric Priorities,* 184, 217–59.

52. McKeown, Record, and Turner, "Decline in mortality in England and Wales"; McKeown, *Modern Rise of Population,* 142, 153–54.

53. Davies et al., "Historical declines in tuberculosis."

54. Daniels et al., *Tuberculosis in Young Adults.*

55. Anderson et al.," Control of tuberculosis."

56. Kallman and Reisner, "Significance of genetic factors in tuberculosis."

57. Woods, *Demography of Victorian England and Wales,* 340.

58. Stocks and Lewis-Faning, "Wartime incidence and mortality."

59. Hardy, *Epidemic Streets,* 235–36, 255–58, 260–62.

60. Ibid., 241.

61. Newsholme, "Causes of the reduction in the death rate from phthisis."

62. Hardy, *Epidemic Streets,* 260.

63. Phillip, "Outlook on tuberculosis," 44.

64. Dubos and Dubos, *White Plague,* 211–16.

65. Frieden, Lerner, and Rutherford, "Lessons from the 1800s."

66. Hardy, *Epidemic Streets,* 264.

67. Phillip, "Outlook on tuberculosis," 44.

68. Wilson, "Commentary: medicine, population, and tuberculosis."

69. McKeown, *Modern Rise of Population,* 93.

70. Dahlberg, "Mortality from tuberculosis." See also Cronje, "Tuberculosis and mortality decline," 81–82.

71. Vynnycky and Fine, "Interpreting the decline in tuberculosis."

Chapter Ten

1. Marks and Burney, "Diseases of the respiratory system," 98–100.

2. Ibid., 110.

3. Ibid., 103.

4. Preston, *Mortality Patterns in National Populations.*

5. Tromp, *Medical Biometeorology*; Daw, "Mortality from degenerative heart disease," 85–86; Caselli, "Health transition and cause-specific mortality," 88.

6. Szreter, "Social intervention in Britain's mortality decline," 27.

7. Howe, *National Atlas of Disease Mortality*, 240–41; Gartner et al., "Rural-urban mortality differences."

8. Gore and Shaddick, "Atmospheric pollution and mortality"; Fairbairn and Reid, "Air pollution and other local factors"; Daly, "Air pollution and causes of death."

9. Melia, Florey, and Swan, "Respiratory illness in British schoolchildren."

10. The smog affecting London in December 1952 resulted in a large increase in the number of deaths from bronchitis, pneumonia, and heart disease. This focused attention on the deleterious effects of air pollution and eventually led to passage of the Clean Air Act of 1956. See Gore and Shaddick, "Atmospheric pollution and mortality"; Fairbairn and Reid, "Air pollution and other local factors."

11. Howard, "Changing face of chronic bronchitis."

12. Barker and Osmond, "Childhood respiratory infection," 1273.

13. Fletcher et al., *Chronic Bronchitis and Emphysema*, 144.

14. Colley and Reid, "Urban and social origins of chronic bronchitis"; Anonymous, "Chronic bronchitis and occupation."

15. Anonymous, "Natural history of chronic bronchitis"; Fletcher, "Natural history of chronic bronchitis."

16. Ebi-Kryston, "Predicting 15-year chronic bronchitis mortality."

17. Colley and Reid, "Urban and social origins of chronic bronchitis."

18. Davey Smith, Gunnell, and Ben-Schlomo, "Life course approaches to socio-economic differentials," 110–11, presenting data from Strachan, "Respiratory and allergic diseases."

19. Colley, Douglas, and Reid, "Respiratory disease in young adults."

20. Davey Smith, Gunnell, and Ben-Schlomo, "Life course approaches to socio-economic differentials," 111–12.

21. Britten, Davies, and Colley, "Early respiratory experience and subsequent cough."

22. Shaheen et al., "Birth weight, childhood lower respiratory tract infection"; Davey Smith, Gunnell, and Ben-Schlomo, "Life course approaches to socioeconomic differentials."

23. Barker and Osmond, "Childhood respiratory infection."

24. Burnet and White, *Natural History of Infectious Diseases*, 74–75.

25. Gladstone et al., "Continued control of pneumococcal disease."

26. Perry and Halsey, "Clinical significance of measles."

27. Hussey and Clements, "Clinical problems in measles case management."

28. Flick, "Pulmonary complications of measles"; Hussey and Clements, "Clinical problems in measles case management."

29. Morley, "Severe measles in the tropics," 299.

30. Bwibo, "Measles in Uganda."

31. Wilson, "Measles."

32. Oswald, "Collapse of the lungs in children."

33. Fawcett and Parry, "Lung changes in pertussis and measles."

34. Linnemann et al., "Use of pertussis vaccine"; Kurt et al., "Spread of pertussis"; Lambert, "Epidemiology of a small pertussis outbreak."

35. Warner and Marshall, "Crippling lung disease."

36. Reves, "Declining fertility in England and Wales"; Mercer, "Relative trends in mortality."

37. Brimblecombe et al., "Family studies of respiratory infections"; Longini et al., "Estimating household and community transmission parameters."

38. Longini et al., "Estimating household and community transmission parameters."

39. Badger et al., "Illness in a group of Cleveland families"; Dingle, Badger, and Jordan, "Common respiratory diseases"; Leeder et al., "Influence of family factors"; Gardner, Frank, and Taber, "Effects of social and family factors."

40. Watkins, Leeder, and Corkhill, "Breast- and bottle-feeding and respiratory illness."

41. Burnet and White, *Natural History of Infectious Diseases*, 204.

42. Ibid., 205.

43. Ibid., 206.

44. Ewald, *Plague Time*, 22–24.

45. Burnet and White, *Natural History of Infectious Diseases*, 207.

46. Ibid.

47. Ibid., 210.

48. Ibid.

49. Ewald, *Plague Time*, 23.

50. Morens, Tauenberger, and Fauci, "Pandemic influenza viruses."

51. Ibid.

Chapter Eleven

1. De Flora et al., "The epidemiological revolution of the 20th century," 892.

2. Sandison and Tapp, "Disease in ancient Egypt," 47–48; Magee, "Arterial disease in antiquity"; Crimmins and Finch, "Infection, inflammation, height, and longevity," 498.

3. Black, *Mortality of the Human Species.*

4. Pound, Bury, and Ebrahim, "From apoplexy to stroke," 335.

5. Preston and Nelson, "Structure and change in cause of death," 28–30.

6. Registrar General, *Annual Report*, 1855; United Nations, *Population Bulletin, No. 6.*

7. Clayton, Taylor, and Shaper, "Trends in heart disease," 5–6; Haberman, Capideo, and Rose, "Diverging trends in cerebrovascular disease," 586; Heasman and Lipworth, "Accuracy of certification," 110–28.

8. Waldron and Vickerstaff, *Intimations of Quality*, 14–21.

9. Britton, "Diagnostic errors discovered at autopsy," 205, 208.

10. Shojania et al., "Rates of autopsy-detected diagnostic errors."

11. Office for National Statistics, *Death Certification Reform.*

12. Adelstein, "Certification of cause of death," 80–81; Lillienfeld, *Foundations of Epidemiology*, 52–57; Manton and Poss, "Dependency among causes of death," 313–14, 325.

13. In 1926 about one-fifth of all deaths were assigned to the heart disease category, undefined (ICD 90–99); respiratory disease (mainly bronchitis) was stated as an associated cause of death in 19.5% of these deaths. Registrar General, *Statistical Review* (1931), supplement.

14. Uemura and Pisa, "Trends in cardiovascular disease mortality," 167–68; Nikiforov and Mamaev, "Sex differences in cardiovascular disease mortality," 1350.

15. Davey Smith, Gunnell, and Ben-Schlomo, "Life course approaches to socioeconomic differentials," 100–101.

16. Barker and Osmond, "Infant mortality, child nutrition," 1077–81; Barker et al., "Growth in utero," 567; Barker and Martyn, "Maternal and fetal origins of cardiovascular disease," 10–11.

17. Crimmins and Finch, "Infection, inflammation, height, and longevity," 500–502; Danesh et al., "Low grade inflammation and coronary heart disease," 199.

18. Barker, "Childhood causes of adult diseases," 868.

19. Fleming, Cross, and Pannell, "Influenza and circulatory disorders," 261; Warren-Gash, Smeeth, and Hayward, "Influenza as a trigger," 607–8; Corrales-Medina, Madjid, and Musher, "Role of acute infection," 89.

20. Charlton et al., "Cardiovascular diseases," 66–67.

21. Yates, "Cerebrovascular disease."

22. Lawlor et al., "Secular trends in mortality," 1818–23.

23. Kuller et al., "Trends in cerebrovascular disease mortality."

24. Wylie, "Recent trends in mortality"; Whisnant, "Decline of stroke"; Centers for Disease Control, "Achievements in public health," 649.

25. Clayton, Taylor, and Shaper, "Trends in heart disease."

26. Anderson and Le Riche, "Ischaemic heart disease and sudden death," 8.

27. Florey, Melia, and Darby, "Mortality from ischemic heart disease," 635.

28. Nikiforov and Mamaev, "Sex differences in cardiovascular disease mortality," 1349–50.

29. Doll et al., "Mortality in relation to smoking: 50 years' observations."

30. Preston, "International comparison of excessive adult mortality"; Retherford, *Changing Sex Differential in Mortality*, 71–82.

31. Davey Smith, Gunnell, and Ben-Schlomo, "Life course approaches to socioeconomic differentials," 101. See also Wild and Byrne, "Risk factors for diabetes and coronary heart disease."

32. Cummins et al, "Smoking and drinking."

33. Halliday and Anderson, "Sex differential in ischemic heart disease," 75; Rose and Marmot, "Social class and coronary heart disease," 14. The socio-economic categories used to assess mortality differentials were based on the scheme adopted by the Registrar General in 1913. Occupations were classified into five or six social classes broadly consisting of professional and similar occupations (I), intermediate (II), skilled occupations, subdivided into manual and nonmanual (III), partly skilled (IV), and unskilled occupations (V). See Heath, "Sociology of social class," 3; and Goldblatt, "Social class mortality differences" for a comparison with other socio-economic categories used to asses mortality differentials.

34. Marmot et al., "Social-class distribution of heart disease," 1110.

35. Goldblatt, "Social class mortality differences," 31.

36. Le Grand, "Inequalities in health"; Illsey, "Occupational class selection"; Illsey and Le Grand, "Measurement of inequality in health."

37. Goldblatt, "Social class mortality differences," 45–55. See, for example, Moser, Pugh, and Goldblatt, "Inequalities in women's health."

38. Ibid., 46, 49.

39. Doll et al., "Mortality in relation to smoking: 50 year's observations"; Doll and Peto, "Mortality in relation to smoking: 20 year's observations," 1534.

40. Morris et al., "Ischemic heart disease in London busmen"; Ragland et al., "Prevalence of hypertension in bus drivers."

41. Hubert et al., "Obesity as an independent risk factor"; Wilson et al., "Overweight and obesity as determinants."

42. Popkin and Doak, "Obesity epidemic"; Gregg et al., "Cardiovascular disease risk factors"; Rosengren, "Declining cardiovascular mortality"; Stamatakis et al., "Overweight and obesity trends."

43. Pi-Sunyer, "Health implications of obesity."

44. Marmot et al., "Employment grade and coronary heart disease"; Marmot, Shipley, and Rose, "Inequalities in death."

45. Marmot and Theorell, "Social class and cardiovascular disease."

46. Marmot et al., "Job control and other risk factors"; Bosma et al., "Low job control."

47. Brunner et al., "Childhood social circumstances."

48. Bosma et al., "Two alternative job stress models."

49. Kivimäki et al., "Work stress and risk of cardiovascular mortality."

50. Toivanen and Hemström, "Income differences in cardiovascular disease."

51. Lynch et al., "Workplace conditions, socioeconomic status, and risk of mortality."

52. Moser et al., "Stress and heart disease."

53. Campbell, "Main cause of increased death rate"; "Death rates from diseases of the heart: 1876–1959."

54. Magnus and Beaglehole, "Major risk factors and coronary epidemics."

55. Stamler et al., "Low risk-factor profile."

56. Howe, *National Atlas of Disease Mortality*; Gardner, Winter, and Barker, *Atlas of Mortality from Selected Diseases.*

57. Yusuf et al., "Global burden of cardiovascular diseases," 2746.

58. United Nations, *Levels and Trends of Mortality*; World Health Organization, *World Health Statistics* (1982–85).

59. Mirzaei et al., "Coronary heart disease epidemics: not all the same," 745.

60. Mackenbach et al., "Geographical variation," 1621.

61. Brenner, "Economic changes"; "Mortality and the national economy"; Eyer, "Hypertension as a disease"; "Does unemployment cause death rate peak?"

62. Guberan, "Surprising decline in cardiovascular mortality," 119.

63. Salonen and Valonen, "Longitudinal cross-national analysis of coronary mortality"; Byington et al., "Coronary risk factors and CHD mortality," 346.

64. De Looper and Bhatia, *International Health*, 87–89; Uemura and Pisa, "Trends in cardiovascular disease mortality," 159.

65. See data on cigarette smoking in the United States for 1950 and 1960 from the Framingham Study, Sytkowski et al, "Trends in cardiovascular disease," 346.

66. Kannel and Thom, "Declining cardiovascular mortality," 332.

67. Ibid.; Walker, "Changing United States life-style"; US Surgeon General, *Smoking and Health.*

68. Stamler, "Decline in coronary heart disease mortality rates."

69. Uemura and Pisa, "Trends in cardiovascular disease mortality," 159.

70. Kesteloot et al, "Cardiovascular and all-cause mortality."

71. Leon et al., "Variation in Russian mortality rates"; McKee, "Health consequences," 19, 24.

72. Kesteloot et al, "Cardiovascular and all-cause mortality."

73. Levi et al., "Trends in mortality," 120–21.

74. Vartiainen et al., "Changes in risk factors"; Magnus and Beaglehole, "Major risk factors and coronary epidemics."

75. Sigfusson et al., Decline in ischemic heart disease."

76. Unal, Critchley, and Capewell, "Decline in coronary heart disease mortality."

77. Ford et al., "Decrease in US deaths from coronary disease."

78. Goldman and Cook, "Decline in ischemic heart disease mortality rates"; Bots and Grobbe, "Decline of coronary heart disease mortality"; Huninck et al., "Recent decline in mortality from coronary heart disease"; Capewell et al., "Decline in coronary heart disease mortality rates"; Capewell, Morrison, and McMurray, "Contribution of modern cardiovascular treatment"; Bjorck et al., "Modelling decreasing coronary heart disease mortality."

79. Charlton et al., "Cardiovascular diseases," 70–76.

80. Charlton and Quaife, "Trends in diet 1841–1993," 98, 104–9.

81. Centers for Disease Control, "Achievements in public health," 649.

82. Sytkowski et al., "Trends in cardiovascular disease," 346.

83. Whisnant, "Decline of stroke," 164.

84. La Vechia and Levi, "Trends in cerebrovascular mortality."

85. Gale and Martyn, "Conundrum of time trends in stroke."

86. Centers for Disease Control, "Achievements in public health," 649; Haberman, Capideo, and Rose, "Diverging trends in cerebrovascular disease," 587; Kannel et al., "Role of blood pressure in stroke."

87. Bonita and Beaglehole, "Does treatment of hypertension explain the decline?"; Bonita and Beaglehole, "Increased treatment of hypertension does not explain the decline."

88. Wing, "Decline of hypertension-related mortality."

89. Ebrahim, "Stroke mortality"; Wolfe and Burney, "Is stroke mortality on the decline?"

90. Charlton et al., "Cardiovascular diseases," 80; Wolfe and Burney, "Is stroke mortality on the decline?"

91. National Heart, Lung, and Blood Institute, *Report on Epidemiology and Cardiovascular Diseases*; Epstein, "Cardiovascular disease epidemiology"; Centers for Disease Control, "Achievements in public health."

92. Marmot et al., "Social-class distribution of heart disease"; Marmot et al., "Employment grade and coronary heart disease"; Marmot, Shipley, and Rose, "Inequalities in death"; CSDH, *Closing the Gap.*

93. Nieto. "Infections and atherosclerosis."

94. Burch and Giles, "Role of viruses in heart disease."

95. Bisno, "Group A streptococcal infections"; Quinn, "Review of morbidity and mortality trends."

96. Lu, "Agglutination of human platelets"; Jerushalmy, Kohn, and de Vries, "Interaction of myxoviruses"; Mustard et al., "Platelets and atherosclerosis"; Morat et al., "Platelet aggregation and release"; Terada et al., "Interaction of influenza virus"; Packham, Nishizawa, and Mustard, "Response of platelets."

97. Mustard, "Platelets and thromboembolic disease"; Genton, Weily, and Steck, "Platelets, thrombosis and coronary diseases."

98. Mustard et al., "Platelets and atherosclerosis"; Mustard, "Platelets and thromboembolic disease."

99. Benditt and Benditt, "Monoclonal origin of human atherosclerotic plaques."

100. Ross, "Atherosclerosis—an inflammatory disease"; Nieto, "Infections and atherosclerosis."

101. Ngeh, Anand, and Gupta, "*Chlamydia pneumoniae* and atherosclerosis."

102. Charlton et al., "Cardiovascular diseases," 64.

103. Nieto, "Infections and atherosclerosis," 941.

104. Kiechl et al., "Chronic infections and carotid atherosclerosis."

105. Morré et al., "Microorganisms," 651–52.

106. Campbell, Kuo, and Grayston, "*Chlamydia pneumoniae* and cardiovascular disease," 571; Grayston, "Knowledge of *Chlamydia pneumoniae* and atherosclerosis."

107. Mussa et al., "*Chlamydia pneumoniae* and vascular disease"; Ridker, "On evolutionary biology, inflammation, infection."

108. Ewald, *Plague Time*, 110–11, 125.

109. Patel et al., "Association of *Helicobacter pylori* and *Chlamydia pneumoniae* infections."

110. Markus and Mendall, "*Helicobacter pylori* infection"; Grau et al., "Recent infection as a risk factor."

111. Danesh, Collins, and Peto, "Chronic infections and coronary heart disease"; Danesh et al., "Low grade inflammation and coronary heart disease."

112. Wald et al., "*Chlamydia pneumoniae* infection and mortality."

113. Smeeth et al., "Risk of myocardial infarction and stroke," 2617.

114. Heltai et al., "Elevated antibody levels," 339.

115. Ibid., 340; Taylor-Robinson and Boman, "Failure of antibiotics."

116. Madjid, "Acute infections, vaccination and prevention."

117. Corrales-Medina, Madjid, and Musher, "Role of acute infection."

118. Warren-Gash, Smeeth, and Hayward, "Influenza as a trigger."

119. Bainton, Jones, and Hole, "Influenza and ischemic heart disease"; Madjid et al., "Influenza epidemics and acute respiratory disease."

120. Madjid et al., "Influenza and cardiovascular disease—Is there a causal relationship?

121. Keller et al., "Influenza vaccines"; Warren-Gash, Smeeth, and Hayward, "Influenza as a trigger."

122. Bull, "Meteorological correlates"; West, Lloyd, and Roberts, "Mortality from ischemic heart diseases"; West and Lowe, "Mortality from ischemic heart diseases"; Alling, Blackwelder, and Stuart-Harris, "Study of excess mortality"; Tillett, Smith, and Gooch, "Excess deaths attributable to influenza"; Fleming, Cross, and Pannell, "Influenza and circulatory disorders."

123. Lu, "Agglutination of human platelets"; Terada et al., "Interaction of influenza virus"; Mustard, "Platelets and thromboembolic disease."

124. Madjid et al., "Influenza and cardiovascular disease: Is there a causal relationship?"; Warren-Gash, Smeeth, and Hayward, "Influenza as a trigger."

125. Madjid et al., "Influenza epidemics and acute respiratory disease."

126. Madjid et al., "Influenza and cardiovascular disease—a new opportunity for prevention"; "Influenza and cardiovascular disease: Is there a causal relationship?"; "Influenza epidemics and acute respiratory disease"; Madjid, "Acute infection, vaccination and prevention"; Lamontagne et al., "Pneumonococcal vaccination and myocardial infarction."

127. Reichert et al., "Japanese experience with vaccinating schoolchildren."

Chapter Twelve

1. Capasso, "Antiquity of cancer."

2. Sandison and Tapp, "Disease in ancient Egypt," 46, 51.

3. Capasso, "Antiquity of cancer," 8–9.

4. Dobson, *Disease*, 224.

5. Onuigbo, "Links between tuberculosis and cancerous diseases."

6. Pearl, "Cancer and tuberculosis."

7. Burnet, *Immunology, Aging and Cancer*, 358–60; "Immunological approach to aging."

8. Weinberg, "How cancer arises."

9. Ibid., 70.

10. Soto and Sonnenschein, "Regulation of cell proliferation"; Sonnenschein and Soto, "Theories of carcinogenesis."

11. Ewald and Swain Ewald, "General evolutionary theory of oncogenesis."

12. Jensen, "International and urban-rural variation."

13. Doll, "Urban and rural factors in the aetiology of cancer."

14. Quinn et al., *Cancer Trends*, 15.

15. Rachet et al., "Cancer survival."

16. Barker, "Time trends in cancer mortality."

17. Blythe and Beral, "Monitoring cancer trends."

18. Coleman et al., "Trends in socioeconomic inequalities"; Rachet et al., "Cancer survival."

19. Osmond, Gardner, and Acheson, "Trends in cancer mortality," 1006.

20. Davey Smith, Gunnell, and Ben-Schlomo, "Life course approaches to socioeconomic differentials," 105; Leon et al., "Adult height and mortality."

21. Case, "Cohort analysis of cancer mortality." It should be noted that long series of data for Italy and New Zealand published in Preston et al, *Causes of Death: Life Tables* do not indicate that any cohort-related influence predominated in the mortality trends.

22. Cramer, "Antagonism in development of malignancy."

23. Institute of Cancer Research, *Serial Mortality Tables.*

24. Doll and Peto, "Avoidable risks of cancer," 1258.

25. Ibid., 1226–35.

26. Coley, "Fight against food adulteration"; Charlton and Quaife, "Trends in diet 1841–1993," 98–106.

27. Davey Smith, Gunnell, and Ben-Schlomo, "Life course approaches to socio-economic differentials," 109.

28. Doll, "Tobacco."

29. Doll and Peto, "Mortality in relation to smoking: 50 years' observations," 8.

30. Todd, *Cigarette Smoking Characteristics.*

31. Preston, "International comparison of excessive adult mortality"; *Mortality Patterns in National Populations*; Retherford, *Changing Sex Differential in Mortality.*

32. Retherford, *Changing Sex Differential in Mortality.*

33. Preston, "International comparison of excessive adult mortality"; *Mortality Patterns in National Populations.*

34. Doll and Hill, "Smoking and carcinoma"; Doll and Peto, "Mortality in relation to smoking"; Doll et al., "Mortality in relation to smoking: 40 years' observations"; US Surgeon General, *Smoking and Health: Report of the Advisory Committee*; US Surgeon General, *Smoking and Health: Report of Surgeon General.*

35. Doll and Peto, "Avoidable risks of cancer," 125.

36. Epstein, *Politics of Cancer*; Epstein and Swartz, "Fallacies of lifestyle cancer theories."

37. International Agency for Research on Cancer, *Tobacco Smoke and Involuntary Smoking.*

38. Sasco, Secretan, and Straif, "Tobacco smoking and cancer."

39. Taylor, Najafi, and Dobson, "Passive smoking and lung cancer."

40. Swerdlow, Doll, and dos Santos Silva, "Cancer incidence and mortality," 31–43.

41. Doll, Darby, and Whitley, "Mortality from smoking-related diseases," 134–36.

42. Royal College of Physicians, *Smoking or Health?*

43. Townsend and Davidson, *Inequalities in Health*, 69.

44. Davey Smith, Gunnell, and Ben-Schlomo, "Life course approaches to socio-economic differentials," 114.

45. Ibid., 115; Hart et al., "Class differences in lung cancer mortality."

46. Davey Smith, et al., "Socioeconomic differentials in cancer."

47. Davey Smith, Gunnel, and Ben-Schlomo, "Life course approaches to socioeconomic differentials," 89.

48. Davey Smith, Shipley, and Rose, "Magnitude and causes."

49. Leon, "Common threads," 78.

50. Coglan, *International Medical Congress of Australasia*, 203.

51. Cherry, "Cancer and acquired resistance to tuberculosis," pts. 1 and 2; "Cancer and tuberculosis: The development of malignancy"; "Cancer and tuberculosis."

52. Cherry, "Cancer and tuberculosis: development of malignancy"; *Cancer and Tuberculosis*; *Cancer and Tubercle Bacillus.*

53. Cruikshank, "Association of tuberculosis and cancer"; "Distribution of cancer and tuberculosis"; Paxon, "Tuberculosis and cancer mortality rates"; Campbell and Guilfoyle, "Pulmonary tuberculosis"; Campbell, "Cancer and tuberculosis mortality."

54. Haybittle, "Mortality rates."

55. Mercer, "Dying from tuberculosis and cancer."

56. Ibid., 379.

57. Zheng et al., "Lung cancer and prior tuberculosis infection"; Aoki, "Excess incidence of lung cancer"; Wu et al., "Previous lung disease"; Wu et al, "Pulmonary tuberculosis increases lung cancer"; Yu et al., "Increased lung cancer risk." A retrospective study in England also found raised lung cancer mortality among tuberculosis patients followed up for eight years. Tocque et al, "Elevated mortality."

58. Zheng et al., "Lung cancer and prior tuberculosis infection," 504.

59. Engels et al., "Tuberculosis and lung cancer."

60. Shiels et al., "Increased risk of lung cancer."

61. Liang et al., "Facts and fiction."

62. Auerbach, Garfinkel, and Parks, "Scar cancer of the lung"; Bobba et al., "Scar carcinoma of the lung." See also Doll, *Prevention of Cancer*, 90–92. Doll pointed out that "microcancers" were commonly found with tubercular scars, but not all would develop into cancer.

63. Yu et al., "Lung cancer risk."

64. Wu et al., "Previous lung disease"; Brenner et al., "Previous pulmonary diseases."

65. Mayne, Buenconsejo, and Janerich, "Previous lung diseases"; Littman et al., "Prior lung disease and risk of lung cancer."

66. Bae et al., "Pulmonary tuberculosis and lung cancer risk."

67. Brenner et al., "Previous lung diseases."

68. Brenner et al., "Previous pulmonary diseases," 121.

69. World Health Organization, "Disease and injury regional estimates, 2000–2011."

70. Askling and Ekbom, "Risk of non-Hodgkin's lymphoma."

71. Davignon et al., "BCG vaccination and leukemia mortality," 638; Davignon et al., "BCG vaccination and leukemia mortality," 80–81.

72. Rosenthal et al., "BCG vaccination and leukemia mortality."

73. Hoover, "Bacillus Calmette-Guérin vaccination."

74. Clemens and Stanton, "BCG prophylaxis against cancer."

75. Grange, Stanford, and Stanford, "Campbell de Morgan's 'Observations on cancer,'" 298.

76. Ibid.; Fine, "Variation in protection by BCG."

77. Grange, Stanford, and Rook, "Tuberculosis and cancer"; Grange and Stanford, "BCG vaccination and cancer."

78. Grange, Stanford, and Rook, "Tuberculosis and cancer"; Grange, Stanford, and Stanford, "Campbell de Morgan's 'Observations on cancer,'" 298.

79. Pfahlberg et al., "Melanoma and previous vaccinations"; Krone et al., "Protection against melanoma by vaccination."

80. Kölmel et al., "Prior immunization of patients."

81. Villumsen et al., "Risk of lymphoma and leukemia."

82. Burnet, "Immunological aspects of malignant disease"; *Immunology, Aging and Cancer*; "Immunological approach to aging"; *Immunological Surveillance.*

83. Brenner et al., "Previous pulmonary diseases," 121.

84. Burnet, *Immunology, Aging and Cancer*, 136–41.

85. Doll and Kinlen, "Immunosurveillance and cancer"; Kinlen, "Immunosuppressive therapy and cancer."

86. Bouvard et al., "Review of human carcinogens"; Maupas and Melnick, "Hepatitis B and liver cancer"; Millan et al., "DNA sequences of human papillomavirus."

87. Crawford, *The Invisible Enemy*, 180–83; Doll and Peto, "Avoidable risks of cancer," 1254.

88. Lawson, "Do viruses cause breast cancer?"; Amarante and Watanabe, "Involvement of virus in breast cancer"; Lawson and Heng, "Viruses and breast cancer."

89. Al-Sumidaie et al., "Particles with properties of retroviruses."

90. Lawson, "Do viruses cause breast cancer?"

91. Davey Smith, Gunnell, and Ben-Schlomo, "Life course approaches to socioeconomic differentials," 106–8.

92. Forman et al., "*Helicobacter pylori* and gastric cancer"; Helicobacter and Cancer Collaborative Group, "Gastric cancer and *Helicobacter pylori*."

93. Eurogast Study Group, "*Helicobacter pylori* infection and gastric cancer."

94. Wong et al., "Differential *Helicobacter pylori* infection rates"; Wong et al., "*Helicobacter pylori* eradication."

95. You et al., "Gastric dysplasia and gastric cancer," 1611.

96. International Agency for Research on Cancer, *Shistosomes, Liver Flukes and Helicobacter Pylori*, 177–240.

97. Barker et al., "Poor housing in childhood"; Mendall et al., "Childhood living conditions and *Helicobacter pylori*."

98. Davey Smith, Gunnell, and Ben-Schlomo, "Life course approaches to socioeconomic differentials," 109.

99. Banatvala et al., "Cohort effect and *Helicobacter pylori*."

100. Graham, "*Helicobacter pylori* infection"; Sugiyama and Asaka, "*Helicobacter pylori* infection."

101. Helicobacter and Cancer Collaborative Group, "Gastric cancer and *Helicobacter pylori*," 352.

102. Asaka and Dragosics, "*Helicobacter pylori* and gastric malignancies," 35, 39. On the possibilities for prevention, see Malfertheiner, Bornschein, and Selgrad, "A chance for prevention."

103. Wong et al., "*Helicobacter pylori* eradication," 194.

104. Littman, Jackson, and Vaughan, "*Chlamydia pneumoniae* and lung cancer."

105. Chaturvedi et al., "*Chlamydia pneumoniae* infection."

106. Zhan et al., "*Chlamydia pneumoniae* infection."

107. Bouvard et al., "Review of human carcinogens."

108. Martel et al., "Global burden of cancers"; Danaei, "Global burden of infection-related cancer."

109. Ewald, *Plague Time*, 55.

110. Burnett-Hartman, Newcomb, and Potter, "Infectious agents and colorectal cancer."

Chapter Thirteen

1. Armitage and Doll, "Age distribution of cancer"; "Two-stage theory of carcinogenesis"; Burch, *Enquiry Concerning Growth Disease and Aging*; *Biology of Cancer*, 91, 393.
2. Auerbach et al, "Smoking in relation to atherosclerosis"; Auerbach et al., "Cigarette smoking and coronary artery disease."
3. Mustard et al., "Platelets and atherosclerosis."
4. Doll and Peto, "Avoidable risks of cancer," 1255.
5. Nguyen-Van-Tam and Logan, "Digestive diseases," 137.
6. Sonnenberg, "Smoking and mortality."
7. Kurata et al., "Sex and smoking differences."
8. Susser and Stein, "Civilisation and peptic ulcer."
9. Marshall, "Helicobacter as the 'environmental factor.'"
10. Susser and Stein, "Civilisation and peptic ulcer."
11. Sonnenberg, Cucino, and Bauerfeind, "Unresolved mystery of birth-cohort phenomena."
12. Marshall and Warren, "Unidentified curved bacilli."
13. Langman, "Peptic ulcer, Susser and Stein."
14. Marshall, "Helicobacter as the 'environmental factor.'"
15. Haruma et al., "Incidence of *Helicobacter pylori* infection."
16. Marshall, "Helicobacter as the 'environmental factor'"; Barker et al., "Poor housing in childhood."
17. Sonnenberg, Cucino, and Bauerfeind, "Unresolved mystery of birth-cohort phenomena."
18. Marshall, "Helicobacter as the 'environmental factor.'"
19. Lau et al., "Epidemiology of complicated peptic ulcer disease."
20. Pounder and Ng, "Prevalence of *Helicobacter pylori* infection"; World Gastroenterology Organization, "*Helicobacter pylori* in developing countries."
21. Plant, "Alcohol and illicit drug-related diseases," 115–6.
22. Leon and McCambridge, "Liver cirrhosis mortality rates," 645.
23. Corrao et al., "Amount and duration of alcohol intake."
24. Norström, *Alcohol in Postwar Europe*, 62.
25. Corrao et al., "Liver cirrhosis mortality in Europe."
26. Crombie and Precious, "Social class gradient of cirrhosis mortality."
27. Ibid., 82.
28. Morrison, Boyd, and Richardson, "Liver cirrhosis mortality rates," 1899.
29. Corrao and Arico, "Hepatitis C virus infection and alcohol consumption."
30. Corrao et al., "Liver cirrhosis mortality in Europe."
31. World Health Organization, *Hepatitis C.*
32. Crawford, "Death rates from diabetes mellitus."
33. Trowell, "Diabetes mellitus death rates."
34. Yeung, Rawlinson, and Craig, "Enterovirus infection"; Hober and Sauter, "Type 1 diabetes mellitus"; Gamble, "Epidemiology of insulin-dependent diabetes."
35. Goldacre et al., "Underlying-cause and multiple-cause coding."
36. Goldacre et al., "Death-certificate-coded diabetes mellitus."
37. Masso Gonzales et al., "Diabetes in the UK."
38. Gregg et al., "Men and women with diabetes."

39. Preis et al., "All-cause and cardiovascular disease mortality."

40. Gu, Cowie, and Harris, "Mortality in adults with and without diabetes"; Roper et al., "Excess mortality."

41. Seidell, "Obesity, insulin resistance and diabetes."

42. The recent dramatic increase in the prevalence of diabetes among hunter-gatherer populations and in Asia and Africa has been linked with the adoption of "western lifestyle" behaviors. See Diamond, *World until Yesterday*, 437–49.

43. Pollard, *Western Diseases*, 32–49.

44. Ibid., 125–30; Dunne and Cooke, "Worm's eye view of the immune system."

45. Maahs et al., "Epidemiology of type 1 diabetes."

46. Goldberg and Krause, "Infection and type 1 diabetes."

47. Gamble et al., "Viral antibodies in diabetes mellitus."

48. Barrett-Connor, "Is insulin-dependent diabetes mellitus caused by coxsackie virus B infection?"

49. Wagenknecht, Roseman, and Herman, "Incidence of insulin-dependent diabetes mellitus."

50. Dotta et al., "Coxsackie B4 virus infection."

51. Fohlman and Friman, "Is juvenile diabetes a viral disease?"

52. Dotta et al., "Coxsackie B4 virus infection."

53. Yeung, Rawlinson, and Craig, "Enterovirus infection."

54. White, Ratziu, and El-Serag, "Hepatitis C infection and diabetes."

55. Mehta et al., "Hepatitis C virus infection."

56. Wang et al., "Hepatitis C virus infection," 201.

57. Negro and Alaei, "Hepatitis C virus."

58. Ibid., 1537; Alberti et al., "Review article: Chronic hepatitis C."

59. Symmons, "Musculoskeletal diseases," 156.

60. Swingler and Martyn, "Neurological diseases," 89.

61. Roderick, "Renal diseases," 123.

62. Schiffrin, Lipman, and Mann, "Chronic kidney disease"; Eknoyan et al, "Burden of kidney disease."

63. Haroun et al., "Chronic kidney disease"; Stengel et al., "Lifestyle risk factors"; Centers for Disease Control, "Prevalence of chronic kidney disease."

64. Atkins, "Epidemiology of chronic kidney disease," S15.

65. Ibid.; El Nahas and Bello, "Chronic kidney disease."

66. Feest, "Chronic renal failure," 441.

67. Kessner and Florey, "Mortality trends for nephritis."

68. Roderick, "Renal diseases," 126.

69. Waters, "Trends in mortality from nephritis."

70. Hansen and Susser, "Deaths from chronic kidney disease," 422.

71. Ibid.

72. Ewald, *Plague Time*, 49–50.

73. Hansen and Susser, "Deaths from chronic kidney disease," 423.

74. Carbonne, Luftig, and Buckley, *Microbial Triggers of Chronic Human Illness.*

75. Ibid., 2.

76. Lowe, Yansouni, and Behr, "Causality and gastrointestinal infections."

77. Carbonne, Luftig, and Buckley, *Microbial Triggers of Chronic Human Illness*, 5.

78. Ibid., 2.

79. Ibid., 8.
80. Barker et al., "Poor housing in childhood."
81. Carbonne, Luftig, and Buckley, *Microbial Triggers of Chronic Human Illness*, 9.
82. Hadley, "Infection connection."
83. Ewald, "Evolution of virulence," 10.
84. Rosenau and Schur, "Association of measles virus with rheumatoid arthritis."
85. Kaplan, "Pathogenesis of acute rheumatic fever."
86. Kazmierski et al., "Association of influenza incidence with multiple sclerosis."
87. Martyn, "Infection in childhood," 36–37.
88. Ibid., 34.
89. Pedro-Cuesta et al., "Whooping cough and Parkinson's disease."
90. Martyn, "Infection in childhood," 30.
91. Carbonne, Luftig, and Buckley, *Microbial Triggers of Chronic Human Illness*, 2.
92. Crow, "Is schizophrenia an infectious disease?"
93. Munk-Jorgensen and Ewald, "Epidemiology in neurobiological research."
94. Ledgerwood, Ewald, and Cochran, "Genes, germs, and schizophrenia."
95. Ibid.; Cochran, Ewald, and Cochran, "Infectious causation of disease."
96. Ewald, *Plague Time*, 155–56.
97. Balin et al., "Identification and localization of *Chlamydia pneumoniae*"; Hammond et al., "Immunohistological detection of *Chlamydia pneumoniae*."
98. Balin and Appelt, "Role of infection in Alzheimer's disease."
99. Ewald, *Plague Time*, xviii.

Chapter Fourteen

1. Derrick, "Changes in generation mortality"; Kermack, McKendrick, and McKinlay, "Death rates"; Jones, "Aging, disease and life expectancy."
2. Costa, "Understanding the twentieth-century decline."
3. Barker, "Childhood causes of adult diseases"; Barker and Osmond, "Infant mortality, childhood nutrition."
4. Doll, Darby, and Whitley, "Mortality from smoking-related diseases."
5. Rachet et al., "Cancer survival."
6. Coley, "The fight against food adulteration"; Charlton and Quaife, "Trends in diet 1841–1993," 100–101.
7. Griffiths and Brock, "Twentieth century mortality trends in England and Wales"; Charlton and Murphy, "Trends in causes of mortality," 47–51.
8. In view of the focus here on long-term trends in death rates, the arithmetic contribution of particular causes to a unit of change in the overall death rate has been used as a crude indicator, as this allows comparison with changes before registration began. More sophisticated methods for assessing the contribution to increasing life expectancy at birth made by changes in age-, sex-, and cause-specific mortality in different countries were developed by Arriaga and applied in studies of mortality change in the second half of the twentieth century. Arriaga, "Change in life expectancies"; "Changing trends in mortality decline." See also Yoshinaga and Une, "Contributions of mortality changes"; and Yang et al., "Life expectancy in South Korea."

9. Susser and Susser, "Choosing a future for epidemiology," pt. 1, 672; Pearce, "Traditional epidemiology, modern epidemiology, and public health."

10. Ewald, *Plague Time*, 44.

11. Susser and Susser, "Choosing a future for epidemiology," pt. 1, 670.

12. Loomis and Wing, "Is molecular epidemiology a germ theory for the end of the twentieth century?"

13. Susser and Susser, "Choosing a future for epidemiology," pt. 1, 670.

14. Ibid., 671.

15. Townsend and Davidson, *Inequalities in Health*, 160–63; Davey Smith, Gunnell, and Ben-Schlomo, "Life course approaches to socioeconomic differentials," 90.

16. The damage caused by the tobacco industry and the issue of control have been a focus of attention for many years. See for example Peto, "Distorting the epidemiology of cancer."

17. Susser and Susser, "Choosing a future for epidemiology," pt. 1, 671; pt. 2, 674.

18. Cochran, Ewald, and Cochran, "Infectious causation of disease," 439.

19. Ewald, *Plague Time*, 49–50.

20. Ibid., 50–51.

21. Ibid., 53–54.

22. Ibid., 55; Bouvard et al., "Review of human carcinogens."

23. Carbonne, Luftig, and Buckley, *Microbial Triggers of Chronic Human Illness*, 4.

24. Susser and Susser, "Choosing a future for epidemiology," pts. 1–2; Pearce, "Traditional epidemiology, modern epidemiology, and public health"; March and Susser, "Eco- in eco-epidemiology."

25. Loomis and Wing, "Is molecular epidemiology a germ theory for the end of the twentieth century?"; Susser and Susser, "Choosing a future for epidemiology," pt. 1, 668; pt. 2, 674.

26. Manollo et al., "Missing heritability of complex diseases," 9–10.

27. Cochran, Ewald, and Cochran, "Infectious causation of disease," 407–8.

28. Ledgerwood, Ewald, and Cochran, "Genes, germs, and schizophrenia."

29. Susser and Susser, "Choosing a future for epidemiology," pt. 2, 674.

30. Preston, "Mortality and level of economic development"; Preston and Haines, *Fatal Years.*

31. Costa, "Understanding the twentieth-century decline."

32. Preston, "Mortality and level of economic development," 243; *Mortality Patterns in National Populations.*

33. Gwatkin and Guillot, *Burden of disease.*

34. Beaglehole and Yach, "Globalisation and non-communicable disease," 903; Beaglehole et al., "Non-communicable disease crisis," 1438–39.

35. Ewbank and Preston, "Personal health behaviour"; Marmot, "Affluence, urbanisation and heart disease."

36. Kunitz, "Value of particularism."

37. Beaglehole, "Poverty and human development," 1871.

38. Daar et al., "Grand challenges," 494.

39. Ibid.; World Health Organization, *Preventing Chronic Diseases.*

40. McKeown, *Modern Rise of Population*; *Role of Medicine.*

41. Beaglehole and Yach, "Globalisation and non-communicable disease," 903.

42. Beaglehole et al., "Non-communicable disease crisis," 1438–39.

43. Ibid., 1439.

44. Wilkinson, *Unhealthy Societies*, 76–92.

45. Dorling, Mitchell, and Pearce, "Global impact of income inequality."

46. CSDH, *Closing the Gap.*

47. Grundy, "McKeown debate," 532.

48. Colgrove, "McKeown thesis," 729.

49. Link and Phelan, "McKeown," 731.

50. Beaglehole and Yach, "Globalisation and non-communicable disease," 904.

51. Beaglehole et al., "Non-communicable disease crisis," 1438.

52. Siegel, "Mass media antismoking campaigns"; Siegel and Biener, "Impact of an antismoking media campaign."

53. Beaglehole et al., "Non-communicable disease crisis,"1440.

54. Popkin, "Symposium: Obesity in developing countries."

55. Beaglehole and Yach, "Globalisation and non-communicable disease," 906.

56. Elo and Preston, "Effects of early life conditions"; Mosley and Gray, "Childhood precursors of adult morbidity and mortality," 71–77.

57. Mosley and Gray, "Childhood precursors of adult morbidity and mortality," 76; World Health Organization, "Cervical cancer prevention and control."

58. Pollard, "Childhood immunization."

59. Ewald, *Plague Time*, 80.

60. Nichol et al., "Influenza vaccination and reduction in hospitalizations"; Lamontagne et al., "Pneumonococcal vaccination and myocardial infarction"; Keller et al., "Influenza vaccines"; Madjid, "Acute infections, vaccination and prevention"; Madjid et al., "Influenza and cardiovascular disease—a new opportunity for prevention."

61. Madjid et al., "Influenza and cardiovascular disease: Is there a causal relationship?," 7–8.

62. Ibid., 10; Reichert et al., "Japanese experience with vaccinating schoolchildren."

63. Madjid et al., "Influenza and cardiovascular disease: Is there a causal relationship?"; Warren-Gash, Smeeth, and Hayward, "Influenza as a trigger."

64. Ewald, *Plague Time*, 80, 243.

65. Lorber, "Infectious causes of chronic illness."

66. Bjerke, "Impact of infectious disease," 52–54.

67. Morens, Folkers, and Fauci, "Emerging and re-emerging infectious diseases"; Krause, "Microbes and emerging infections"; Garrett, *Coming Plague*; Armelagos, Barnes, and Lin, "Disease in human evolution"; Barrett et al., "Emerging and re-emerging infectious diseases."

Bibliography

Aaby, P., J. Bukh, I. M. Lisse, and A. J. Smits. "Overcrowding and intensive exposure as determinants of measles mortality." *American Journal of Epidemiology* 120 (1984): 49–63.

———. "Severe measles in Sunderland, 1885: A European-African comparison of causes of severe infection." *International Journal of Epidemiology* 15, no. 1 (1986): 101–7.

Aaby, P., J. Bukh, I. M. Lisse, A. J. Smits, J. Gomes, M. A. Fernandes, I. Francisco, and M. Soares. "Determinants of measles mortality in a rural area of Guinea-Bissau: Crowding, age and malnutrition." *Journal of Tropical Paediatrics* 30 (1984): 164–67.

Ackland, M., B. C. K. Choi, and P. Puska. "Rethinking the terms non-communicable disease and chronic disease." *Journal of Epidemiology and Community Health* 58 (2004): 838–39.

Adelstein, A. "Certification of cause of death." *Health Trends* 9, no. 4 (1977): 78–79.

Albert, A., A. Vario, A. Ferrari, and R. Pistis. "Review article: Chronic hepatitis C—natural history and cofactors." *Alimentary Pharmacology & Therapeutics* 22, supplement 2 (November 2005): 74–78.

Alling, D. W., W. C. Blackwelder, and C. H. Stuart-Harris. "A study of excess mortality during influenza epidemics in the United States, 1968–1976." *American Journal of Epidemiology* 113 (1981): 30–42.

Al-Sumidaie, A. M., C. A. Hart, S. J. Levisher, C. D. Green, and K. McCarthy. "Particles with properties of retroviruses in monocytes from patients with breast cancer." *Lancet* 1 (1988): 5–9.

Amarante, M. K., and M. A. Watanabe. "The possible involvement of virus in breast cancer." *Journal of Research in Clinical Oncology* 135, no. 3 (2009): 329–37.

Anderson, A. W., B. Benjamin, R. Grenville-Mathers, and H. J. Trenchard. "Control of tuberculosis: Importance of heredity and environment." *British Journal of Preventive and Social Medicine* 11 (1957): 1–6.

Anderson, R. M. "Transmission dynamics and control of infectious disease agents." In Anderson and May, *Population Biology of Infectious Diseases*, 149–76.

Anderson, R. M., and R. M. May. "Population biology of infectious diseases: Part I." *Nature* 280 (1979): 361–67.

———. *Population Biology of Infectious Diseases*. West Berlin: Dahlem Konferenzen, Springer-Verlag, 1982.

Anderson, T. W., and W. H. Le Riche. "Ischaemic heart disease and sudden death: 1960–1." *British Journal of Preventive and Social Medicine* 24 (1970): 1–9.

Anonymous. "Chronic bronchitis and occupation." *British Medical Journal* 1 (1966): 101–2.

———. "Pathogenesis of measles." *British Medical Journal* 29 (1973): 187–88.

———. "Natural history of chronic bronchitis." *British Medical Journal* 1 (1976): 1297.

———. "Pulmonary complications of measles." *British Medical Journal* 2 (1976): 777–78.

Aoki, K. "Excess incidence of lung cancer among pulmonary tuberculosis patients." *Japanese Journal of Clinical Oncology* 23, no. 4 (1993): 205–20.

Appleby, A. B. "Famine, mortality and epidemic disease—a comment." *Economic History Review* 30, no. 3 (1977): 508–10.

———. "Nutrition and disease: The case of London, 1550–1750." *Journal of Interdisciplinary History* 6 (1975): 1–22.

Armelagos, G. J., K. C. Barnes, and J. Lin. "Disease in human evolution: The re-emergence of infectious disease in the third epidemiological transition." *National Museum of Natural History Bulletin for Teachers* 18, no. 3 (1996): 1–6.

Armitage, P., and R. Doll. "The age distribution of cancer and a multistage theory of carcinogenesis." *British Journal of Cancer* 8 (1954): 1–12.

———. "A two-stage theory of carcinogenesis in relation to the age distribution of human cancer." *British Journal of Cancer* 11 (1957): 161–69.

Armstrong, W. A. "The trend of mortality in Carlisle between the 1780s and the 1840s: A demographic contribution to the standard-of-living debate." *Economic History Review* 34, no. 1 (1981): 94–114.

Arriaga, E. E. "Changing trends in mortality decline during the last decades." In *Differential Mortality: Methodological Issues and Biosocial Factors,* edited by L. T. Ruzicka, G. J. Wunsch, and P. Kane, 105–29. Oxford: Clarendon Press, 1989.

———. "Measuring and explaining the change in life expectancies." *Demography* 21, no. 1 (1984): 83–96.

Arriaga, E. E., and K. Davis. "The pattern of mortality change in Latin America." *Demography* 6, no. 3 (1969): 223–42.

Asaka, M., and B. A. Dragosics. "*Helicobacter pylori* and gastric malignancies." *Helicobacter* 9, supplement 1 (2004): 35–41.

Askling, J., and A. Ekbom. "Risk of non-Hodgkin's lymphoma following tuberculosis." *British Journal of Cancer* 84 (2001): 113–15.

Atkins, R. C. "The epidemiology of chronic kidney disease." *Kidney International* 67, supplement 94 (2005): S14–S18.

Auerbach, O., H. Carter, L. Garfinkel, and E. C. Hammond. "Cigarette smoking and coronary artery disease." *Chest* 70, no. 6 (1976): 697–705.

Auerbach, O., L. Garfinkel, and V. R. Parks. "Scar cancer of the lung, increase over a 21-year period." *Cancer* 43 (1979): 636.

Auerbach O., E. C. Hammond, and L. Garfinkel. "Smoking in relation to atherosclerosis of the coronary arteries." *New England Journal of Medicine* 273 (1965): 775–9.

Badger, F. F., J. H. Dingle, A. E. Feller, R. G. Hodges, W. S. Jordan Jr., and C. H. Rammelkamp. "A study of illness in a group of Cleveland families, II: Incidence of the common respiratory diseases." *American Journal of Hygiene* 58 (1953): 31–40.

Bae, J., Z. Li, M. Shin, D. Kim, M. Lee, and Y. Ahn. "Pulmonary tuberculosis and lung cancer risk in current smokers: The Seoul Male Cancer Cohort Study." *Journal of Korean Medical Sciences* 28 (2013): 896–900.

Bainton, D., G. R. Jones, and D. Hole. "Influenza and ischemic heart disease—a possible trigger for acute myocardial infarction?" *International Journal of Epidemiology* 7, no. 3 (1978): 231–39.

Balin, B. J., and D. M. Appelt. "Role of infection in Alzheimer's disease." *Journal of the American Osteopathic Association* 101, no. 12, supplement (2001): S1–S6.

Balin, B. J., H. C. Gerard, E. J. Arking, D. M. Appelt, P. J. Branigan, J. T. Abrams, J. A. Whittum-Hudson, and A. P. Hudson. "Identification and localization of *Chlamydia pneumoniae* in the Alzheimer's brain." *Medical Microbiology and Immunology* 187 (1998): 25–42.

Banatvala, N., K. Mayo, F. Megraud, R. Jennings, J. J. Deeks, and R. A. Feldman. "The cohort effect and *Helicobacter pylori*." *Journal of Infectious Diseases* 168, no. 1 (1993): 219–21.

Barker, D. J. P. "Childhood causes of adult diseases." *Archives of Diseases in Childhood* 63 (1988): 867–69.

———. "Time trends in cancer mortality in England and Wales." *British Medical Journal* 288 (1984): 1325–26.

Barker, D. J. P., D. Coggon, C. Osmond, and C. Wickham. "Poor housing in childhood and high rates of stomach cancer in England and Wales." *British Journal of Cancer* 61 (1990): 575–78.

Barker, D. J. P. and C. N. Martyn. "The maternal and fetal origins of cardiovascular disease." *Journal of Epidemiology and Community Health* 46, no. 1 (1992): 8–11.

Barker, D. J. P., and C. Osmond. "Childhood respiratory infection and adult chronic bronchitis in England and Wales." *British Medical Journal* 293 (1986): 1271–75.

———. "Infant mortality, childhood nutrition, and ischemic heart disease in England and Wales." *Lancet* 10 (1986): 1077–81.

Barker D. J. P., C. Osmond, J. Golding, D. Kuh, and M. E. J. Wadsworth. "Growth in utero, blood pressure in childhood and adult life, and mortality from cardiovascular disease." *British Medical Journal* 298 (1989): 564–67.

Barker, T., and M. Drake. *Population and Society in Britain, 1850–1980.* London: Batsford, 1982.

Barrett, R., C. W. Kuzawa, T. McDade, and G. J. Armelagos. "Emerging and re-emerging infectious diseases: The third epidemiologic transition." *Annual Review of Anthropology* 27 (1998): 247–71.

Barrett-Connor, E. "Is insulin-dependent diabetes mellitus caused by coxsackievirus B infection? A review of the epidemiologic evidence." *Review of Infectious Diseases* 7, no. 2 (1985): 207–15.

Bartlett, M. S. "Measles periodicity and community size." *Journal of the Royal Statistical Society* 120 (1957): 48–62.

Beaglehole, R. "Poverty and human development: The global implications of cardiovascular disease." *Circulation* 116 (2007): 1871–73.

Beaglehole, R., R. Bonita, R. Horton, C. Adams, G. Alleyne, P. Asaria, and V. Baugh. "Priority actions for the non-communicable disease crisis." *Health Policy* 377 (2011): 1438–47.

Beaglehole, R., and D. Yach. "Globalisation and the prevention and control of non-communicable disease: The neglected chronic diseases of adults." *Public Health* 362 (2003): 903–8.

Beaver, M. W. "Population, infant mortality and milk." *Population Studies* 27 (1973): 243–54.

Behar, M. "A deadly combination." *World Health* (February–March 1974): 28–33.

Benditt, E. P., and J. M. Benditt. "Evidence for a monoclonal origin of human atherosclerotic plaques." *Proceedings of the National Academy of Science in the USA* 70 (1973): 1753–56.

Bengtsson, T., G. Fridlizius, and R. Ohlsson, eds. *Pre-industrial Population Change: The Mortality Decline and Short-Term Population Movements.* Stockholm: Almquist and Wiksell International, 1985.

Bengtsson, T., and M. Lindström. "Airborne infectious diseases during infancy and mortality in later life in southern Sweden, 1766–1894." *International Journal of Epidemiology* 32 (2003): 286–94.

Bentzon, J. W. "The effect of certain infectious diseases on tuberculin allergy." *Tubercle* 34 (1953): 34–41.

Biraben, J. N. "Current medical and epidemiological views on plague." In *The Plague Reconsidered. Local Population Studies* supplement, 25–36. Cambridge: Cambridge Group for the History of Population and Social Structure, 1977.

Bisno, A. L. "Group A streptococcal infections and acute rheumatic fever." *New England Journal of Medicine* 325 (1991): 783–93.

Bjerke, W. "The impact of infectious disease on chronic disease: A review of contemporary findings." *Journal of Social, Behavioural, and Health Sciences* 5, no. 1 (2011): 45–57.

Bjorck, L., A. Rosengren, K. Bennett, G. Lappas, and S. Capewell. "Modelling the decreasing coronary heart disease mortality in Sweden between 1986 and 2002." *European Heart Journal* 30, no. 9 (2009): 1046–56.

Black, W. *A Comparative View of the Mortality of the Human Species at all Ages.* London: C. Dilly, 1788.

Blythe, F., and V. Beral. "Monitoring cancer trends." *British Journal of Cancer* 63 (1991): 479–80.

Bobba, R. K., J. S. Holly, T. Loy, and M. C. Perry. "Scar carcinoma of the lung: A historical perspective." *Clinical Lung Cancer* 12, no. 3 (2011): 148–54.

Bonita, R., and R. Beaglehole. "Does treatment of hypertension explain the decline in mortality from stroke?" *British Medical Journal* 292 (1986): 191–92.

———. "Increased treatment of hypertension does not explain the decline in stroke mortality in the United States, 1970–1980." *Hypertension* 13, no. 5, supplement (1989): I69–I73.

Booth, C. *Life and Labour of the People in London.* London, 1902.

Bosma, H., M. G. Marmot, H. Hemingway, A. C. Nicholson, E. Brunner, and S. A. Stansfeld. "Low job control and risk of coronary heart disease in Whitehall II (prospective cohort) study." *British Medical Journal* 314 (1997): 558–65.

Bosma, H., R. Peter, J. Siegrist, and M. Marmot. "Two alternative job stress models and the risk of coronary heart disease." *American Journal of Public Health* 88, no. 1 (1998): 68–74.

Bots, M. L., and D. E. Grobbe. "Decline of coronary heart disease mortality in the Netherlands from 1978 to 1985: Contribution of medical care and changes over time in presence of major cardiovascular risk factors." *Journal of Cardiovascular Risk* 3 (1996): 271–76.

Bourdelais, P. "Cholera: A victory for medicine?" In Schofield, Reher, and Bideau, *Decline of Mortality in Europe*, 118–30.

Boutayeb, A. "The double burden of communicable and non-communicable diseases in developing countries." *Transactions of the Royal Society of Tropical Medicine and Hygiene* 100, no. 3 (2006): 191–99.

Bouvard, V., R. Baan, K. Straif, Y. Grosse, B. Secretan, F. El Ghissassi, and L. Benbrahim-Tallaa. "A review of human carcinogens—part B: Biological agents. *Lancet Oncology* 10 (2009): 321–22.

Bradley, L. "Reply to a review." *Local Population Studies* 10 (1973): 67–68.

Brenner, A. V., Z. Wang, R. A. Kleinerman, L. Wang, S. Zhang, C. Metayer, K. Chen, S. Lei, H. Cui, and J. H. Lubin. "Previous pulmonary diseases and risk of lung cancer in Gansu Province, China." *International Journal of Epidemiology* 30 (2001): 118–24.

Brenner, D. R., P. Boffetta, E. J. Duell, H. Blickeboller, A. Rosenberger, V. McCormack, and J. E. Muscat. "Previous lung diseases and lung cancer risk: A pooled analysis from the International Lung Cancer Consortium." *American Journal of Epidemiology* 176, no. 7 (2012): 573–85.

Brenner, M. H. "Economic changes and heart disease mortality." *American Journal of Public Health* 61, no. 3 (1971): 606–10.

———. "Mortality and the national economy: A review, and the experience of England and Wales, 1936–76." *Lancet* 314 (1979): 568–73.

Brimblecombe, F. S. W., R. Cruikshank, P. L. Masters, D. D. Reid, and G. T. Stewart. "Family studies of respiratory infections." *British Medical Journal* 1 (1958): 119–28.

Britten, N., J. M. C. Davies, and J. R. T. Colley. "Early respiratory experience and subsequent cough and peak expiratory flow rate in 36 year old men and women." *British Medical Journal* 294 (1987): 1317–20.

Britton, M. "Diagnostic errors discovered at autopsy." *Acta Medica Scandinavica* 196 (1974): 203–19.

Brownlee, J. "History of birth and death rates in England and Wales taken as a whole, from 1750 to the present time." *Public Health* 29 (1916): 228–38.

Bruneel, C. *La Mortalité dans les Campagnes, Le Duché de Brabant aux XVII et XVIII Siècles.* Leuven, Belgium: Bureau du Recueil, Bibliothèque de l'Université; Éditions Nauwelaerts, 1977.

Brunner, E., G. Davey Smith, M. Marmot, R. Canner, M. Belinska, and J. O'Brien. "Childhood social circumstances and psychosocial and behavioural factors as determinants of plasma fibrinogen." *Lancet* 347 (1996): 1008–13.

Brunton, D. "Smallpox inoculation and demographic trends in eighteenth-century Scotland. *Medical History* 36 (1992): 403–29.

Bull, G. M. "Meteorological correlates with myocardial and cerebral infarction and respiratory diseases." *British Journal of Preventive and Social Medicine* 27 (1973): 108–13.

Burch, G. E., and T. D. Giles. "The role of viruses in the production of heart disease." *American Journal of Cardiology* 29 (1972): 231–39.

Burch, P. R. J. *The Biology of Cancer—a New Approach.* Lancaster: MTP, 1976.

———. *An Enquiry Concerning Growth Disease and Aging.* Edinburgh: Oliver and Boyd, 1968.

Burnet, F. M. *Cellular Immunology*. Carlton, Australia: Melbourne University Press, 1969.

———. "An immunological approach to aging." *Lancet* 2 (1970): 358–60.

———. "Immunological aspects of malignant disease." *Lancet* 2 (1967): 1171–74.

———. *Immunological Surveillance*. Oxford: Pergammon, 1970.

———. *Immunology, Aging and Cancer*. San Francisco: Freeman, 1970.

Burnet, F. M., and D. O. White. *Natural History of Infectious Diseases*. Cambridge: Cambridge University Press, 1972.

Burnett, J. "Housing and the decline in mortality." In Schofield, Reher, and Bideau, *Decline of Mortality in Europe*, 158–76.

———. *Plenty and Want: A Social History of Diet in England from 1815 to the Present Day*. London: Scolar Press, 1979.

Burnett, A. N., P. A. Newcomb, and J. D. Potter. "Infectious agents and colorectal cancer: A review of *Helicobacter pylori, Streptococcus bovis,* JC virus, and human papillomavirus." *Cancer Epidemiology, Biomarkers & Prevention* 17, no. 11 (2008): 2970–79.

Bwibo, N. "Measles in Uganda: An analysis of children with measles admitted to Mulago Hospital." *Tropical Geographical Medicine* 22 (1970): 167–71.

Byington, R., A. R. Dyer, D. Garside, K. Liu, D. Moss, J. Stamler, and Y. Tsong. "Recent trends of major coronary risk factors and CHD mortality in the United States and other industrialized countries." In *Proceedings of the Conference on the Decline in Coronary Heart Disease Mortality. NIH Publication No. 79,* edited by J. R. Havlick and M. Fenleib, 340–80. Washington, DC: US Department of Health, Education, and Welfare, 1979.

Caldwell, J. C. *Demographic Transition Theory*. Dordrecht, Netherlands: Springer, 2006.

———. "Education as a factor in mortality decline: An examination of Nigerian data." *Population Studies* 33 (1979): 395–413.

———. "Health transition: The cultural, social and behavioural determinants of health in the Third World." *Social Science and Medicine* 36, no. 2 (1993): 125–35.

———. "Major new evidence on health transition and its interpretation." *Health Transition Review* 1, no. 2 (1991): 221–33.

———. "Mortality in relation to economic development." *Bulletin of the World Health Organization* 81, no. 11 (2003): 831–32.

———. "Old and new factors in health transitions." *Health Transition Review* 2, supplementary issue (1992): 205–16.

———. "Population health in transition." *Bulletin of the World Health Organization* 79, no. 2 (2001). doi:10.1590/S0042-96862001000200011.

———. "Routes to low mortality in poor countries." *Population and Development Review* 12 (1986): 171–220.

Caldwell, J. C., and P. Caldwell. "What have we learnt about the cultural, social and behavioural determinants of health? From selected readings to the first health transition workshop." *Health Transition Review* 1, no. 1 (1991): 3–17.

Caldwell, J. C., S. Findley, P. Caldwell, M. G. Santow, W. H. Cosford, J. Braid, and D. Broers-Freeman. *What We Know about Health Transition: The Cultural, Social and Behavioural Determinants of Health. The Proceedings of an International Workshop, Canberra, May 1989,* Health Transition Series No. 2. Canberra: Australian National University, 1990.

Caldwell, J. C., P. H. Reddy, and P. Caldwell. "The social component of mortality decline: An investigation in South India employing alternative methodologies." *Population Studies* 37 (1983): 185–205.

Campbell, A. H. "The relationship between cancer and tuberculosis mortality rates." *British Journal of Cancer* 15 (1961): 10–18.

Campbell, A. H., and P. Guilfoyle. "Pulmonary tuberculosis, isoniazid and cancer." *British Journal of Diseases of the Chest* 64, no. 3 (1970): 141–49.

Campbell, L. A., C. Kuo, and J. T. Grayston. "*Chlamydia pneumoniae* and cardiovascular disease." *Emerging Infectious Diseases* 4 (1998): 571–79.

Campbell, M. "Death rates from diseases of the heart: 1876–1959." *British Medical Journal* 2 (1963): 528–35.

———. "The main cause of increased death rate from diseases of the heart 1920–1959." *British Medical Journal* 2 (1963): 712–17.

Capasso, L. L. "Antiquity of cancer." *International Journal of Cancer* 113, no. 1 (2005): 2–13.

Capewell, S., R. Beaglehole, M. Seddon, and J. McMurray. "Explanation for the decline in mortality from coronary heart disease in Auckland, New Zealand, between 1982 and 1993." *Circulation* 102 (2000): 1511–16.

Capewell, S., C. E. Morrison, and J. J. McMurray. "Contribution of modern cardiovascular treatment and risk factor changes to the decline in coronary heart disease mortality in Scotland between 1975 and 1994." *Heart* 81 (1999): 380–86.

Carbonne, K. M., R. B. Luftig, and M. R. Buckley. *Microbial Triggers of Chronic Human Illness.* Report on a colloquium sponsored by the American Academy of Microbiology, June 25–27, 2004. Washington, DC: American Academy of Microbiology, 2005.

Cartwright, P. P. *A Social History of Medicine.* London: Longman, 1977.

Case, R. A. M. "Cohort analysis of cancer mortality in England and Wales, 1911–54, by site and sex." *British Journal of Preventive and Social Medicine* 10 (1956): 172–99.

Caselli, G. "Health transition and cause-specific mortality." In Schofield, Reher, and Bideau, *Decline of Mortality in Europe,* 68–96.

Centers for Disease Control and Prevention. "Achievements in public health, 1900–1999: Decline in deaths from heart disease and stroke—United States, 1900–1999." *MMWR Weekly* 48, no. 30 (1999): 649–56.

———. National Vital Statistics System, *Mortality Database.* National Center for Health Statistics, United States, 2010. http://www.cdc.gov/nchs/nvss/mortality/hist293.htm.

———. "Prevalence of chronic kidney disease and associated risk factors—United States, 1999–2004." *MMWR Weekly* 56, no. 8 (2007): 161–65.

Chadwick, E. *Report on the Sanitary Condition of the Labouring Population of Great Britain.* 1842. Reprint, Edinburgh: Edinburgh University Press, 1965.

Chalmers, A. K. "Infant mortality." *Public Health* 18 (1905): 409–38.

Chambers, J. D. *Population, Economy and Society in Pre-industrial England.* London: Oxford University Press, 1972.

———. "The Vale of Trent, 1670–1800." *Economic History Review,* supplement (1957): 33–57.

Charlton, J., and M. Murphy. "Trends in causes of mortality: 1841–1994—an overview." In Charlton and Murphy, *Health of Adult Britain*, 1:30–57.

Charlton, J., and M. Murphy, eds. *The Health of Adult Britain 1841–1994*. 2 vols. London: The Stationery Office, 1997.

Charlton, J., M. Murphy, K. Khaw, S. Ebrahim, and G. Davey Smith. "Cardiovascular diseases." In Charlton and Murphy, *Health of Adult Britain*, 2:60–81.

Charlton, J., and K. Quaife. "Trends in diet 1841–1994." In Charlton and Murphy, *Health of Adult Britain*, 1:93–113.

Chaturvedi, A. K., C. A. Gaydos, P. Agreda, J. P. Holden, N. Chatterjee, J. J. Goedert, N. E. Caporaso, and E. A. Engels. "*Chlamydia pneumoniae* infection and risk for lung cancer." *Cancer Epidemiology, Biomarkers and Prevention* 19, no. 6 (2010): 1498–1505.

Cherry, S. "The hospitals and population growth: The voluntary and general hospitals, mortality and local population in the English provinces in the 18th and 19th centuries. Part 1." *Population Studies* 34, no. 1 (1980): 59–75.

———. "The hospitals and population growth: The voluntary and general hospitals, mortality and local populations in the English provinces in the 18th and 19th centuries. Part 2." *Population Studies* 35, no. 2 (1980): 251–65.

Cherry, T. "Cancer and acquired resistance to tuberculosis, part 1." *Medical Journal of Australia* 2 (1924): 372–78.

———. "Cancer and acquired resistance to tuberculosis, part 2." *Medical Journal of Australia* 1 (1925): 581–98.

———. *Cancer and Tubercle Bacillus*. Melbourne: Melbourne Cancer Causation Research Committee, 1945.

———. "Cancer and tuberculosis." *Medical Journal of Australia* 2 (1933): 197–217.

———. *Cancer and Tuberculosis*. Melbourne: Patterson, 1935.

———. "Cancer and tuberculosis: The development of malignancy." *Lancet* 217 (1931): 285–88.

Choi, B. C. K., H. Morrison, T. Wong, J. Wu, Y. Yan. "Bringing chronic disease epidemiology and infectious disease epidemiology back together." *Journal of Epidemiology and Community Health* 61, no. 9 (2007): 802.

Clay, J. *Report of the Commission for Enquiry into the State of Large Towns and Population Districts*. London, 1844.

Clayton, D. G., D. Taylor, and A. G. Shaper. "Trends in heart disease in England and Wales, 1950–73." *Health Trends* 9 (1977): 1–6.

Cleland, J. G. "Maternal education and child survival: Further evidence and explanations." In Caldwell et al., *What We Know about Health Transition*, 400–419.

Cleland, J. G., and J. K. van Ginneken. "Maternal education and child survival in developing countries: The search for pathways of influence." *Social Science and Medicine* 27, no. 12 (1988): 1357–67.

Clemens, J. D., and B. F. Stanton. "BCG prophylaxis against cancer: Methodological evaluation of a continuing controversy." *Journal of Chronic Diseases* 37, no. 1 (1984): 45–54.

Cochran, G. M., P. W. Ewald, and K. D. Cochran. "Infectious causation of disease: An evolutionary perspective." *Perspectives in Biology and Medicine* 43, no. 3 (2000): 406–48.

Cockburn, T. A. *The Evolution and Eradication of Infectious Diseases.* Baltimore: Johns Hopkins University Press, 1963.

———. *Infectious Diseases: Their Evolution and Eradication.* Springfield, IL: Charles C. Thomas, 1967.

———. "Infectious disease in ancient populations." *Current Anthropology* 12, no. 1 (1971): 45–62.

Coglan, T. A. *International Medical Congress of Australasia, Transactions of the 6th Session.* Hobart: IMCA, 1902.

Cohen, M. N. *Health and the Rise of Civilization.* New Haven, CT: Yale University Press, 1989.

Coleman, M. P., B. Rachet, L. M. Woods, E. Mitry, M. Riga, N. Cooper, and M. J. Quinn. "Trends in socioeconomic inequalities in cancer survival in England and Wales." *British Journal of Cancer* 90 (2004): 1367–73.

Coley, N. G. "The fight against food adulteration." *Education in Chemistry,* 42 (2005): 46–49.

Colgrove, J. "The McKeown thesis: A historical controversy and its enduring influence." *Health Policy and Ethics* 92, no. 5 (2002): 725–29.

Colley, J. R. T., J. W. B. Douglas, and D. D. Reid. "Respiratory disease in young adults: Influences of early childhood respiratory tract illness, social class, air pollution and smoking." *British Medical Journal* 364, no. 3 (1973): 195–98.

Colley, J. R. T., and D. D. Reid. "Urban social origins of childhood bronchitis in England and Wales." *British Medical Journal* 2 (1970): 213–18.

Comstock, G. W. "Identification of an effective vaccine against tuberculosis." *American Review of Respiratory Diseases* 138 (1988): 479–80.

Condran, G. A., and R. A. Cheney. "Mortality trends in Philadelphia: Age- and cause-specific death rates 1870–1930." *Demography* 19, no. 1 (1982): 97–123.

Condrau, F., and M. Worboys. "Epidemics and infections in nineteenth century Britain." *Social History of Medicine* 22, no. 1 (2010): 165–71.

Cook, S. E., and W. Borah. *Mexico and the Caribbean.* Vol. 2. Berkeley: University of California Press, 1974.

Corrales-Medina, V. F., M. Madjid, and D. M. Musher. "Role of acute infection in triggering acute coronary syndromes." *Lancet Infectious Diseases* 10 (2010): 83–92.

Corrao, G., and S. Arico. "Independent and combined action of Hepatitis C virus infection and alcohol consumption on the risk of symptomatic liver cirrhosis." *Hepatology* 27, no. 4 (1998): 914–19.

Corrao, G., S. Arico, R. Lepore, M. Valenti, P. Torchio, G. Galatola, M. Tabone, and F. Di Orio. "Amount and duration of alcohol intake as risk factors of symptomatic liver cirrhosis: A case-control study." *Journal of Clinical Epidemiology* 46, no. 7 (1993): 601–7.

Corrao, G., P. Ferrari, A. Zambon, P. Torchio, S. Arico, and A. Decarli. "Trends of liver cirrhosis mortality in Europe, 1970–1989: Age-period-cohort analysis and changing alcohol consumption." *International Journal of Epidemiology* 26, no. 1 (1997): 100–109.

Costa, D. L. "Understanding the twentieth-century decline in chronic conditions among older men." *Demography* 37 (2000): 53–72.

Cramer, W. "On antagonism in development of malignancy in two different organisms." *Journal of Pathological Bacteriology* 43 (1936): 73–89.

Crawford, D. H. *The Invisible Enemy: A Natural History of Viruses*. Oxford: Oxford University Press, 2000.

Crawford, E. M. "Death rates from diabetes mellitus in Ireland 1833–1983: A historical commentary." *Ulster Medical Journal* 56, no. 2 (1987): 109–15.

Creighton, C. *The History of Epidemics in Britain*. Cambridge: Cambridge University Press, 1894.

Crimmins, E. M., and C. E. Finch. "Infection, inflammation, height, and longevity." *Proceedings of the National Academy of Sciences* 103, no. 2 (2006): 498–503.

Crombie, I. K., and E. Precious. "Changes in the social class gradient of cirrhosis mortality in England and Wales across the 20th century." *Alcohol and Alcoholism* 46, no. 1 (2011): 80–82.

Cronje, G. "Tuberculosis and mortality decline in England and Wales, 1851–1910." In Woods and Woodward, *Urban Disease and Mortality*, 79–101.

Crow, T. J. "Is schizophrenia an infectious disease?" *Lancet* 1 (1983): 173–75.

Cruikshank, D. B. "The association of tuberculosis and cancer." *Papworth Research Bulletin* 2 (1939): 1.

———. "The topography of the relative distribution of cancer and tuberculosis." *Tubercle* 21, no. 9 (1940): 281–91.

CSDH. *Closing the Gap in a Generation: Health Equity through Action on the Social Determinants of Health: Final Report of the Commission on Social Determinants of Health*. Geneva: World Health Organization, 2008.

Cummins, R. O., A. G. Shaper, M. Walker, and C. J. Wale. "Smoking and drinking by middle-aged British men: Effects of social class and town residence." *British Medical Journal* 283 (1981): 1497–1502.

Cutler, D., and G. Miller. "The role of public health improvements in health advances: The 20th century United States." *Demography* 42, no. 1 (2005): 1–22.

Daar, A. S., P. A. Singer, D. L. Parsad, S. K. Pramming, D. R. Matthews, R. Beaglehole, and A. Bernstein. "Grand challenges in chronic non-communicable diseases." *Nature* 450, no. 22 (2007): 494–96.

Dahlberg, G. "Mortality from tuberculosis in some countries." *British Journal of Preventive and Social Medicine* 4 (1949): 220–27.

Daly, C. "Air pollution and causes of death." *British Journal of Preventive and Social Medicine* 13 (1959): 14–27.

Danaei, G. "Global burden of infection-related cancer revisited." *Lancet Oncology* 13, no. 6 (2012): 564–65. Published online May 9, 2012. doi:10.1016/S1470-2045(12)70176-6.

Danesh, J., R. Collins, and R. Peto. "Chronic infections and coronary heart disease: Is there a link?" *Lancet* 350 (1997): 430–36.

Danesh, J., P. Whincup, M. Walker, L. Lennon, A. Thomson, P. Appleby, J. R. Gallimore, and M. B. Pepys. "Low grade inflammation and coronary heart disease: Prospective study and updated meta-analyses." *British Medical Journal* 321 (2000): 199–204.

Daniels, M., F. Ridehalgh, V. H. Springett, and I. M. Hall. *Tuberculosis in Young Adults: Report on the Prophit Tuberculosis Survey 1935–44*. London: Lewis, 1948.

Davey Smith, G., D. Gunnell, and Y. Ben-Schlomo. "Life course approaches to socioeconomic differentials in cause-specific adult mortality." In Leon and Walt, *Poverty, Inequality and Health*, 88–124.

Davey Smith, G., D. Leon, M. Shipley, and G. Rose. "Socioeconomic differentials in cancer." *International Journal of Epidemiology* 20, no. 2 (1991): 339–45.

Davey Smith, G., M. J. Shipley, and G. Rose. "Magnitude and causes of socioeconomic differentials in mortality: Further evidence from the Whitehall study." *Journal of Epidemiology and Community Health* 44 (1990): 265–70.

———. "Socioeconomic differentials in cancer among men." *International Journal of Epidemiology* 20 (1991): 339–45.

Davies, R. P. O., K. Tocque, M. A. Bellis, T. Rimmington, and P. D. O. Davies. "Historical declines in tuberculosis in England and Wales: Improving social conditions or natural selection?" *International Journal of Lung Diseases* 3, no. 12 (1999): 1051–54.

Davignon, L., P. Lemonde, P. Robillard, and A. Frappier. "BCG vaccination and leukemia mortality." *Lancet* 2 (1970): 638.

Davignon, L., P. Lemonde, J. St. Pierre, and A. Frappier. "BCG vaccination and leukemia mortality." Letter to the editor. *Lancet* 1 (1971): 80–81.

Daw, R. H. "Some statistical aspects of mortality from degenerative heart disease." *Journal of the Institute of Actuaries* 354, no. 1 (1954): 69–100.

De Flora, S., A. Quaglia, C. Benicelli, and M. Vercelli. "The epidemiological revolution of the 20th century." *FASEB Journal* 19 (2005): 892–97.

De Looper, M., and K. Bhatia. *International Health—How Australia Compares.* Canberra: Australian Institute of Health and Welfare, 1998.

Derrick, V. P. A. "Changes in generation mortality: England and Wales." *Journal of the Institute of Actuaries* 58 (1927): 117–59.

Diamond, J. *The World until Yesterday: What Can We Learn from Traditional Societies?* London: Penguin Books, 2013.

Diaz-Briquets, S. "Determinants of mortality transition in developing countries before and after the 2nd World War: Some evidence from Cuba." *Population Studies* 35, no. 3 (1981): 399–411.

Dickens, Charles. *Hard Times.* 1854. Reprint, Harmondsworth: Penguin, 1983.

Dingle, J. H., G. F. Badger, and W. S. Jordan Jr. "Common respiratory diseases: Incidence by family size." In *Illness in the Home. A Study of 25,000 Illnesses in a Group of Cleveland Families,* edited by J. H. Dingle, G. F. Badger, and W. S. Jordan Jr., 39–40. Cleveland: Press of Western Reserve University, 1964.

Dixon, C. W. *Smallpox.* London: Churchill, 1962.

Dobson, M. *Disease.* London: Qurecus, 2007.

Doll, R. *Prevention of Cancer—Pointers from Epidemiology.* London: Nuffield Provincial Hospitals Trust, 1967.

———. "Tobacco: A medical history." *Journal of Urban Health* 76 (1999): 289–313.

———. "Urban and rural factors in the aetiology of cancer." *International Journal of Cancer* 47, no. 6 (1991): 803–10.

Doll, R., S. Darby, and E. Whitley. "Trends in mortality from smoking-related diseases." In Charlton and Murphy, *Health of Adult Britain,* 1:128–55.

Doll, R., and A. B. Hill. "Smoking and carcinoma of the lung." *British Medical Journal* 221, no. 2 (1950): 739–48.

Doll, R., and L. Kinlen. "Immunosurveillance and cancer—epidemiological evidence." *British Medical Journal* 4 (1970): 420–22.

Doll, R., and R. Peto. "Avoidable risks of cancer in the United States." *Journal of the National Cancer Institute* 66, no. 6 (1981): 1191–1265.

———. "Mortality in relation to smoking: 20 years' observations on male British doctors." *British Medical Journal* 2 (1976): 1525–36.

Doll, R., R. Peto, J. Boreham, and I. Sutherland. "Mortality in relation to smoking: 50 years' observations on male British doctors." *British Medical Journal* 328 (2004): 1519–33. Published online June 24, 2004. doi:10.1136/bmj.38142.554479.AE.

Doll, R., R. Peto, K. Wheatley, R. Gray, and I. Sutherland. "Mortality in relation to smoking: 40 years' observations on male British doctors." *British Medical Journal* 309 (1994): 901–11.

Dorling, D., R. Mitchell, and J. Pearce. "The global impact of income inequality on health by age: An observational study." *British Medical Journal* 335 (2008): 873–75. doi:10.1136/bmj.39349.507315.DE.

Dotta, F., S. Censini, A. G. S. van Halteren, L. Marselli, M. Masini, S. Dionisis, and F. Mosca. "Coxsackie B4 virus infection of β cells and natural killer cell insulitis in recent-onset type 1 diabetic patients." *Proceedings of the National Academy of Sciences* 104, no. 12 (2007): 5115–20.

Draper, E. *Birth Control in the Modern World.* Harmondsworth: Penguin, 1972.

Dubos, R., and J. Dubos. *The White Plague.* London: Gollanz, 1952.

Duncan, C. J., S. R. Duncan, and S. Scott. "The dynamics of scarlet fever epidemics in England and Wales in the 19th century." *Epidemiology of Infectious Diseases* 117 (1996): 493–99.

Duncan, S. R., S. Scott, and C. J. Duncan, "The dynamics of smallpox epidemics in Britain, 1550–1800." *Demography* 30, no. 3 (1993): 405–23.

Dunne, D. W., and A. Cooke. "A worm's eye view of the immune system: Consequences for evolution of human autoimmune disease." *Nature* 5 (2005): 420–26.

Dwork, D. *War Is Good for Babies and Other Young Children.* London: Taylor and Francis, 1987.

Easterlin, R. A. "How beneficent is the market? A look at the modern history of mortality." *European Review of Economic History* 3, no. 3 (1999): 257–94.

Ebi-Kryston, K. "Predicting 15-year chronic bronchitis mortality in the Whitehall Study." *Journal of Epidemiology and Community Health* 43 (1989): 168–72.

Ebrahim, S. "Stroke mortality—secular and geographic trends: Comment on papers by Maheswaram and colleagues." *Journal of Epidemiology and Community Health* 51 (1997): 132–33.

Edwardes, E. J. *A Concise History of Smallpox and Vaccination in Europe.* London: Lewis, 1902.

Eknoyan, G., N. Lameire, R. Barsoum, K. Eckhardt, A. Levin, N. Levin, and F. Locatelli. "The burden of kidney disease: Improving global outcomes." *Kidney International* 66 (2004): 1310–14.

El Nahas, A. M., and A. K. Bello. "Chronic kidney disease: The global challenge." *Lancet* 365 (2005): 331–40.

Elo, I. T., and S. H. Preston. "Effects of early life conditions on adult mortality: A review." *Population Index* 58, no. 2 (1992): 186–212.

Engels, E. A., M. Shen, R. S. Chapman, R. M. Pfeiffer, Y. Yu, X. He, and Q. Lan. "Tuberculosis and subsequent risk of lung cancer in Xuanwei, China." *International Journal of Cancer* 124, no. 5 (2009): 1183–87. doi:10.1002/ijc.24042.

Engels, F. *The Conditions of the Working Class in England.* 1845. Reprint, London: Grenada, 1982.

Epstein, F. H. "Cardiovascular disease epidemiology: A journey from the past into the future." *Circulation* 93 (1996): 1755–64.

Epstein, S. S. *The Politics of Cancer.* New York: Anchor Doubleday, 1979.

Epstein, S. S., and J. B. Swartz. "Fallacies of lifestyle cancer theories." *Nature* 289 (1981): 127–30.

Eurogast Study Group. "An international association between *Helicobacter pylori* infection and gastric cancer." *Lancet* 341 (1993): 1359–62.

Ewald, P. W. "Evolution of virulence." *Infectious Disease Clinics of North America* 18, no. 1 (2004): 1–15.

———. *Plague Time—the New Germ Theory of Disease.* New York: Anchor Books, 2002.

Ewald, P. W., and H. A. Swain Ewald. "Toward a general evolutionary theory of oncogenesis." *Evolutionary Applications* 6 (2012): 70–81. doi:10.1111/eva.12023.

Ewbank, D. E., and S. H. Preston. "Personal health behaviour and the decline in infant and child mortality: The United States, 1900–1930." In Caldwell et al. *What We Know about Health Transition,* 116–49. Canberra: Australian National University, 1990.

Eyer, J. "Does employment cause the death rate peak in each business cycle?" *International Journal of Health Services* 7, no. 4 (1977): 625.

———. "Hypertension as a disease of modern society." *International Journal of Health Services* 5, no. 4 (1975): 539.

Eyler, J. M. *Victorian Social Medicine: The Ideas and Methods of William Farr.* Baltimore: Johns Hopkins University Press, 1979.

Fairbairn, A. S., and D. O. Reid. "Air pollution and other local factors in respiratory disease." *British Journal of Preventive and Social Medicine* 12 (1958): 94–103.

Farr, W. *Vital Statistics or the Statistics of Health, Sickness and Death.* First published in 1837. Reprinted in *Mortality in Mid 19th Century Britain,* edited by R. Wall. London: Gregg International, 1974.

Fawcett, J., and H. E. Parry. "Lung changes in pertussis and measles in childhood." *British Journal of Radiology* 30 (1957): 76–82.

Feest, T. "Epidemiology and causes of chronic renal failure." *Medicine* 35, no. 8 (2007): 438–41.

Feinstein, C. "A new look at the cost of living 1870–1914." In *New Perspectives on the Late Victorian Economy: Essays in Quantitative Economic History 1860–1914,* edited by F. Foreman-Peck, 151–79. Cambridge: Cambridge University Press, 1991.

Fenner, F., D. A. Henderson, I. Arita, Z. Jezek, and I. D. Ladnyi. *Smallpox and Its Eradication.* Geneva: World Health Organization, 1988.

Fildes, V. A. *Breasts, Bottles and Babies.* Edinburgh: Edinburgh University Press, 1986.

Fine, P. E. M., J. L. Aron, J. Berger, D. J. Bradley, H. J. Bürger, E. G. Knox, H. P. R. Seeliger. "The control of infectious disease." In Anderson and May, *Population Biology of Infectious Diseases,* 121–47.

———. "Variation in protection by BCG: Implications of and for heterologous immunity." *Lancet* 346 (1995): 1339–45.

Fine, P. E. M., and J. A. Clarkson. "Measles in England and Wales, III. Assessing published predictions of the impact of vaccination on incidence." *International Journal of Epidemiology* 12, no. 3 (1980): 332–39.

Fleming, D. M., K. W. Cross, and R. S. Pannell. "Influenza and its relationship to circulatory disorders." *Epidemiology and Infection* 133 (2005): 255–62.

Fletcher, C. M. "The natural history of chronic bronchitis." *British Medical Journal* 1 (1976): 1297–98.

Fletcher, C. M., R. Peto, C. M. Tinker, and F. S. Speizer. *The Natural History of Chronic Bronchitis and Emphysema*. London: Oxford University Press, 1976.

Flick, J. A. "Does measles really predispose to tuberculosis?" *American Review of Respiratory Diseases* 114 (1976): 257–65.

Flinn, M. *British Population Growth 1700–1850*. London: Macmillan, 1970.

———. *The European Demographic System, 1500–1820*. Brighton: Harvester, 1981.

———. *Scottish Population History from the 17th Century to the 1920s*. Cambridge: Cambridge University Press, 1977.

Florey, C. du V., R. J. W. Melia, and S. C. Darby. "Changing mortality from ischemic heart disease in Great Britain, 1968–76." *British Medical Journal* 1 (1978): 635–37.

Floud, R. "Medicine and the decline of mortality: Indicators of nutritional status." In Schofield, Reher, and Bideau, *Decline of Mortality in Europe*, 146–57.

———. "The heights of Europeans since 1750: A new source for European economic history." In *Stature, Living Standards, and Economic Development: Essays in Anthropometric History*, edited by J. Komlos, 9–24. Chicago: University of Chicago Press, 1994.

Floud, R., and B. Harris. "Health, height and welfare: Britain, 1700–1980." In *Health and Welfare during Industrialization*, edited by R. H. Steckel and R. Floud, 91–126. Chicago: University of Chicago Press, 1997.

Floud, R., and K. W. Wachter. "Poverty and physical stature." *Social Science History* 4 (1982): 422–52.

Floud, R., K. Wachter, and A. Gregory. *Height, Health and History: Nutritional Status in the United Kingdom, 1750–1980*. Cambridge: Cambridge University Press, 1990.

Fogel, R. W. "Changes in the disparities in chronic disease during the course of the 20th century." *NBER Working Paper 10311*. Cambridge, MA: National Bureau of Economic Research, 2004.

———. *The Escape from Hunger and Premature Death, 1700–2100*. Cambridge: Cambridge University Press, 2004.

———. *Explaining Long-Term Trends in Health and Longevity*. Cambridge: Cambridge University Press, 2012.

———. "New findings about trends in life expectation and chronic diseases: The implications for health costs and pensions." *Selected Paper Number 76*. University of Chicago Graduate School of Business, 1996.

Fogel, R. W., and D. L. Costa, "A theory of technophysio evolution, with some implications for forecasting population, health care costs, and pension costs." *Demography* 34, no. 1 (1997): 49–66.

Fogel, R. W., S. L. Engerman, and J. Trussell. "Exploring the uses of data on height: The analysis of long-term trends in nutrition, labour welfare, and labour productivity." *Social Science History* 4 (1982): 401–21.

Fohlman, J., and G. Friman. "Is juvenile diabetes a viral disease?" *Annals of Medicine* 25, no. 6 (1993): 569–74.

Ford, E. S., U. A. Ajani, J. B. Croft, J. A. Critchley, D. R. Labarthe, T. E. Kottke, W. H. Giles, and S. Capewell. "Explaining the decrease in US deaths from coronary disease, 1980–2000." *New England Journal of Medicine* 356, no. 23 (2007): 2388–98.

Forman, D., D. G. Newell, F. Fullerton, J. W. G. Yarnell, A. R. Stacey, N. Wald, and F. Sitas. "Association between infection with *Helicobacter pylori* and risk of gastric cancer: Evidence from a prospective investigation." *British Medical Journal* 302 (991): 1302–5.

Fraser, S. "Leicester and the smallpox." *Medical History* 24 (1980): 315–32.

Frenk, J., J. L. Bobadilla, C. Stern, T. Frejka, and R. Lozano. "Elements for a theory of the health transition." *Health Transition Review* 1 (1991): 21–38.

Fridlizius, G. "The mortality decline in the first phase of the demographic transition: Swedish experiences." In Bengtsson, Fridlizius, and Ohlsson, *Pre-industrial Population Change*, 17–40.

Fridlizius, G., and R. Ohlsson. "Mortality patterns in Sweden, 1751–1820: A regional analysis." In Bengtsson, Fridlizius, and Ohlsson, *Pre-industrial Population Change*, 299–328.

Frieden, T. R., B. H. Lerner, and B. R. Rutherford. "Lessons from the 1800s: Tuberculosis control in the new millennium." *Lancet* 355 (2000): 1088–92.

Gale, A. H. *Epidemic Diseases.* Harmondsworth: Penguin, 1959.

Gale, C. R. and C. N. Martyn. "The conundrum of time trends in stroke." *Journal of the Royal Society of Medicine* 90, no. 3 (1997): 138–43.

Galloway, P. R. "Basic patterns in annual variations in fertility, nuptiality, mortality and prices in pre-industrial Europe." *Population Studies* 42 (1988): 275–303.

Galvani, A. P., and M. Slatkin. "Evaluating plague and smallpox as historical selective pressures for the CCR5-delta 32 HIV-resistance allele." *Proceedings of the National Academy of Sciences* 100, no. 25 (2003): 15276–79.

Gamble, D. R. "The epidemiology of insulin-dependent diabetes, with particular reference to the relationship of virus infection to its aetiology." *Epidemilogic Review* 2 (1980): 49–70.

Gamble, D. R., M. L. Kinsley, M. G. FitzGerald, R. Bolton, and K. W. Taylor. "Viral antibodies in diabetes mellitus." *British Medical Journal* 3 (1969): 627–30.

Gardner, G., A. L. Frank, and L. H. Taber. "Effects of social and family factors on viral respiratory infection and illness in the first year of life." *Journal of Epidemiology and Community Health* 38 (1984): 42–48.

Gardner, M. J., P. O. Winter, and D. J. P. Barker. *Atlas of Mortality from Selected Diseases in England and Wales: 1968–1978.* Chichester, England: Wiley, 1984.

Garrett, L. *The Coming Plague.* New York: Penguin Books, 1995.

Gartner, A., D. Farewell, P. Roach, and F. Dunstan. "Rural-urban mortality differences in England and Wales and the effect of deprivation adjustment." *Social Science and Medicine* 72, no. 10 (2011): 1685–94.

Gaylin, D. S., and J. Kates. "Refocusing the lens: Epidemiologic transition theory, mortality differentials, and the AIDS pandemic." *Social Science and Medicine* 44, no. 5 (1997): 609–21.

Gaziano, J. M. "Fifth phase of the epidemiologic transition." *Journal of the American Medical Association* 303, no. 3 (2010): 275–76.

Genton, E., H. S. Weily, and P. P. Steck. "Platelets, thrombosis and coronary diseases." *Advances in Cardiology* 9 (1973): 29.

Gladstone, R. A., J. M. Jefferies, S. N. Faust, and S. C. Clarke. "Continued control of pneumococcal disease in the UK—the impact of vaccination." *Journal of Medical Microbiology* 60 (2011): 1–8.

Glass, D. V. *Numbering the People.* Farnborough: Saxon House, 1973.

———. "Socioeconomic status and occupation in the city of London at the end of the 17th century." In *Studies in London History,* edited by A. E. J. Hollaender and W. Kellerway, 373–89. London: Hodder and Stoughton, 1969.

Goldacre, M. J., M. E. Duncan, P. Cook-Mozaffari, and M. Griffith. "Trends in mortality rates comparing underlying-cause and multiple-cause coding in an English population 1979–1998." *Journal of Public Health Medicine* 25, no. 3 (2003): 249–53.

Goldacre, M. J., M. E. Duncan, P. Cook-Mozaffari, and H. A. Neil. "Trends in mortality rates for death-certificate-coded diabetes mellitus in an English population 1979–99." *Diabetic Medicine* 21, no. 8 (2004): 936–39.

Goldblatt, P. O. "Social class mortality differences." In *Biosocial Aspects of Social Class,* edited by N. Mascie-Taylor, 24–58. Oxford: Oxford University Press, 1990.

Goldberg, E., and I. Krause. "Infection and type 1 diabetes mellitus—a two edged sword?" *Autoimmunity Reviews* 8, no. 8 (2009): 682–86.

Goldman, L., and E. Cook. "The decline in ischemic heart disease mortality rates: An analysis of the comparative effects of medical interventions and changes in lifestyle." *Annals of Internal Medicine* 101 (1984): 825–36.

Goldstein, H. "Factors influencing the height of seven year old children—results from the National Child Development Study." *Human Ecology* 6, no. 2 (1978): 27–54.

Goldstone, J. A. "The demographic revolution in England: A re-examination." *Population Studies* 49 (1986): 5–33.

Gordon, T., and T. Thom. "The recent decrease in CHD mortality." *Preventive Medicine* 4, no. 2 (1975): 115–25.

Gore, A. T., and C. W. Shaddick. "Atmospheric pollution and mortality in the county of London." *British Journal of Preventive and Social Medicine* 12 (1958): 104–13.

Goubert, J. P. *Malades et Médicins en Bretagne, 1770–1970.* Paris: Klincksieck, 1974.

Graham, D. Y. "*Helicobacter pylori* infection is the primary cause of gastric cancer." *Journal of Gastroenterology* 35, supplement 12 (2000): 90–97.

Grange, J. M., and C. H. Collins. "Bovine tubercle bacilli and disease in animals and man." *Epidemiology and Infection* 92 (1987): 221–34.

Grange, J. M., and J. L. Stanford. "BCG vaccination and cancer." *Tubercle* 71 (1990): 61–64.

Grange, J. M., J. L. Stanford, and G. A. W. Rook. "Tuberculosis and cancer parallels in host responses and therapeutic approaches?" *Lancet* 345 (1995): 1350–52.

Grange, J. M., J. L. Stanford, and C. A. Stanford. "Campbell de Morgan's 'Observations on cancer' and their relevance today." *Journal of the Royal Society of Medicine* 95 (2002): 296–99.

Grau, A. J., F. Buggle, S. Heindl, C. Steichen-Wiehn, T. Banerjee, M. Maiwald, and M. Rohlfs. "Recent infection as a risk factor for cerebrovascular ischaemia." *Stroke* 26 (1995): 373–79.

Grayston, J. T. "Background and current knowledge of *Chlamydia pneumoniae* and atherosclerosis." *Journal of Infectious Diseases* 181, supplement 3 (2000): S402–S410.

Great Britain, Department of Health and Social Security. *Inequalities in Health: A Report of a Research Working Group.* London: Department of Health and Social Security, 1980.

Great Britain, Royal Commission on Vaccination. *Royal Commission on Vaccination: 1889. Reports with minutes of evidence and appendices.* London: HMSO, 1889–97.

Greenwood, M., W. W. C. Topley, and G. S. Wilson. *Experimental Epidemiology. Medical Research Council, Special Report Series No. 29.* London: MRC, 1936.

Gregg, E. W., Y. J. Cheng, B. L. Caldwell, G. Imperatore, D. E. Williams, K. M. Flegal, and K. M. Venkat Narayan. "Secular trends in cardiovascular disease risk factors according to body mass index in US adults." *Journal of the American Medical Association* 293, no. 15 (2009): 1868–75.

Gregg, E. W., Q. Gu, Y. J. Cheng, K. M. Venkat Narayan, and C. C. Cowie. "Mortality trends in men and women with diabetes, 1971 to 2000." *Annals of Internal Medicine* 147 (2007): 149–55.

Griffith, G. T. *Population Problems in the Age of Malthus.* Cambridge: Frank Cass, 1926.

Griffiths, C., and A. Brock. "20th century mortality trends in England and Wales." *Health Statistics Quarterly* 18 (2003): 5–17.

Grundy, E. "Commentary: The McKeown debate: Time for burial." *International Journal of Epidemiology* 34 (2005): 529–33.

Gu, K., C. C. Cowie, and M. I. Harris. "Mortality in adults with and without diabetes in a national cohort of the US population, 1971–1993." *Diabetes Care* 7 (1998): 1138–45.

Guberan, E. "Surprising decline in cardiovascular mortality in Switzerland 1951–76." *Journal of Epidemiology and Community Health* 33 (1979): 114–20.

Guha, S. "The importance of social intervention in England's mortality decline: The evidence reviewed." *Social History of Medicine* 7, no. 1 (1994): 89–113.

Guy, W. A. "250 years of smallpox in London." *Journal of the Royal Statistical Society* 45 (1882): 399–443.

Gwatkin, D. R. "Poverty and inequalities in health within developing countries: Filling the information gap." In Leon and Walt, *Poverty, Inequality and Health,* 217–46.

Gwatkin, D. R., and M. Guillot. *The Burden of Disease among the World's Poor, Current Situation, Future Trends, and Implications for Policy.* Washington, DC: World Bank and Global Forum for Health Research, 1999.

Gwatkin, D. R., M. Guillot, and P. Heuveline. "The burden of disease among the global poor." *Lancet* 354 (1999): 586–89.

Haberman, S., R. Capideo, and F. C. Rose. "Diverging trends in cerebrovascular disease and ischemic heart disease mortality." *Stroke* 13 (1982): 582–89.

Hadley, C. "The infection connection." *Science and Society* 7, no. 5 (2006): 470–73.

Halliday, M. L., and T. W. Anderson. "The sex differential in ischemic heart disease: Trends by social class 1931 to 1971." *Journal of Epidemiology and Community Health* 33 (1979): 74–77.

Halsey, N. A., D. L. Eddins, and A. R. Henman. "Measles mortality in the United States 1971–1975." *American Journal of Public Health* 70, no. 2 (1980): 1166–69.

Hammond, C. J., L. R. Hallock, R. J. Howanski, D. M. Appelt, C. S. Little, and B. J. Balin. "Immunohistological detection of *Chlamydiae pneumonia* in the Alzheimer's disease brain." *BMC Neuroscience* 11 (2010): 121–32. doi:10.1186/1471-2202-11-121.

Hansen, H., and M. Susser, "Historic trends in deaths from chronic kidney disease in the United States and Britain." *American Journal of Hygiene* 93, no. 6 (1971): 413–23.

Hardy, A. "Diagnosis, death and diet: The case of London, 1750–1909." *Journal of Interdisciplinary History* 18 (1988): 387–401.

———. *The Epidemic Streets: Infectious Disease and the Rise of Preventive Medicine, 1856–1900.* Cambridge: Cambridge University Press, 1993.

———. "Smallpox in London: Factors in the decline of the disease in the 19th century." *Medical History* 27 (1983): 111–38.

Haroun, M. K., B. G. Jaar, S. C. Hoffman, G. W. Comstock, M. J. Klag, and J. Coresh. "Risk factors for chronic kidney disease: A prospective study of 25,534 men and women in Washington County, Maryland." *Journal of the American Society of Nephrology* 14 (2003): 2934–41.

Harper, K., and G. Armelagos. "The changing disease-scape in the third epidemiological transition." *International Journal of Environmental Research and Public Health* 7 (2010): 675–97.

Harris B. "Health, height and history: An overview of recent developments in anthropometric history." *Social History of Medicine* 7 (1994): 297–320.

Hart, C. L., D. J. Hole, C. R. Gillis, G. Davey Smith, G. C. M. Watt, and V. M. Hawthorne. "Social class differences in lung cancer mortality: Risk factor explanations using two Scottish cohort studies." *International Journal of Epidemiology* 30 (2001): 268–74.

Haruma, K., S. Okamoto, H. Kawaguchi, T. Gotoh, T. Kamada, M. Yoshihara, S. Koji, and G. Kajiyama. "Reduced incidence of *Helicobacter pylori* infection in young Japanese persons between the 1970s and 1990s." *Journal of Clinical Gastroenterology* 25 (1997): 583–86.

Hatcher, J. *Plague, Population and the English Economy 1348–1530.* London: Macmillan, 1977.

Haybittle, J. L. "Mortality rates from cancer and tuberculosis." *British Journal of Preventive and Social Medicine* 16 (1962): 93–104; 17 (1963): 23–28.

Haygarth, J. "Observations on the population and disease of Chester in the year, 1774." A paper presented to the Royal Society. *Philosophical Transactions and Observations, Royal Society,* January 1777. Original in Chester Town Hall.

Health Protection Agency. *HIV in the United Kingdom: 2012 Report.* London: Health Protection Services, Colindale.

Heasman, M. A., and L. Lipworth. "Accuracy of certification of cause of death." *Medical and Population Subjects No. 20,* 110–28. London: HMSO, 1966.

Heath, A. "The sociology of social class." In *Biosocial Aspects of Social Class,* edited by C. G. N. Mascie-Taylor, 1–23. Oxford: Oxford University Press, 1990.

Heberden, W. *Observations on the Increase and Decline of Different Diseases,* 1801. Reprinted in *Population and Disease in Early Industrial England,* edited by B. Benjamin. Farnborough, England: Gregg International, 1973.

Hedrich, A. W. "The corrected average attack rate for measles among city children." *American Journal of Hygiene* 11 (1930): 576–600.

Helicobacter and Cancer Collaborative Group. "Gastric cancer and *Helicobacter pylori*: A combined analysis of 12 case control studies nested within prospective cohorts." *Gut* 49 (2001): 347–53.

Heltai, K., Z. Kis, K. Burian, V. Endresz, A. Veres, E. Ludwig, E. Gönczöl, and I. Valvy-Nagi. "Elevated antibody levels against *Chlamydia pneumoniae*, human HSP60 and mycobacterial HSP65 are independent risk factors in myocardial infarction and ischemic heart disease." *Atherosclerosis* 173 (2004): 339–46.

Henry, L., and Y. Blayo. "La population de la France de 1740 à 1860." *Population*, Numéro Special (November 1975): 71–122.

Heysham, J. *Observations on the Bills of Mortality in Carlisle for the Year 1779*. Carlisle: Mililieu, 1782.

Hill, A. B. "The environment and disease: Association or causation?" *Proceedings of the Royal Society of Medicine* 58 (1965): 295–300.

Hobcraft, J. N., W. McDonald, and S. O. Rutstein. "Demographic determinants of infant and early child mortality: A comparative analysis." *Population Studies* 39 (1985): 363–85.

Hober, D., and P. Sauter, "Pathogenesis of type 1 diabetes mellitus: Interplay between enterovirus and host." *Nature Reviews Endocrinology* 6 (2010): 279–89. doi:10.1038/nrendo.2010.27.

Hobsbawm, E. J. "The British standard of living, 1790–1850." *Economic History Review*, 2nd ser., 10, no. 1 (1957): 46–68.

Hofsten, E., and G. Lundström. *Swedish Population History: Main Trends from 1750–1970*. Urval No. 8. Stockholm: Statistiska Centralbyran, 1977.

Hollingsworth, T. H. "A demographic study of the British ducal families." *Population Studies* 11 (1957): 1–26.

———. "The demography of the British peerage." *Population Studies*, supplement 18, no. 2 (1965).

Holy Trinity Parish, Whitehaven. Parish registers for 1752–80. County Records Office, Carlisle.

Hoover, R. N. "Bacillus Calmette-Guérin vaccination and cancer prevention: A critical review of the human experience." *Cancer Research* 36 (1976): 652–54.

Howard, P. "The changing face of chronic bronchitis with airways obstruction." *British Medical Journal* 2 (1974): 89–93.

Howe, G. M. *Man, Environment and Disease in Britain: A Medical Geography through the Ages*. Harmondsworth: Penguin, 1976.

———. *A National Atlas of Disease Mortality in the UK*. London: Nelson, 1970.

Howie, P., and A. S. McNeilly. "Effect of breast-feeding patterns on human birth intervals." *Journal of Reproduction and Fertility* 65 (1982): 545–57.

Howie, P., A. S. McNeilly, M. J. Huston, A. Cook, and H. Boyle. "Effect of supplementary food on suckling patterns and ovarian activity during lactation." *British Medical Journal* 283 (1981): 757–59.

Hubert, H. B., M. Feinleib, P. M. McNamara, and W. P. Castelli. "Obesity as an independent risk factor for cardiovascular disease: A 26-year follow-up of participants in the Framingham Heart Study." *Circulation* 67, no. 5 (1983): 968–77.

Huck, P. "Shifts in the seasonality of infant deaths in nine English towns during the 19th century: A case for reduced breast feeding?" *Explorations in Economic History* 34, no. 3 (1997): 368–86.

Huninck, M. G., L. Goldman, A. N. Tosteson, M. A. Mittleman, P. A. Goldman, L. W. Williams, J. Tseval, and M. C. Weinstein. "The recent decline in mortality from coronary heart disease, 1980–1990." *Journal of the American Medical Association* 277, no. 7 (1997): 535–42.

Hunt, R. H., S. D. Xiao, F. Megraud, R. Leon-Barua, F. Bazzoli, S. van der Merwe, L. G. Vaz Coelho. "*Helicobacter Pylori* in Developing Countries. World Gastroenterology Organisation Global Guideline." *Journal of Gastrointestinal and Liver Diseases* 20, no. 3 (2011): 299–304.

Hussey, G. D., and C. J. Clements, "Clinical problems in measles case management." *Annals of Tropical Paediatrics* 16 (1996): 307–17.

Illsey, R. "Occupational class, selection and the production of inequalities." *Quarterly Journal of Social Affairs* 2 (1986): 151–61; 3 (1987): 213–23.

Illsey, R., and J. Le Grande. "Measurement of inequality in health." London School of Economics and Political Science Paper, February 1987.

Institute of Cancer Research. *Serial Mortality Tables.* London: Institute of Cancer Research, 1976.

International Agency for Research on Cancer. *Schistosomes, Liver Flukes, and Helicobacter pylori—IARC Monographics on the Evolution of Carcinogenic Risks to Humans.* Vol. 61. Lyon, France: IARC, 1994, 177–240.

———. *Tobacco Smoke and Involuntary Smoking—IARC Monographs on the Evaluation of Carcinogenic Risks to Humans.* Vol. 83. Lyon, France: IARC, 2004.

Italy, Central Institute of Statistics. *Annuaria di Statistiche Sanitarie.* Rome: Republica Italiana, 1956–.

———. *Cause di Morte.* Rome: Republica Italiana, 1887–1955.

Jacob J. T., A. K. Mehta, and M. K. Leonard. "Acute forms of tuberculosis in adults." *American Journal of Medicine* 122, no. 1 (2009): 12–17.

Jensen, O. M. "International and urban-rural variation in cancer." In *Changing Disease Patterns and Human Behaviour,* edited by N. F. Stanley and R. A. Joske, 107–26. London: Academic Press, 1980.

Jerushalmy, Z., A. Kohn, and A. de Vries. "Interaction of myxoviruses with human blood platelets in vitro." *Proceedings of the Royal Society for Experimental Biology* 106 (1961): 462–66.

Jones, H. B. "Aging, disease and life expectancy." *Advances in Biological and Medical Physics* 4 (1956): 281–337.

Jones, P. E., and A. V. Judges. "London population in the late 17th century." *Economic History Review* 6 (1935): 45–63.

Jones, R. E. "Further evidence on the decline in infant mortality in North Shropshire 1561–1810." *Population Studies* 34, no. 2 (1980): 239–50.

Kallman, F. J., and D. Reisner. "Twin studies on the significance of genetic factors in tuberculosis." *American Review of Tuberculosis* 47 (1943): 549–74.

Kannel, W. B., and T. J. Thom. "Declining cardiovascular mortality." *Circulation* 70, no. 3 (1984): 331–36.

Kannel, W. B., P. A. Wolf, J. Verter, and P. M. McNamara. "Epidemiologic assessment of the role of blood pressure in stroke: The Framingham Study, 1970." *Journal of the American Medical Association* 276, no. 15 (1996): 1269–78.

Kaplan, E. L. "Pathogenesis of acute rheumatic fever and rheumatic heart disease: Evasive after half a century of clinical, epidemiological, and laboratory investigation." *Heart* 91 (2005): 3–4. doi:10.1136/hrt.2004.034744.

Karlen, A., *Plague's Progress.* London: Indigo, 1996.

Katz, A. R., and D. M. Morens. "Severe streptococcal infections in historical perspective." *Clinical Infectious Diseases* 14, no. 1 (1992): 298–307.

Kazmierski, R., M. Wender, P. Guzik, and D. Zielonka. "Association of influenza incidence with multiple sclerosis onset." *Folia Neuropathologica* 42, no. 1 (2004): 19–24.

Keller, T., V. B. Weeda, C. J. van Dongen, and M. Levi. "Influenza vaccines for preventing coronary heart disease." *Cochrane Database of Systematic Reviews*, no. 3 (2008). doi:10.1002/14651858.CD005050.pub2.

Kermack, M. A., A. G. McKendrick, and P. L. McKinlay. "Death rates in Great Britain and Sweden: Some general regularities and their significance." *International Journal of Epidemiology* 30 (2001): 678–83.

Kessner, D. M., and C. du V. Florey. "Mortality trends for acute and chronic nephritis and infections of the kidney." *Lancet* 2 (1967): 979–82.

Kesteloot, H., S. Sans, and D. Kromhout. "Dynamics of cardiovascular and all-cause mortality in western and eastern Europe between 1970 and 2000." *European Heart Journal* 27, no. 1 (2006): 107–13.

Keusch, G. T. "The history of nutrition: Malnutrition, infection and immunity." *Journal of Nutrition* 133 (2003): 336S–340S.

Kiechl, S., G. Egger, M. Mayr, C. J. Wiedermann, E. Bonora, F. Oberhollenzer, and M. Muggeo. "Chronic infections and the risk of carotid atherosclerosis." *Circulation* 103 (2001): 1064–70.

Kinlen, L. J. "Immunosuppressive therapy and cancer." *Cancer Surveys* 1, no. 4 (1982): 565–83.

Kirk, D. "Demographic transition theory." *Population Studies* 50, no. 3 (1996): 361–87.

Kivimäki, M., P. Leino-Arjas, R. Luukkonen, H. Riihimäki, J. Vahtera, and J. Kirjonen. "Work stress and risk of cardiovascular mortality: Prospective cohort study of industrial employees." *British Medical Journal* 325 (2002): 857–60.

Knobler, S. L., S. O'Connor, S. M. Lemon, and M. Najafi, eds. *The Infectious Etiology of Chronic Diseases: Defining the Relationship, Enhancing the Research, and Mitigating the Effects—Workshop Summary.* Forum on Emerging Infections, Institute of Medicine. Washington, DC: The National Academy Press, 2004.

Kölmel, K. F., J. M. Grange, B. Krone, G. Mastrangelo, C. R. Rossi, B. M. Henz, and C. Seebacher. "Prior immunization of patients with malignant melanoma with vaccinia or BCG is associated with better survival: An European Organization for Research and Treatment of Cancer cohort study on 542 patients." *European Journal of Cancer* 41 (2005): 118–25.

Konner, M., and C. Worthman. "Nursing frequency, gonadal function and birth spacing among !Kung hunter-gatherers." *Science* 207 (1980): 788–91.

Krause, J. T. "Changes in English fertility and mortality, 1781–1850." *Economic History Review* 11 (1958): 52–70.

Krause, R. M. "Evolving microbes and re-emerging streptococcal disease." *Clinical Laboratory Medicine* 22, no. 4 (2002): 835–48.

———. "Microbes and emerging infections: The compulsion to become something new." *American Society for Microbiology, ASM News* 67, no. 1 (2001): 15–19.

Krone, B., K. F. Kölmel, B. M. Hengz, and J. M. Grange. "Protection against melanoma by vaccination with Bacille Calmette Guérin (BCG) and/or vaccinia: An epidemiology-based hypothesis on the nature of a melanoma risk factor and its immunological control." *European Journal of Cancer* 41 (2005): 104–17.

Kuller, L., R. Seltser, R. Paffenberger, and D. Krueger. "Trends in cerebrovascular disease mortality based on multiple cause tabulation of death certificates 1930–1960: A comparison of trends in Memphis and Baltimore." *American Journal of Epidemiology* 88 (1968): 307–17.

Kunitz, S. J. "Mortality change in America, 1620–1920." *Human Biology* 56, no. 3 (1984): 559–82.

———. "Speculations on the European mortality decline." *Economic History Review* 36, no. 3 (1983): 349–64.

———. "The value of particularism in the study of the cultural, social and behavioural determinants of mortality." In Caldwell et al, *What We Know About Health Transition*, 92–109.

Kurata, J. H., J. D. Elashoff, A. N. Nogawa, and B. M. Haile. "Sex and smoking differences in duodenal ulcer mortality." *American Journal of Public Health* 76, no. 6 (1986): 700–702.

Kurt, T. L., A. S. Yeager, S. Guerette, and S. Dunlop. "Spread of pertussis by hospital staff." *Journal of the American Medical Association* 221 (1972): 264–67.

Lambert, H. J. "Epidemiology of a small pertussis outbreak in Kent County, Michigan." *Public Health Report* 80 (1965): 365–69.

Lamontagne, F., M. Garant, J. Carvalho, L. Lanthier, M. Smieja, and D. Pilon. "Pneumonococcal vaccination and risk of myocardial infarction." *Canadian Medical Association Journal* 179, no. 8 (2008): 773–77.

Landers, J. "Historical epidemiology and the structural analysis of mortality." *Health Transition Review* 2, supplement (1992): 47–75.

———. "Mortality and metropolis: The case of London 1675–1825." *Population Studies* 41 (1987): 59–76.

Langford, C. M. "Reasons for the decline in mortality in Sri Lanka immediately after the Second World War: A re-examination of the evidence." *Health Transition Review* 6 (1996): 3–23.

Langman, M. "Peptic ulcer, Susser and Stein and the cohort phenomenon." *International Journal of Epidemiology* 31 (2002): 27–28.

Larsen, I. *Eighteenth Century Diseases, Diagnostic Trends and Mortality*. Oslo: University of Oslo Press, 1979.

Lau, J. Y., J. Sung, C. Hill, C. Henderson, C. W. Howden, and D. C. Metz. "Systematic review of the epidemiology of complicated peptic ulcer disease: Incidence, recurrence, risk factors and mortality." *Digestion* 84 (2011): 102–13.

La Vecchia, C., and F. Levi. "Trends in cerebrovascular mortality in western and eastern Europe." *European Neurology* 34 (1994): 301–5.

Lawlor, D. A., G. Davey Smith, D. A. Leon, J. A. C. Sterne, and S. Ebrahim. "Secular trends in mortality by stroke subtype in the 20th century: A retrospective analysis." *Lancet* 360 (2002): 1818–23.

Lawn, J. E., S. Cousens, J. Zupan. "4 million neonatal deaths: When? Where? Why?" *Lancet* 365 (2005): 891–900.

Lawson, J. S. "Do viruses cause breast cancer?" *Methods in Molecular Biology* 471 (2009): 421–38.

Lawson, J. S., and B. Heng. "Viruses and breast cancer." *Cancers* 2 (2010): 752–72. doi:10.3390/cancers2020752.

Ledgerwood, L. G., P. Ewald, and G. M. Cochran. "Genes, germs, and schizophrenia: An evolutionary perspective." *Perspectives in Biology and Medicine* 46, no. 3 (2003): 317–48.

Lee, R. "The demographic transition: Three centuries of fundamental change." *Journal of Economic Perspectives* 17, no. 4 (2003): 167–90.

Lee, W. R. *Population Growth, Economic Development and Social Change in Bavaria, 1750–1850.* New York: Arno, 1977.

Leeder, S. R., R. Corkhill, L. M. Irwig, and W. W. Holland. "Influence of family factors on the incidence of lower respiratory illness during the first year of life." *British Journal of Preventive and Social Medicine* 30 (1976): 203–12.

Le Grand, J. "Inequalities in health: Some international comparisons." *European Economic Review* 31, no. 1 (1987): 182–91.

Leon, D. A. "Common threads: Underlying components of inequalities in health between and within countries." In Leon and Walt, *Poverty, Inequality and Health,* 58–87.

Leon, D. A., L. Chenet, V. M. Shkolnikov, S. Zakharov, J. Shapiro, G. Rakhmanova, S. Vassin, and M. McKee. "Huge variation in Russian mortality rates 1984–1994: Artefact, alcohol or what?" *Lancet* 350 (1997): 383–88.

Leon, D. A., G. Davey Smith, M. Shipley, and D. Strachan. "Adult height and mortality in London: Early life, socioeconomic confounding, or shrinkage?" *Journal of Epidemiology and Community Health* 45 (1995): 5–9.

Leon, D. A., and J. McCambridge. "Liver cirrhosis mortality rates in Britain from 1950 to 2002: An analysis of routine data." *Lancet* 367 (2006): 52–56; 645.

Leon, D. A., and G. Walt, eds. *Poverty, Inequality and Health: An International Perspective.* Oxford: Oxford University Press, 2001.

Lerner, M. "Modernization and health: A model of the health transition." Paper presented at the annual meeting of the American Public Health Association, San Francisco, November 1973.

Levi, F., F. Lucchini, E. Negri, and C. La Vecchia. "Trends in mortality from cardiovascular and cerebrovascular diseases in Europe and other areas of the world." *Heart* 88 (2002): 119–24.

Liang, H., X. Li, X. Yu, P. Guan, Z. Yin, Q. He, and B. Zhou. "Facts and fiction of the relationship between pre-existing tuberculosis and lung cancer risk: A systematic review." *International Journal of Cancer* 125 (2009): 2936–44.

Lillienfeld, A. M. *Foundations of Epidemiology.* New York: Oxford University Press, 1976.

Lindert, P. H., and J. G. Williamson. "English workers' living standards during the industrial revolution: A new look." *Economic History Review* 36 (1983): 1–25.

Lindskos, B. I. "Mortalitaetsdiagnosen in Suedschweden 1749–1801." In *Medizinische Diagnostik in Geschichte and Gesenwart*, edited by H. Goerke, J. H. Wolf, F. Marguth, and C. Habrich, 583–606. Munich: Fritsch, 1978.

Link, B. G., and J. C. Phelan. "McKeown and the idea that social conditions are fundamental causes of disease." *Health Policy and Ethics* 92, no. 5 (2002): 730–32.

Linnemann, C. C., Jr., P. H. Perlstein, N. Ramundo, S. D. Minton, G. S. Englender, J. B. McCormick, and P. S. Hayes. "Use of pertussis vaccine in an epidemic involving hospital staff." *Lancet* 2 (1975): 540–45.

Littman, A. J., L. A. Jackson, and T. L. Vaughan. "*Chlamydia pneumoniae* and lung cancer: Epidemiologic evidence." *Cancer Epidemiology, Biomarkers and Prevention* 14 (2005): 773–78.

Littman, A. J., M. D. Thornquist, E. White, L. A. Jackson, G. E. Goodman, and T. L. Vaughan. "Prior lung disease and risk of lung cancer in a large prospective study." *Cancer Causes and Control* 15, no. 8 (2004): 819–27.

Longini, I. M., J. S. Koopman, A. S. Monto, and J. P. Fox. "Estimating household and community transmission parameters for influenza." *American Journal of Epidemiology* 115 (1982): 736–51.

Longmate, N. *King Cholera*. London: Hamish Hamilton, 1966.

Lonsdale, H. *The Life of John Heysham MD*. London: Longmans Green, 1870.

Loomis, D., and S. Wing. "Is molecular epidemiology a germ theory for the end of the 20th century?" *International Journal of Epidemiology* 19, no. 1 (1990): 1–3.

Lorber, B., "Infectious causes of chronic illness: An overview." *Microbe* 7, no. 2 (2012): 59–63.

Loschky, D. J. "Urbanisation and England's eighteenth century crude birth and death rates." *Journal of European Economic History* 1 (1972): 697–712.

Loudon, I. "Maternal mortality in the past and its relevance to developing countries today." *American Journal of Nutrition* 72, supplement (2000): 241S–246S.

Lowe, A., C. P. Yansouni, and M. A. Behr. "Causality and gastrointestinal infections: Koch, Hill and Crohn's." *Lancet Infectious Diseases* 8, no. 1 (2008): 720–26.

Lu, W. C. "Agglutination of human platelets by influenza PR8 strain virus and mumps virus." *Federation Proceedings* 17 (1958): 446.

Luckin, B. "Evaluating the sanitary revolution: Typhus and typhoid in London, 1851–1900." In Woods and Woodward, *Urban Disease and Mortality*, 102–19.

Luckin, W. "The decline of smallpox and the demographic revolution of the 18th century." *Social History* 6 (1977): 793–97.

Lunn, P. G. "Nutrition, immunity and infection." In Schofield, Reher, and Bideau, *Decline of Mortality in Europe*, 131–45.

Lynch, J., N. Krause, G. A. Kaplan, J. Tuomilehto, and J. T. Salonen. "Workplace conditions, socioeconomic status, and the risk of mortality and acute myocardial infarction: the Kuopio Ischaemic Heart Disease Risk Factor Study." *American Journal of Public Health* 87, no. 4 (1997): 617–22.

Lynch, J., and G. D. Smith. "A life course approach to chronic disease epidemiology." *Annual Review of Public Health* 26 (2005): 1–35.

Maahs, D. M., N. A. West, J. H. M. Lawrence, and E. J. Mayer-Davis. "Epidemiology of type 1 diabetes." *Endocrinology and Metabolism Clinics of North America* 39, no. 3 (2010): 481–97.

Mackenbach, J. P. "The epidemiologic transition theory." *Journal of Epidemiology and Community Health* 48 (1994): 329–32.

Mackenbach, J. P., W. N. Casper, W. N. Looman, and A. E. Kunst. "Geographic variation in the onset of decline of male ischemic heart disease mortality in the Netherlands." *American Journal of Public Health* 79, no. 12 (1989): 1621–27.

Madjid, M. "Acute infections, vaccination and prevention of cardiovascular disease." *Journal of the Canadian Medical Association* 179, no. 8 (2008): 749–50.

Madjid, M., I. Aboshady, I. Awan, S. Litovsky, and S. W. Casscells. "Influenza and cardiovascular disease: Is there a causal relationship?" *Texas Heart Institute Journal* 31 (2004): 4–13.

Madjid, M., C. C. Miller, V. V. Zarubaev, I. G. Marinich, O. I. Kiselev, Y. V. Lobzin, A. E. Filippov, and S. W. Casscells. "Influenza epidemics and acute respiratory disease activity are associated with a surge in autopsy-confirmed coronary heart disease deaths: Results from 8 years of autopsies in 34,892 subjects." *European Heart Journal*. Published online April 17, 2007. doi:10.1093/eurheartj/ehm035.

Madjid, M., M. Nahghavi, S. Litovsky, and S. W. Casscells. "Influenza and cardiovascular disease—a new opportunity for prevention and the need for further studies." *Circulation* 108 (2003): 2730–36.

Magee, R. "Arterial disease in antiquity." *Medical Journal of Australia* 169 (1998): 663–66.

Magill, T. P. "The immunologist and the evil spirits." *Journal of Immunology* 4 (1955): 1–8.

Magnus, P., and R. Beaglehole. "The real contribution of the major risk factors to the coronary epidemics." *Archives of Internal Medicine* 161 (2001): 2657–60.

Malferheiner, P., J. Bomschein, and M. Seigrad. "Role of *Helicobacter pylori* infection in gastric cancer pathogenesis: A chance for prevention." *Journal of Digestive Diseases* 11, no. 1 (2010): 2–11.

Malthus, T. R. *An Essay on the Principle of Population.* 1798. Reprint, edited by A. Flew, Harmondsworth: Penguin, 1970.

Mandle, J. R. "The decline in mortality in British Guyana, 1911–1960." *Demography* 7, no. 3 (1970): 301–15.

Manollo, T. A., F. S. Collins, N. J. Cox, D. B. Goldstein, L. A. Hindorff, D. J. Hunter, and M. I. McCarthy. "Finding the missing heritability of complex diseases." *Nature* 461 (2009): 747–53. doi:10.1038/nature08494.

Manton, K. G., and S. S. Poss. "Effects of dependency among causes of death for cause-elimination life-table strategies." *Demography* 16, no. 2 (1979). 313–26.

March, D., and E. Susser. "The eco- in eco-epidemiology." *International Journal of Epidemiology* 35 (2006): 1379–83.

Marks, G., and P. Burney. "Diseases of the respiratory system." In Charlton and Murphy, *Health of Adult Britain,* 2:93–113.

Markus, H. S., and M. A. Mendall. "*Helicobacter pylori* infection: A risk factor for ischemic cerebrovascular disease and carotid atheroma." *Journal of Neurology and Neurosurgery* 64 (1998): 104–7.

Marmot, M. G. "Affluence, urbanisation and coronary heart disease." In *Disease and Urbanisation,* edited by E. J. Clegg and J. P. Garlick, 127–43. London: Taylor Francis, 1980.

Marmot, M. G., A. M. Adelstein, N. Robinson, and G. A. Rose. "Changing social-class distribution of heart disease." *British Medical Journal* 2 (1978): 1109–12.

Marmot M. G., H. Bosma, H. Hemingway, E. Brunner and S. Stansfeld. "Contribution of job control and other risk factors to social variations in coronary heart disease incidence." *Lancet* 350 (1997): 235–39.

Marmot, M. G., G. Rose, M. Shipley, and P. J. S. Hamilton. "Employment grade and coronary heart disease in British civil servants." *Journal of Epidemiology and Community Health* 32 (1978): 244–49.

Marmot, M. G., M. Shipley, and G. Rose. "Inequalities in death—specific explanations of a general pattern?" *Lancet* 1 (1984): 1003–6.

Marmot, M., and T. Theorell. "Social class and cardiovascular disease: the contribution of work." *International Journal of Health Sciences* 18, no. 4 (1988): 659–74.

Marshall, B. "Commentary: Helicobacter as the 'environmental factor' in Susser and Stein's cohort theory of peptic ulcer disease." *International Journal of Epidemiology* 31 (2002): 21–22.

Marshall, B. J., and J. R. Warren. "Unidentified curved bacilli in the stomach of patients with gastritis and peptic ulceration." *Lancet* 323 (1984): 1311–15.

Marshall, J. *Mortality in the Metropolis.* London, 1832.

Martel, C. de, J. Ferlay, S. Franceschi, J. Vignat, F. Bray, D. Forman, and M. Plummer. "Global burden of cancers attributable to infections in 2008: A review and synthetic analysis." *Lancet Oncology* 13, no. 6 (2012): 607–15.

Martyn, C. N. "Infection in childhood and neurological diseases in adult life." *British Medical Bulletin* 53, no. 1 (1997): 24–39.

Masso Gonzales, E. L., S. Johansson, M. A. Wallander, and L. A. Garcia Rodrigues. "Trends in the prevalence and incidence of diabetes in the UK: 1996–2005." *Journal of Epidemiology and Community Health* 63 (2009): 332–36.

Mathers, C. D., and D. Loncar. "Projections of global mortality and burden of disease from 2002 to 2030." *PLoS Medicine* 3, no. 11 (2006): e442. doi:10.1371/journal.pmed.0030442.

Maupas, P., and J. L. Melnick. "Hepatitis B and primary liver cancer." *Progress in Medical Virology* 27 (1981): 1–5.

Mayne, S. T., J. Buenconsejo, and D. T. Janerich. "Previous lung diseases and risk of lung cancer among men and women." *American Journal of Epidemiology* 149, no. 1 (1999): 13–20.

McCormick, A., D. Fleming, and J. Charlton. *Morbidity Statistics from General Practice: Fourth National Study 1991–1992.* London: HMSO, 1995.

McKee, M. "The health consequences of the collapse of the Soviet Union." In Leon and Walt, *Poverty, Inequality and Health,* 17–36.

McKeown, R. E. "The epidemiologic transition: Changing patterns of mortality and population dynamics." *American Journal of Lifestyle Medicine* 3, supplement 1 (2009): 19S–26S. doi:10.1177/1559827609335350.

McKeown, T. "Fertility, mortality and cause of death." *Population Studies* 32, no. 3 (1978): 535–42.

———. *The Modern Rise of Population.* London: Edward Arnold, 1976.

———. *The Role of Medicine: Dream, Mirage or Nemesis?* London: Nuffield Provincial Hospitals Trust, 1976.

McKeown, T., and R. G. Brown. "Medical evidence related to English population changes in the eighteenth century." *Population Studies* 9 (1955): 119–41.

McKeown, T., and R. G. Record. "Reasons for the decline in mortality in England and Wales during the nineteenth century." *Population Studies* 16 (1962): 94–122.

McKeown, T., R. G. Record, and R. G. Brown. "An interpretation of the modern rise of population in Europe." *Population Studies* 26, no. 3 (1972): 345–82.

McKeown, T., R. G. Record, and R. D. Turner. "An interpretation of the decline in mortality in England and Wales during the 20th century." *Population Studies* 29 (1975): 391–422.

McMichael, A. J. "Population, environment, disease, and survival: Past patterns, uncertain futures." *Lancet* 359 (2002): 1145–48.

McNeill, W. H. "Migration patterns and infection in traditional societies." In *Changing Disease Patterns and Human Behaviour,* edited by N. F. Stanley and R. A. Joske, 27–36. London: Academic Press, 1980.

———. *Plagues and Peoples.* Harmondsworth: Penguin, 1976.

McNeilly, A. S. "Effects of lactation on fertility." *British Medical Bulletin* 35 (1979): 151–54.

Mehta, S. H., F. L. Brancati, S. A. Strathdee, J. S. Pankow, D. Netski, J. Coresh, M. Szklo, and D. L. Thomas. "Hepatitis C virus infection and incident type 2 diabetes." *Hepatology* 38, no. 1 (2003): 50–56.

Melia, R. J. W., C. du V. Florey, and A. V. Swan. "Respiratory illness in British schoolchildren and atmospheric smoke and sulphur dioxide, 1973–7." *Journal of Epidemiology and Community Health* 35 (1981): 161–67.

Mendall, M. A., P. M. Goggin, N. Molineaux, J. Levy, T. Toosy, D. Strachan, and T. C. Northfield. "Childhood living conditions and *Helicobacter pylori* seropositivity in adult life." *Lancet* 339 (1992): 896–97.

Mensch, B., H. Lentzner, and S. H. Preston, *Socioeconomic Differentials in Child Mortality in Developing Countries.* New York: United Nations Department of International Economic and Social Affairs, 1985.

Mercer, A. *Disease, Mortality and Population in Transition.* London: Leicester University Press; Pinter, 1990.

———. "Relative trends in mortality from related respiratory and airborne infectious diseases." *Population Studies* 40, no. 1 (1986): 129–45.

———. "Risk of dying from tuberculosis and cancer: Further aspects of a possible association." *International Journal of Epidemiology* 10, no. 4 (1981): 377–80.

———. "Smallpox and epidemiological-demographic change in Europe in the 18th and 19th centuries: The importance of vaccination." *Population Studies* 39, no. 2 (1985): 287–307.

Merle, C. S. C., S. S. Cunha, and L. C. Rodrigues. "BCG vaccination and leprosy protection: Review of current evidence and status of BCG in leprosy control." *Expert Review of Vaccines* 9 (2010): 209–22. doi:101586/erv.09.161.

Middleton, N., and S. Weitzman. *A Place for Everyone: A History of State Education from the 18th Century to the 1970s.* London: Gollanz, 1976.

Mielke, J. H., L. B. Jorde, P. G. Trapp, D. L. Anderton, K. Pitkänen, and A. W. Eriksson. "Historical epidemiology of smallpox in Åland, Finland: 1751–1890." *Demography* 21, no. 3 (1984): 271–95.

Millan, D. W. M., J. A. Davis, T. E. Torbet, and M. S. Campo. "DNA sequences of human papillomavirus types 11, 16 and 18 in lesions of uterine cervix in the west of Scotland." *British Medical Journal* 293 (1986): 93–96.

Miller, G. *The Adoption of Inoculation for Smallpox in England and France.* London: Oxford University Press, 1957.

Mirzaei, M., A. S. Truswell, R. Taylor, and S. R. Leeder. "Coronary heart disease epidemics: Not all the same." *Heart* 95 (2009): 740–46.

Mitchell, B. R. *European Historical Statistics 1750–1970.* London: Macmillan, 1971.

Mooney, G. "Infectious diseases and epidemiologic transition in Victorian Britain? Definitely." *Social History of Medicine* 20 (2007): 595–606.

———. "Public health versus private practice: The contested development of compulsory infectious disease notification in late nineteenth century Britain." *Bulletin of the History of Medicine* 73 (1999): 238–67.

Morat, H. Z., J. E. Mustard, N. S. Taichman, and T. Uriuhara. "Platelet aggregation and release of ADP, serontinin and histamine associated with phagocytosis of antigen-antibody complexes." *Proceedings of the Society for Experimental Biology* 120 (1966): 232–37.

Morens, D. M., G. K. Folkers, and A. S. Fauci. "The challenge of emerging and re-emerging diseases." *Nature* 430 (2004): 242–49.

Morens, D. M., J. K. Tauenberger, and A. S. Fauci. "Pandemic influenza viruses—hoping for the road not taken." *New England Journal of Medicine* 368, no. 25 (2013): 2345–47.

———. *Paediatric Priorities in the Developing World.* London: Butterworth, 1973.

———. "Severe measles in the tropics." *British Medical Journal* 1 (1969): 297–301, 363–65.

Morré, S. A., W. Stooker, W. K. Lagrand, A. J. C. van den Brule, and H. W. M. Niessen. "Microorganisms in the aetiology of atherosclerosis." *Journal of Clinical Pathology* 53 (2000): 647–54.

Morris, J. N., A. Kagan, D. C. Pattison, M. J. Gardner, and P. Raffle. "Incidence and prediction of ischemic heart diseases in London busmen." *Lancet* 288 (1966): 553–59.

Morris, N. *Uses of Epidemiology.* London: Livingstone, 1964.

Morrison, D. S., A. A. Boyd, and T. Richardson, "Correspondence: Liver cirrhosis mortality rates in Britain." *Lancet* 367 (2006): 1899.

Moser, K. A., A. J. Fox, P. O. Goldblatt, and P. R. Jones. "Stress and heart disease: Evidence of associations between unemployment and heart disease from the OPCS Longitudinal Study." *Postgraduate Medical Journal* 62 (1986): 797–99.

Moser, K. A., H. S. Pugh, and P. O. Goldblatt. "Inequalities in women's health: Looking at mortality differentials using an alternative approach." *British Medical Journal* 296 (1988): 1221–24.

Mosley, W. H., and L. C. Chen. "An analytical framework for the study of child survival in developing countries." In *Child Survival: Strategies for Research,* edited by W. H. Mosley and L. C. Chen. *Population and Development Review* 10, supplement (1984): 25–45.

Mosley, W. H., and R. Gray. "Childhood precursors of adult morbidity and mortality in developing countries: Implications for health programmes." In *The Epidemiological Transition: Policy and Planning Implications for Developing Countries,* edited by J. N. Gribble and S. H. Preston, 69–100. Washington, DC: National Academy Press, 1993.

Munk-Jorgensen, P., and H. Ewald. "Epidemiology in neurobiological research: Exemplified by the influenza-schizophrenia theory." *British Journal of Psychiatry* 178, supplement (2001): S30–S32.

Murray, C. J., and A. D. Lopez, eds. *The Global Burden of Disease: A Comprehensive Assessment of Mortality from Diseases, Injuries and Risk Factors in 1990 and Projected to 2020.* Cambridge, MA: Harvard University Press, 1996.

Mussa, F. F., C. Hong, W. Xinwen, Y. Qizhi, A. B. Lumsden, and C. Changyi. "*Chlamydia pneumoniae* and vascular disease: An update." *Journal of Vascular Surgery* 43 (2006): 1301–7.

Mustard, J. F. "Platelets and thromboembolic disease." *Advances in Cardiology* 4 (1970): 131–42.

Mustard, J. F., E. A. Murphy, H. C. Rowsell, and H. G. Downie. "Platelets and atherosclerosis." *Journal of Atherosclerosis Research* 4 (1964): 1–28.

Muthayya S. "Maternal nutrition and low birth weight—what is really important?" *Indian Journal of Medical Research* 130 (2009): 600–608.

National Diet Heart Study. "The National Diet-Heart Study Final Report." *Circulation* 37, supplement 3 (1968).

National Heart, Lung, and Blood Institute. *Report of the Task Force on Research in Epidemiology and Prevention of Cardiovascular Diseases.* Rockville, MD: National Institutes of Health, 1994.

Negro, F., and M. Alaei. "Hepatitis C virus and type 2 diabetes." *World Journal of Gastroenterology* 15, no. 3 (2009): 1537–47.

Nelson, M. C., and J. Rogers. "The right to die? Anti-vaccination activity and the 1874 smallpox epidemic in Stockholm." *Social History of Medicine* 5, no. 3 (1992): 369–88.

Nemir, R. L. "Pertussis pneumonia" In *Pulmonary Disorders,* vol. 1, edited by E. L. Kendig Jr, 732–39. Philadelphia: Saunders, 1972.

Newberne, P. M., and G. Williams. "Nutritional influences on the course of infections." In *Resistance to Infectious Disease,* edited by R. H. Dunlop and H. W. Moon, 93–111. Saskatoon, SK, Canada: Saskatoon Modern Press, 1970.

Newsholme, A. "An inquiry into the principal causes of the reduction in the death rate from phthisis during the last forty years, with special reference to the segregation of phthisical patients in general institutions." *Journal of Hygiene* 6, no. 3 (1906): 304–84.

Ngeh, J., V. Anand, and S. Gupta. "*Chlamydia pneumoniae* and atherosclerosis—what we know and what we don't know." *Clinical Microbiology and Infection* 8 (2002): 2–13.

Nguyen-Van-Tam, J., and R. Logan. "Digestive diseases." In Charlton and Murphy, *Health of Adult Britain,* 2:129–39.

Nichol, K. L., J. Nordin, J. Mullooly, R. Lask, K. Fillbrandt, and M. Iwane. "Influenza vaccination and reduction in hospitalizations for cardiac disease and stroke among the elderly." *New England Journal of Medicine* 348 (2003): 1322–32.

Nieto, F. J. "Infections and atherosclerosis: New clues from an old hypothesis?" *American Journal of Epidemiology* 148, no. 10 (1998): 937–47.

Nikiforov, S. V., and V. B. Mamaev. "The development of sex differences in cardiovascular disease mortality: A historical perspective." *American Journal of Public Health* 88 (1998): 1348–53.

Norström, T., ed. *Alcohol in Postwar Europe: Consumption, Drinking Patterns, Consequences and Policy Responses in 15 European Countries.* Stockholm: Almqvist and Wiksell International, National Institute of Public Health, 2002.

Northampton Bills of Mortality. *Bills for All Saints Parish.* 1779–87. Held in the British Library, London.

Norway, Central Bureau of Statistics. *Health Statistics.* Oslo, 1880–.

Noymer, A., and B. Jarosz. "Causes of death in 19th century New England: The dominance of infectious disease." *Social History of Medicine* 21 (2008): 573–78.

O'Connor S., D. Fairweather, B. D. Pearce, and S. Rasmussen. "Infectious etiologies of chronic diseases: focus on women." *Emerging Infectious Diseases* 10, no. 11 (2004): 2028–29.

O'Connor, S. M., C. E. Taylor, and J. M. Hughes. "Emerging infectious determinants of chronic diseases." *Emerging Infectious Diseases* 12, no. 7 (2006): 1051–57.

Oddy, J. D. "The health of the people." In *Population and Society in Britain,* edited by T. Barker and M. Drake, 121–39. London: Batsford, 1982.

Office for National Statistics, UK Statistics Authority. *Death Certification Reform: A Case Study on the Potential Impact on Mortality Statistics, England and Wales.* Statistical Bulletin, November 26, 2012.

———. "Decennial life tables—period expectations of life from English life tables, nos. 1–16." Released June 25, 2009. http://www.ons.gov.uk/ons/publications/re-reference-tables.html?edition=tcm%3A77-224936.

———. *Mortality Statistics: Deaths Registered in England and Wales (Series DR).* London: HMSO, 2006–10.

———. "Report: Decennial life tables (2000–02)." *Population Trends* 136, Summer (2009): 108–11.

———. *Twentieth Century Mortality.* CD-ROM. Norwich: Stationery Office Books, 2004.

Office of Population Censuses and Surveys. *Mortality Statistics: Cause, Series DH2.* London: HMSO, 1974–2005.

Olshansky, S. J., and A. B. Ault. "The fourth stage of the epidemiologic transition: The age of degenerative diseases." *Millbank Memorial Quarterly* 64, no. 3 (1986): 355–91.

Omran, O. R. "A century of epidemiologic transition in the United States." *Preventive Medicine* 6 (1977): 30–51.

———. "Epidemiologic transition." In *International Encyclopedia of Population,* edited by J. A. Ross, 172–83. London: The Free Press, 1982.

———. "The epidemiologic transition." *Milbank Quarterly* 49, no. 4 (1971): 509–38.

———. "The epidemiologic transition: A theory of the epidemiology of population change." *Milbank Quarterly* 83, no. 4 (2005): 731–57.

———. "Epidemiologic transition in the United States." *Population Bulletin* 32 (1977): 3–42.

———. "The epidemiologic transition theory: A preliminary update." *Journal of Tropical Paediatrics* 29 (1983): 305–16.

Onuigbo, W. I. B. "Some 19th-century ideas on links between tuberculosis and cancerous diseases of the lung." *British Journal of Diseases of the Chest* 169 (1975): 207–10.

Orubuloye, I. O., and J. C. Caldwell. "The impact of public health services on mortality: A study of mortality differentials in a rural area of Nigeria." *Population Studies* 29, no. 2 (1975): 259–72.

Osmond, C., M. J. Gardner, and E. D. Acheson. "Analysis of trends in cancer mortality in England and Wales during 1951–80, separating changes associated with period of birth and period of death." *British Medical Journal* 284 (1982): 1005–8.

Oswald, N. C. "Collapse of the lower lobes of the lungs in children." *Proceedings of the Royal Society of Medicine* 40 (1947): 736–37.

Packham, M. A., E. E. Nishizawa, and J. F. Mustard. "Response of platelets to tissue injury." *Biochemical Pharmacology* 17, supplement (1968): 171–84.

Parish, H. J. *Victory with Vaccines.* Edinburgh: Livingstone, 1968.

Parry, W. H. *Infectious Diseases.* London: English Universities Press, 1969.

Patel, P., M. A. Mendall, D. Carrington, D. P. Strachan, E. Leatham, N. Molineaux, and J. Levy. "Association of *Helicobacter pylori* and *Chlamydia pneumoniae* infections with coronary heart disease and cardiovascular risk factors." *British Medical Journal* 311 (1995): 711–14.

Paxon, T. G. "A study of tuberculosis and cancer mortality rates with special reference to lung cancer rates." *British Journal of Cancer* 10 (1956): 623–33.

Pearce, N. "Traditional epidemiology, modern epidemiology, and public health." *American Journal of Public Health* 86, no. 5 (1996): 678–83.

Pearl, R. "Cancer and tuberculosis." *American Journal of Hygiene* 9 (1929): 97–159.

Pearson, T. A. "Education and income: Double-edged swords in the epidemiologic transition of cardiovascular disease." *Ethnicity & Disease* 13 (Spring 2003): S2-158–S2-163.

Pedro-Cuesta, J. de, G. Gudmundsson, V. Abraira, G. Gudmundsson, A. Löve, H. Tunius, J. Veiga, J. Almazán, and I. J. Petersen. "Whooping cough and Parkinson's disease." *International Journal of Epidemiology* 25, no. 6 (1996): 1301–11.

Percival, T. *Essays on the Smallpox and Measles.* 1798. Reprinted in *Population and Disease in Early Industrial England,* edited by B. Benjamin. Farnborough, England: Gregg International, 1973.

Perrenoud, A. "La mortalité à Genève de 1625 à 1825." *Annales de Demographic Historique* (1978): 209–33.

———. "Mortality decline in its secular setting." In Bengtsson, Fridlizius, and Ohlsson, *Pre-industrial Population Change,* 41–70.

———. *La Population de Genève du Seizième au début du Dix-neuvième Siècle.* Geneva: A. Jullien, 1979.

Perry, R. T., and N. A. Halsey. "The clinical significance of measles: A review." *Journal of Infectious Diseases,* supplement 1 (2004): S4–S16.

Peters, O. H. "Observations upon the natural history of epidemic diarrhea." *Journal of Hygiene* 10, no. 4 (1910): 602–777.

Peto, R. "Distorting the epidemiology of cancer: The need for a more balanced overview." *Nature* 284 (1980): 297–301.

Pfahlberg, A., K. F. Kolme, J. M. Grange, G. Mastrangelo, B. Krone, I. N. Botev, and M. Niin. "Inverse association between melanoma and previous vaccinations against tuberculosis and smallpox: Results of the FEBIM study." *Journal of Investigative Dermatology* 119 (2002): 570–75.

Phadke, A. M., N. R. Samant, and S. D. Dewal. "Smallpox as an etiologic factor in male infertility." *Fertility and Sterility* 24 (1973): 802–4.

Phillip, R. "The outlook on tuberculosis: Changing orientation." *British Medical Journal* 1 (1931): 43–49.

Pi-Sunyer, F. X. "Health implications of obesity." *American Journal of Clinical Nutrition* 53, no. 6 (1991): 1595S–1603S.

Pitkänen, K. J., J. H. Mielke, and L. B. Jorde. "Smallpox and its eradication in Finland: Implications for disease control." *Population Studies* 43 (1989): 95–111.

Plant, M. A. "Trends in alcohol and illicit drug-related diseases." In Charlton and Murphy, *Health of Adult Britain*, 1:114–27.

Pollard, A. J. "Childhood immunization: What is the future?" *Archives of Disease in Childhood* 92 (2007): 426–33. doi:10.1136/adc.2006.095760.

Pollard, T. M. *Western Diseases*. Cambridge Series in Biology and Evolutionary Anthropology. Cambridge: Cambridge University Press, 2008.

Pollitzer, R. *Plague*. World Health Organization Monograph Series 22. Geneva: World Health Organization, 1954.

Pooley, M. E., and C. G. Pooley. "Health, society and environment in 19th-century Manchester." In Woods and Woodward, *Urban Disease and Mortality*, 148–75.

Popkin, B. M. "Symposium: Obesity in developing countries: Biological and ecological factors." *Journal of Nutrition* 131 (2001): 871S–873S.

Popkin, B. M., and C. M. Doak, "The obesity epidemic is a worldwide phenomenon." *Nutrition Reviews* 56, no. 4 (1998): 106–14.

Porter, R. "Cleaning up the Great Wen: Public health in eighteenth-century London." *Medical History* 35, supplement S11 (1991): 61–75.

———. *Disease, Medicine and Society in England 1550–1860*. London: Macmillan, 1987.

Post, J. D. "Famine, mortality and epidemic disease in the process of modernisation." *Economic History Review* 29 (1976): 14–37.

Pound, P., M. Bury, and S. Ebrahim. "From apoplexy to stroke." *Age and Ageing* 26 (1997): 331–37.

Pounder, R. E., and D. Ng. "The prevalence of *Helicobacter pylori* infection in different countries." *Alimentary Pharmacology and Therapeutics* 9, supplement 2 (1995): 33–39.

Preis, S. R., S. Hwang, S. Coady, M. J. Pencina, R. B. D'Agostino, P. J. Savage, D. Levy, and C. S. Fox. "Trends in all-cause and cardiovascular disease mortality among women and men with and without diabetes mellitus in the Framingham Heart Study, 1950 to 2005." *Circulation* 119 (2009): 1728–35.

Preston, S. H. "Causes and consequences of mortality declines in less developed countries during the twentieth century." In *Population and Economic Change in Developing Countries*, edited by R. A. Easterlin, 289–360. Chicago: University of Chicago Press, 1980.

———. "The changing relation between mortality and level of economic development." *Population Studies* 29, no. 2 (1975): 231–45.

———, ed. *The Effects of Infant and Child Mortality on Fertility*. New York: Academic Press, 1977.

———. "An international comparison of excessive adult mortality." *Population Studies* 24 (1970): 5–20.

———. "Mortality in childhood: Lessons from the WFS." In *Reproductive Change in Developing Countries,* edited by J. Cleland and J. Hobcraft, 253–72. Oxford: Oxford University Press, 1985.

———. *Mortality Patterns in National Populations—with Special Reference to Recorded Causes of Death.* New York: Academic Press, 1976.

Preston, S. H., and M. R. Haines. *Fatal Years: Child Mortality in Late Nineteenth Century America.* Princeton: Princeton University Press, 1991.

Preston, S. H., N. Keyfitz, and R. Schoen. *Causes of Death: Life Tables for National Populations.* New York: Seminar Press, 1972.

Preston, S. H., and V. Nelson. "Structure and change in cause of death." *Population Studies* 28, no. 2 (1974): 19–52.

Preston, S. H., and E. Van de Walle. "Urban French mortality in the 19th century." *Population Studies* 32, no. 2 (1978): 275–91.

Pritchett, L., and L. Summers. "Wealthier is healthier." *Journal of Human Resources* 31 (1996): 844–68.

Puranen, B. "Tuberculosis and the decline of mortality in Sweden." In Schofield, Reher, and Bideau, *Decline of Mortality in Europe,* 97–117.

Quinn, R. W. "Comprehensive review of morbidity and mortality trends for rheumatic fever, streptococcal disease, and scarlet fever: The decline of rheumatic fever." *Clinical Infectious Diseases* 11, no. 6 (1989): 928–53.

Quinn, M., P. Babb, A. Brock, L. Kirby, and J. Jones. *Cancer Trends in England and Wales.* Studies on Medical and Population Subjects, No. 66. London: The Stationery Office, 2001.

Rachet, B., L. M. Woods, E. Mitry, M. Riga, N. Cooper, M. J. Quinn, and J. Steward. "Cancer survival in England and Wales at the end of the 20th century." *British Journal of Cancer* 99 (2008): S2–S10.

Ragland, D. R., M. A. Winkleby, J. Schwalbe, B. L. Holman, L. Morse, S. L. Sym, and J. L. Fisher. "Prevalence of hypertension in bus drivers." *International Journal of Epidemiology* 16 (1987): 208–14.

Ratcliffe, J. "Social justice and the demographic transition: Lessons from India's Kerala State." *International Journal of Health Services* 18, no. 1 (1978): 123–44.

Razzell, P. E. *The Conquest of Smallpox.* Firle, Sussex, UK: Caliban Books, 1977.

———. *Edward Jenner's Cowpox Vaccine: The History of a Medical Myth.* Firle, Sussex, UK: Caliban Books, 1977.

———. "An interpretation of the modern rise of population in Europe—a critique." *Population Studies* 28 (1974): 5–17.

———. *Population and Disease: Transforming English Society, 1550–1850.* Firle, Sussex, UK: Caliban Books, 2007.

———. "Population change in 18th-century England—a reinterpretation." *Economic History Review* 18 (1965): 312–32.

———. "The smallpox controversy." *Local Population Studies* 12 (1974): 42–44.

Registrar General. *Annual Report of the Registrar General for England and Wales.* London: HMSO, 1838–1920.

———. *Registrar General's Statistical Review of England and Wales.* London: HMSO, 1921–73.

Reichert, T. A., N. Sugaya, D. S. Fedson, W. P. Glezen, L. Simonsen, and M. Tashiro. "The Japanese experience with vaccinating schoolchildren against influenza." *New England Journal of Medicine* 344 (2001): 889–96.

Retherford, R. D. *The Changing Sex Differential in Mortality.* Studies in Population and Urban Demography No. 1. Westport, CT: Greenwood, 1975.

Reves, R. "Declining fertility in England and Wales as a major cause of the twentieth century decline in mortality. The role of changing family size and age structure in infectious disease mortality in infancy." *American Journal of Epidemiology* 122, no. 1 (1985): 112–28.

Ridker, P. M. "On evolutionary biology, inflammation, infection, and the causes of atherosclerosis." *Circulation* 105 (2002): 2–4.

Riley, J. C. *The Eighteenth-Century Campaign to Avoid Disease.* London: Macmillan, 1987.

———. "From a high mortality regime to a high morbidity regime: Is culture everything in sickness?" *Health Transition Review* 2, no. 1 (1992): 71–78.

———. *Rising Life Expectancy: A Global History.* Cambridge: Cambridge University Press, 2001.

———. *Sickness, Recovery and Death: A History and Forecast of Ill-Health.* Iowa City: University of Iowa Press, 1989.

———. *Sick, Not Dead: The Health of British Workingmen during the Mortality Decline.* Baltimore: Johns Hopkins University Press, 1997.

Roderick, P. "Renal diseases." In Charlton and Murphy, *Health of Adult Britain,* 2:114–28.

Rogers, J., and M. C. Nelson. "The epidemiologic transition revisited: Or what happens if we look beneath the surface?" *Health Transition Review* 7 (1997): 241–55.

Roper, N. A., R. W. Bilous, W. F. Kelly, N. C. Unwin, and V. M. Connolly. "Excess mortality in a population with diabetes and the impact of material deprivation: Longitudinal, population based study." *British Medical Journal* 322 (2001): 1389–93.

Rose, G. "Cold weather and ischaemic heart disease." *British Journal of Preventive and Social Medicine* 20 (1966): 92–100.

Rose, G., and M. G. Marmot. "Social class and coronary heart disease." *British Heart Journal* 45 (1981): 13–19.

Rosen, G. "Disease, debility and death." In *The Victorian City,* edited by H. J. Dyos and M. Wolff, 625–67. London: Routledge, 1973.

———. *A History of Public Health.* 1958. Reprint, Baltimore: Johns Hopkins University Press, 1993.

Rosenau, B. J., and P. H. Schur. "Association of measles virus with rheumatoid arthritis." *Journal of Rheumatology* 36, no. 5 (2009): 893–97.

Rosengren, A. "Declining cardiovascular mortality and increasing obesity: A paradox." *Canadian Medical Association Journal* 181 (2009): 127–28.

Rosenthal, S. R., R. G. Crispen, M. G. Thorpe, N. Piekarski, N. Raisys, and R. G. Rettig. "BCG vaccination and leukemia mortality." *Journal of the American Medical Association* 222, no. 12 (1972): 1543–44.

Ross, R. "Atherosclerosis—an inflammatory disease." *New England Journal of Medicine* 340, no. 2 (1999): 115–25.

Rowntree, B. S. *Poverty: A Study of Town Life.* London: Macmillan, 1901.

Royal College of Physicians. *Smoking or Health? Third Report.* London: Pitman Medical, 1977.

Salonen, J. T., and I. Valonen. "Longitudinal cross-national analysis of coronary mortality." *International Journal of Epidemiology* 11 (1983): 229–38.

Sandbach, F. R. "The history of schistosomiasis research and policy for its control." *Medical History* 20, no. 3 (1976): 259–75.

Sanders, J. W., G. S. Fuhrer, M. D. Johnson, and M. S. Riddle. "The epidemiological transition: The current status of infectious diseases in the developed world versus the developing world." *Science Progress* 91, no. 1 (2008): 1–37.

Sandison, A. T., and E. Tapp. "Disease in ancient Egypt." In *Mummies, Disease and Ancient Cultures,* edited by A. Cockburn, E. Cockburn, and T. A. Reyman, 38–58. 2nd ed. Cambridge: Cambridge University Press, 1998.

Sarti, C., D. Rastenyte, Z. Cepaitis, and J. Tuomilehto. "International trends in mortality from stroke, 1968 to 1994." *Stroke* 31, no. 7 (2000): 1588–1601.

Sasco, A. J., M. B. Secretan, and K. Straif. "Tobacco smoking and cancer: A brief review of recent epidemiological evidence." *Lung Cancer* 45, supplement (2004): S3–S9.

Schiffrin, E. L., M. L. Lipman, and J. F. E. Mann. "Chronic kidney disease: Effects on the cardiovascular system." *Circulation* 116 (2007): 85–97.

Schofield, R. "The Impact of Scarcity and Plenty on Population Change in England, 1541–1871." *Journal of Interdisciplinary History* 14, no. 2 (1983): 265–91.

———. Review of *The Modern Rise of Population,* by T. McKeown. *Population Studies* 31 (1977): 179–81.

———. "Population growth in the century after 1750: The role of mortality decline." In Bengtsson, Fridlizius, and Ohlsson, *Pre-industrial Population Change,* 17–40.

Schofield, R., and D. Reher. "The decline of mortality in Europe." In Schofield, Reher, and Bideau, *Decline of Mortality in Europe,* 1–17.

Schofield, R., D. Reher, and A. Bideau, eds. *The Decline of Mortality in Europe.* Oxford: Clarendon Press, 1991.

Scrimshaw, N. S., C. E. Taylor, and J. E. Gordon. *Interactions of Nutrition and Infection.* World Health Organisation Monograph Series, 57. Geneva: World Health Organization, 1968.

Seidell, J. C. "Obesity, insulin resistance and diabetes—a worldwide epidemic." *British Journal of Nutrition* 83, supplement 1 (2000): S5–S8.

Shaheen, S. O., J. A. C. Sterne, J. S. Tucker, and C. du V. Florey. "Birth weight, childhood lower respiratory tract infection, and adult lung function." *Thorax* 53 (1998): 549–53.

Shiels, M. S., D. Albanes, J. Virtamo, and E. A. Engels. "Increased risk of lung cancer in men with tuberculosis in the alpha-tocopherol, beta-carotene cancer prevention study." *Cancer Epidemiology, Biomarkers and Prevention* 20, no. 4 (2011): 672–78.

Shojania, K. G., E. C. B. Burton, K. M. McDonald, L. Goldman. "Changes in rates of autopsy-detected diagnostic errors over time: A systematic review. *Journal of the American Medical Association* 289, no. 21 (2003): 2849–56.

Short, T. *A History of the Air, Weather, Seasons, etc.* London: T. Longman and A. Millar, 1749.

Siegel, M. "Mass media antismoking campaigns: a powerful tool for health promotion." *Annals of Internal Medicine* 129 (1998): 128–32.

Siegel, M., and L. Biener. "The impact of an antismoking media campaign on progression to established smoking: results of a longitudinal youth study." *American Journal of Public Health* 90, no. 3 (2000): 380–86.

Sigfusson, N., H. Sigvaldason, L. Steingrimsdottir, I. I. Gudmundsdottir, I. Stefansdottir, T. Thorsteinsson, and G. Sigurdsson. "Decline in ischaemic heart disease in Iceland and change in risk factor levels." *British Medical Journal* 302 (1991): 1371–75.

Siljeström, P. A. *En studie i Sjukdomsstatistik.* Stockholm, 1885.

Silverstein, A. M. *A History of Immunology.* London: Academic Press, 1989.

Skold, P. "From inoculation to vaccination: Smallpox in Sweden in the eighteenth and nineteenth centuries." *Population Studies* 50 (1996): 247–62.

———. "Offer and request: Preventive measures against smallpox in Sweden 1750–1900." *Health Transition Review* 7, no. 1 (1997): 75–81.

Slack, P. *The Impact of Plague in Tudor and Stuart England.* London: Routledge, 1985.

———. *Plague: A Very Short Introduction.* Oxford: Oxford University Press, 2012.

Smeeth, L., S. Thomas, A. J. Hall, R. Hubbard, P. Farrington, and P. Vallance. "Risk of myocardial infarction and stroke after acute infection or vaccination." *New England Journal of Medicine* 35, no. 25 (2004): 2611–18.

Smith, C. E. G. "Practical problems in the control of infectious disease." In Anderson and May, *Population Biology of Infectious Diseases,* 177–90.

Smith, F. B. *The People's Health 1830–1910.* London: Croom Helm, 1979.

Smith, T. "The decline of infectious diseases in its relation to modern medicine." *Preventive Medicine* 11 (1928): 345–63.

Snow, J. *On the Mode of Communication of Cholera.* London: John Churchill, 1855.

Sogner, S. *Folkevekst og Flytting: En historisk-demografisk studie i 1700-årenes Øst-Norge.* Oslo: University of Oslo Press, 1979.

Sonnenberg, A. "Smoking and mortality from peptic ulcer in the United Kingdom." *Gut* 27 (1986): 1369–72.

Sonnenberg, A., C. Cucino, and P. Bauerfeind. "The unresolved mystery of birth-cohort phenomena in gastroenterology." *International Journal of Epidemiology* 31 (2002): 23–26.

Sonnenschein, C., and A. M. Soto. "Theories of carcinogenesis: An emerging perspective." *Seminars in Cancer Biology* 18, no. 5 (2008): 372–77. doi:10.1016/j.semicancer.2008.03.012.

Soto, A. M., and C. Sonnenschein. "Regulation of cell proliferation: The negative control perspective." *Annals of the New York Academy of Sciences* 628 (1991): 412–18.

Strachan, D. P., "Respiratory and allergic diseases." In *A Life Course Approach to Chronic Disease Epidemiology,* edited by D. Kuh and Y. Ben-Schlomo, 15–41. Oxford: Oxford University Press, 1997.

Stamatakis, E., P. Primatesta, S. Chinn, R. Rona, and E. Falacheti. "Overweight and obesity trends from 1974 to 2003 in English children: What is the role of socioeconomic factors?" *Archives of Diseases of Childhood* 90 (2005): 999–1004. doi:10.1136/adc.2004.068932.

Stamler, J. "The marked decline in coronary heart disease mortality rates in the United States, 1968–1981: Summary of findings and possible explanations." *Cardiology* 72, nos. 1–2 (1985): 11–22.

Stamler, J., R. Stamler, J. D. Neaton, D. Wentworth, M. L. Daviglus, D. Garside, A. R. Dyer, K. Liu, and P. Greenland. "Low risk-factor profile and long-term cardiovascular and noncardiovascular mortality and life expectancy." *Journal of the American Medical Association* 282, no. 21 (1999): 2012–18.

Starr, S., and S. Berkovich. "Effects of measles, Gamma-globulin-modified measles and vaccine measles on the tuberculin test." *New England Journal of Medicine* 270 (1964): 386–91.

Stead, W. W. "Pathogenesis of a first episode of chronic pulmonary tuberculosis in man." *American Review of Respiratory Diseases* 95 (1967): 729–45.

Steckel, R. H. "Industrialization and health in historical perspective." In Leon and Walt, *Poverty, Inequality and Health,* 37–57.

Stengel, B., M. E. Tarver-Carr, N. R. Powe, M. Eberhardt, and F. L. Brancati. "Lifestyle risk factors, obesity and the risk of chronic kidney disease." *Epidemiology* 14, no. 4 (2003): 479–87.

Stocks, P., and E. Lewis-Faning. "Wartime incidence and mortality from respiratory tuberculosis." *British Medical Journal,* no. 1 (1944): 581–83.

Sugiyama, T., and M. Asaka. "*Helicobacter pylori* infection and gastric cancer." *Medical Electron Microscopy* 37, no. 3 (2004): 149–57.

Sundbärg, G. *Dodligheiten af Lungtuberculos i Sverige dren 1751–1830.* Uppsala, Sweden, 1905.

Susser, E. "Eco-epidemiology: Thinking outside the black box." *Epidemiology* 15, no. 5 (2004): 519–20.

Susser, M., and Z. Stein. "Civilisation and peptic ulcer." *Lancet* 1 (1962): 115–19. Reprinted in *International Journal of Epidemiology* 30 (2001): 13–17.

———. "Commentary: Civilisation and peptic ulcer 40 years on." *International Journal of Epidemiology* 31 (2002): 18–21.

Susser, M., and E. Susser. "Choosing a future for epidemiology, pt. 1: Eras and paradigms." *American Journal of Public Health* 86, no. 5 (1966): 668–73.

———. "Choosing a future for epidemiology, pt. 2: From black box to Chinese boxes and eco-epidemiology." *American Journal of Public Health* 86, no. 5 (1996): 674–77.

Sweden, Statistiska Centralbyrån. *Historisk Statistik för Sverige I, Befolkung: 1720–1950.* Stockholm: Statistiska Centralbyrån, 1955.

Swedlund, A. C., and A. K. Donta. "Scarlet fever epidemics of the nineteenth century: A case of evolved pathogenic virulence?" In *Human Biologists in the Archives: Demography, Health, Nutrition and Genetics in Historical Populations,* edited by D. A. Herring and A. C. Swedlund. Cambridge: Cambridge University Press, 2003, 159–77.

Swerdlow, A., R. Doll, and I. dos Santos Silva. "Time trends in cancer incidence and mortality in England and Wales." In Charlton and Murphy, *Health of Adult Britain,* 2:30–59.

Swingler, R., and C. Martyn. "Neurological diseases." In Charlton and Murphy, *Health of Adult Britain,* 2:82–92.

Symmons, D. "Musculoskeletal diseases." In Charlton and Murphy, *Health of Adult Britain*, 2:140–57.

Sytkowski, P. A., R. B. D'Agostino, A. Belanger, and W. B. Kannal. "Sex and time trends in cardiovascular disease incidence and mortality: The Framingham Heart Study, 1950–1989." *American Journal of Epidemiology* 143, no. 4 (1996): 338–50.

Szreter, S. "Economic growth, disruption, deprivation, disease and death: On the importance of the politics of public health for development." *Population and Development Review* 23, no. 4 (1997): 693–728.

———. "Health, economy, state and society in modern Britain: The long-run perspective." *Population and Development Review* 23, no. 4 (1997): 205–27.

———. "The importance of social intervention in Britain's mortality decline 1850–1914: A re-interpretation of the role of public health." *Social History of Medicine* 1 (1988): 1–38.

———. "The population health approach in historical perspective." *American Journal of Public Health* 93, no. 3 (2003): 421–31.

———. "Rethinking McKeown: The relationship between public health and social change." *American Journal of Public Health* 92, no. 5 (2002): 722–24.

Szreter, S., and G. Mooney. "Urbanization, mortality, and the standard of living debate: New estimates of the expectation of life at birth in nineteenth century British cities." *Economic History Review* 51, no. 1 (1998): 84–112.

Taylor, A. J., ed. *The Standard of Living in Britain in the Industrial Revolution.* London: Methuen, 1975.

Taylor, R., F. Najafi, and A. Dobson. "Meta-analysis of studies of passive smoking and lung cancer: Effects of study type and continent." *International Journal of Epidemiology* 36 (2007): 1048–59. doi:10.1093/ije/dym158.

Taylor-Robinson, D, and J. Boman. "The failure of antibiotics to prevent heart attacks: It's not necessarily the end of the road." *British Medical Journal* 331 (2005): 361–62.

Terada, H., M. Baldini, S. Ebbe, and M. A. Madoff. "Interaction of influenza virus with blood platelets." *Blood* 28 (1966): 213–28.

Thompson, B. "Infant mortality in Bradford." In Woods and Woodward, *Urban Disease and Mortality*, 120–47.

Tillett, H. E., J. W. G. Smith, and C. D. Gooch. "Excess deaths attributable to influenza in England and Wales: Age at death and certified cause." *International Journal of Epidemiology* 12 (1983): 344–52.

Tocque, K., R. P. Convrey, N. J. Beeching, and P. D. Davies. "Elevated mortality following diagnosis with a treatable disease: Tuberculosis." *International Journal of Tuberculosis and Lung Disease* 9, no. 7 (2005): 797–802.

Todd, G. F. *Cigarette Smoking Characteristics in the UK, South Africa and Australia.* Research Paper No. 5. London: Tobacco Research Council, 1963.

Toivanen, S., and O. Hemström. "Income differences in cardiovascular disease: Is the contribution from work similar in prevalence versus mortality outcomes?" *International Journal of Behavioural Medicine* 13, no. 1 (2006): 89–100.

Townsend, P., and N. Davidson. *Inequalities in Health: The Black Report.* Harmondsworth: Penguin, 1982.

Tranter, N. L. *Population and Society 1750–1940.* London: Longman, 1985.

Tromp, S. W. *Medical Biometeorology*. New York: Elsevier, 1963.

Trowell, H. "Diabetes mellitus death rates in England and Wales 1920–70 and food supplies." *Lancet* 304 (1974): 998–1002.

Tucker, R. S. "Real wages of artisans in London, 1729–1935." In *The Standard of Living in Britain in the Industrial Revolution*, edited by A. J. Taylor, 21–35. London: Methuen, 1975.

Turpeinen, O. "Les causes des fluctuations annuelles du taux de mortalité finlandaise entre 1750 et 1806." *Annales de Demographie Historique* (1980): 287–96.

———. "Fertility and mortality in Finland since 1750." *Population Studies* 33, no. 1 (1979): 101–14.

———. "Finnish death rates 1749–1773." *Population Studies* 32, no. 3 (1978): 523–42.

Uemura, K., and Z. Pisa. "Trends in cardiovascular disease mortality in industrialized countries since 1950." *World Health Statistics Quarterly* 41 (1988): 155–78.

Unal, B., J. A. Critchley, and S. Capewell. "Explaining the decline in coronary heart disease mortality in England and Wales between 1981 and 2000." *Circulation* 109 (2004): 1101–7.

United Nations. *Levels and Trends of Mortality since 1950*. New York: United Nations, 1982.

———. *Population Bulletin of the United Nations, No. 6*. New York: United Nations, 1962.

Unwin, N., J. Epping, and R. Bonita. "Rethinking the terms non-communicable disease and chronic disease." *Journal of Epidemiology and Community Health* 58 (2004): 801.

US Bureau of the Census. *Census of the United States. Mortality and Vital Statistics: Population Volumes*. Washington, DC, 1860–.

———. *Historical Statistics of the United States, Colonial Times to 1970*. Bicentennial ed., pt. 2. Washington, DC: Bureau of the Census, 1975.

US Surgeon General. *Smoking and Health: Report of the Advisory Committee to the Surgeon General of the Public Health Service*. Washington, DC: Department of Health, Education, and Welfare, 1964.

———. *Smoking and Health: A Report of the Surgeon General*. Washington, DC: Government Printing Office, 1979.

Ütterström, G. "Some population problems in pre-industrial Sweden." *Scandinavian Economic History Review* 2 (1954): 103–65.

Vallin, J. "Commentary: 'Epidemiologic transition' interrupted or sweep to the second stage of 'health transition.'" *International Journal of Epidemiology* 36 (2007): 384–86.

Vallin, J., and F. Meslé. "Convergences and divergences in mortality: A new approach to health transition." *Demographic Research*, Special Collection 2, Article 2 (2004): 11–44.

Van de Walle, E. "Accounting for population growth." *Science* 197 (1978): 653.

Van Poppell, F., and C. van der Heijden. "The effects of water supply on infant and childhood mortality: A review of historical evidence." *Health Transition Review* 7 (1997): 113–48.

Von Tunzelmann, G. N. "Trends in Real Wages, 1750–1850, Revisited." *Economic History Review* 32, no. 1 (1979): 33–49.

Vartiainen, E., P. Puska, J. Pekkanen, J. Tuomilehto, and P. Jousilahti. "Changes in risk factors explain changes in mortality from ischemic heart disease in Finland." *British Medical Journal* 309 (1994): 23–27.

Villumsen, M., S. Sørup, T. Jess, H. Ravn, T. Relander, J. I. Baker, C. S. Benn, T. L. Sørensen, P. Aaby, and P. A. Roth. "Risk of lymphoma and leukemia after Bacille Calmette-Guérin and smallpox vaccination: A Danish case-cohort study." *Vaccine* 27 (2009): 6950–58.

Von Tunzelmann, G. N. "Trends in real wages, 1750–1850, revisited." *Economic History Review* 32 (1979): 33–49.

Voth, H. and T. Leunig. "Did smallpox reduce height? Stature and the standard of living in London, 1770–1873." *Economic History Review* 49, no. 3 (1996): 541–60.

Vynnycky, E., and P. E. M. Fine. "Interpreting the decline in tuberculosis: The role of secular trends in effective contact." *International Journal of Epidemiology* 28 (1999): 327–34.

Wagenknecht, L. E., J. M. Roseman, and W. H. Herman. "Increased incidence of insulin-dependent diabetes mellitus following an epidemic of Coxsackie virus B5." *American Journal of Epidemiology* 133, no. 10 (1991): 1024–31.

Wald, N. J., M. R. Law, J. K. Morris, X. Zhou, Y. Wong, and M. E. Ward. "*Chlamydia pneumoniae* infection and mortality from ischaemic heart disease: large prospective study." *British Medical Journal* 321 (2000): 204–7.

Waldron, H. A., and L. Vickerstaff. *Intimations of Quality: Ante Mortem and Post Mortem Diagnoses.* London: Nuffield Provincial Hospitals Trust, 1977.

Walker, W. J. "Changing United States life-style and declining vascular mortality: Cause or coincidence?" *New England Journal of Medicine* 297 (1977): 163–65.

Wang, C., S. Wang, W. Yao, T. Chang, and P. Chou. "Hepatitis C virus infection and the development of type 2 diabetes in a community-based longitudinal study." *American Journal of Epidemiology* 166, no. 2 (2007): 196–203.

Warner, J. O., and W. C. Marshall. "Crippling lung disease after measles and adenovirus infection." *British Journal of Diseases of the Chest* 70 (1976): 89–94.

Warren-Gash, C., L. Smeeth, and A. C. Hayward. "Influenza as a trigger for acute myocardial infarction or death from cardiovascular disease: A systematic review." *Lancet Infectious Diseases* 9 (2009): 601–10.

Waters, W. E. "Trends in mortality from nephritis and infections of the kidney in England and Wales." *Lancet* 291 (1968): 241–43.

Watkins, C. J., S. R. Leeder, and R. T. Corkhill. "The relationship between breast- and bottle-feeding and respiratory illness in the first year of life." *Journal of Epidemiology and Community Health* 33 (1979): 180–82.

Watt, R. *Treatise on the History, Nature and Treatment of Chincough.* Glasgow, 1813.

Watterson, P. A. "Environmental factors in infant and early childhood mortality decline in England and Wales, 1895–1910." *Bulletin of the Society for the Social History of Medicine* 35 (December 1984): 37–40.

———. "Infant mortality by father's occupation from the 1911 census of England and Wales." *Demography* 25, no. 2 (1988): 289–306.

Weinberg, R. A. "How cancer arises." *Scientific American* (September 1996): 62–70.

Weisz, G., and J. Olszynko-Gryn. "The theory of epidemiologic transition: The origins of a citation classic." *Journal of the History of Medicine and Allied Sciences* 65, no. 3 (2010): 287–326.

West, R. R., S. Lloyd, and C. J. Roberts. "Mortality from ischemic heart diseases: Association with the weather." *British Journal of Preventive and Social Medicine* 27 (1973): 36–40.

West, R. R., and C. R. Lowe. "Mortality from ischemic heart diseases, inter-town variation and its association with climate in England and Wales." *International Journal of Epidemiology* 6, no. 2 (1976): 195–201.

Whisnant, J. P. "The decline of stroke." *Stroke* 15, no. 1 (1984): 160–68.

White, D. L., V. Ratziu, and H. B. El-Serag, "Hepatitis C infection and risk of diabetes: A systematic review and meta-analysis." *Journal of Hepatology* 49, no. 5 (2008): 831–44.

Widen, L. "Mortality and causes of death in Sweden during the 18th century." *Statistisk Tidskrift* 13 (1975): 93–104.

Wild, S. H., and C. D. Byrne. "Risk factors for diabetes and coronary heart disease." *British Medical Journal* 333 (2006): 1009–11.

Wilkinson, R. G. *Unhealthy Societies: The Afflictions of Inequality*. London: Routledge, 1996.

Wilson, G. N. "Measles: Its prevalence and mortality in Aberdeen." *Public Health* 18 (1905): 65–82.

Wilson, L. G. "Commentary: Medicine, population, and tuberculosis." *International Journal of Epidemiology* 34 (2005): 521–24.

Wilson, P. W., R. B. D'Agostino, L. Sullivan, H. Parise, and W. B. Kannel. "Overweight and obesity as determinants of cardiovascular risk: The Framingham experience." *Archives of Internal Medicine* 162, no. 16 (2002): 1867–72.

Wing, S. "The role of medicine in the decline of hypertension-related mortality." *International Journal of Health Services* 14 (1984): 649–66.

Winter, J. M. "Aspects of the impact of the First World War on infant mortality in Britain." *Journal of European Economic History* 11 (1982): 713–38.

———. "The decline of mortality in Britain 1870–1950." In *Population and Society in Britain, 1850–1980*, edited by T. Barker and M. Drake, 100–120. London: Batsford, 1982.

Wohl, A. S. *Endangered Lives: Public Health in Victorian Times*. London: Dart, 1983.

———. "The Housing of the Artisans and Labourers in 19th-Century London, 1815–1914." PhD diss., Brown University, 1966.

Wolfe, C. D. A., and P. G. J. Burney. "Is stroke mortality on the decline in England? *American Journal of Epidemiology* 136 (1992): 558–65.

Wong, B. C., S. K. Lam, C. K. Ching, W. H. Hu, E. Kwok, J. Ho, and S. T. Yuen. "Differential *Helicobacter pylori* infection rates in contrasting gastric cancer risk regions of south China: China gastric cancer study group." *Journal of Gastroenterological Hepatology* 14, no. 2 (1999): 120–25.

Wong, B. C., S. K. Lam, W. M. Wong, J. S. Chen, T. T. Zheng, R. E. Feng, and K. C. Lai. "*Helicobacter pylori* eradication to prevent gastric cancer in a high-risk region of China. A randomized controlled trial." *Journal of the American Medical Association* 291, no. 2 (2004): 187–94.

Wong, C. K., and L. T. Wu. *History of Chinese Medicine*. Tientsin: Tientsin Press, 1932.

Woods, R. "Approaches to the fertility transition in Victorian England." *Population Studies* 41 (1987): 283–311.

———. *The Demography of Victorian England and Wales.* Cambridge: Cambridge University Press, 2000.

———. "Infant mortality in Britain: A survey of current knowledge on historical trends and variations." In *Infant and Child Mortality in the Past,* edited by A. Bideau, B. Desjardins, and H. P. Brignoli, 74–88. Oxford: Clarendon Press, 1997.

———. "Medical and demographic history: Inseparable?" *Social History of Medicine* 20, no. 3 (2007): 483–503.

———. "Mortality and sanitary conditions in late nineteenth century Birmingham." In Woods and Woodward, *Urban Disease and Mortality,* 176–202.

Woods, R., P. A. Watterson, and J. H. Woodward. "The causes of rapid infant mortality decline in England and Wales, 1861–1921, part 1." *Population Studies* 42 (1988): 343–66.

———. "The causes of rapid infant mortality decline in England and Wales, 1861–1921, part 2." *Population Studies* 43 (1989): 113–32.

Woods, R., N. Williams, and C. Galley. "Differential mortality patterns among infants and other young children: The experience of England and Wales in the nineteenth century." In *The Decline of Infant and Child Mortality,* edited by C. A. Corsini and P. P. Viazzo, 57–72. The Hague: Martinus Nijhoff, 1997.

Woods, R., and J. Woodward. "Mortality, poverty and the environment." In Woods and Woodward, *Urban Disease and Mortality,* 19–36.

Woods, R., and J. Woodward, eds. *Urban Disease and Mortality in Nineteenth Century England.* London: Batsford, 1984.

Woodward, J. "Medicine and the city: The nineteenth-century experience." In Woods and Woodward, *Urban Disease and Mortality,* 65–78.

World Health Organization. "Comprehensive cervical cancer prevention and control: A healthier future for girls and women." WHO Guidance Note. Geneva: WHO Press, 2013.

———. *Hepatitis C: Fact Sheet No. 164.* Updated April 2014. http://www.who.int/mediacentre/factsheets/fs164/en/.

———. *International Classification of Diseases and Related Health Problems. 10th Revision, Volume 2, Instruction Manual, 2010 Edition.* Geneva: WHO, 2011.

———. *Preventing Chronic Diseases: A Vital Investment.* Geneva: WHO, 2005.

———. "Disease and injury regional estimates, 2000–2011: Cause-specific mortality." Accessed May 6, 2014. http://www.who.int/healthinfo/global_burden_disease/estimates_regional_2000_2011/en/index.html.

———. *World Health Report 1999: Making a Difference.* Geneva: WHO, 1999.

———. *World Health Statistics.* Annual. Geneva: WHO, 1948–.

Wrigley, E. A. "Births and baptisms: The use of Anglican baptism registers as a source of information about the numbers of births in England before the beginning of civil registration." *Population Studies* 31, no. 2 (1977): 281–312.

———. "A simple model of London's importance in changing English society and economy 1650–1750." *Past and Present* 37 (1967): 44–70.

Wrigley, E. A., R. Davies, J. Oeppen, and R. Schofield. *English Population History from Family Reconstitution, 1580–1837.* Cambridge: Cambridge University Press, 1997.

Wrigley, E. A., and R. Schofield. "English population history from family reconstitution: Summary results 1600–1799." *Population Studies* 37 (1983): 157–84.

———. *The Population History of England 1541–1871—a Reconstruction.* London: Edward Arnold, 1981.

Wu, A. H., E. T. H. Fontham, P. Reynolds, R. S. Greenberg, P. Buffler, J. Liff, P. Boyd, B. E. Henderson, and P. Correa. "Previous lung disease and risk of lung cancer among lifetime non-smoking women in the United States." *American Journal of Epidemiology* 141, no. 11 (1995): 1023–32.

Wu, C. Y., H. Y. Hu, C. Y. Pu, N. Huang, H. C. Shen, and Y. J. Chou. "Pulmonary tuberculosis increases the risk of lung cancer: A population-based cohort study." *Cancer* 117, no. 3 (2011): 618–24.

Wylie, C. M. "Recent trends in mortality from cerebrovascular accidents in the United States." *Journal of Chronic Diseases* 14 (1961): 213–20.

Wyon, J. B., and J. E. Gordon. *The Khanna Study: Population Problems in the Rural Punjab.* Cambridge, MA: Harvard University Press, 1971.

Yang, S., Y. H. Khang, G. Davey Smith, D. A. Leon, and J. Lynch. "Understanding the rapid increase in life expectancy in South Korea." *American Journal of Public Health* 100, no. 5 (2010): 896–903.

Yates, P. O. "A change in pattern of cerebrovascular disease." *Lancet* 1 (1964): 65–69.

Yelling, J. A. *Slums and Slum Clearance in Victorian London.* London: Allen and Unwin, 1986.

Yeung, W. G., W. D. Rawlinson, and M. E. Craig. "Enterovirus infection and type 1 diabetes mellitus: Systematic review and meta-analysis of observational molecular studies." *British Medical Journal* 342 (2011): d35. doi:10.1136/bmj.d35.

Yoshinaga, K., and H. Une. "Contributions of mortality changes by age group and selected causes of death to the increase in Japanese life expectancy at birth from 1950 to 2000." *European Journal of Epidemiology* 20, no. 1 (2005): 49–57.

You, W., L. Zhang, M. Gail, Y. Chang, W. Liu, J. Ma, and J. Li. "Gastric dysplasia and gastric cancer: *Helicobacter pylori,* serum vitamin C, and other risk factors." *Journal of the National Cancer Institute* 92, no. 19 (2000): 1607–11.

Yu, Y., P. F. Pinsky, N. E. Caporaso, N. Chatterjee, M. Baumgarten, P. Langenberg, J. P. Furuno, Q. Lan, and E. A. Engels. "Lung cancer risk following detection of pulmonary scarring by chest radiography in the prostate, lung, colorectal, and ovarian cancer screening trial." *Archives of Internal Medicine* 168, no. 21 (2008): 2326–32. doi:10.1001/archinte.168.21.2326.

Yu, Y. H., C. C. Liao, W. H. Hsu, W. C. Liao. C. H. Muo, and C. Y. Chen. "Increased lung cancer risk among patients with pulmonary tuberculosis: A population cohort study." *Journal of Thoracic Oncology* 6, no. 1 (2011): 32–37.

Yusuf, S., S. Reddy, S. Ounpuu, and S. Anand. "Global burden of cardiovascular diseases." *Circulation* 104 (2010): 2746–53.

Zhan, P., L. J. Suo, X. K. Shen, L. X. Qiu, L. K. Yu, and Y. Song. "*Chlamydia pneumoniae* infection and lung cancer risk: A meta-analysis." *European Journal of Cancer* 47, no. 5 (2011): 742–47.

Zheng, W., W. J. Blot, M. L. Liao, Z. X. Wang, L. I. Levin, J. J. Zhao, J. F. Fraumeni Jr., and Y. Gao. "Lung cancer and prior tuberculosis infection in Shanghai." *British Journal of Cancer* 56 (1987): 501–4.

Zinsser, H. *Rats, Lice and History.* 1934. Reprint, Basingstoke: Macmillan, 1985.

Zwanenberg, D. "The Suttons and the business of inoculation." *Medical History* 22, no. 1 (1978): 71–82.

Index

www.ingramcontent.com/pod-product-compliance
Lightning Source LLC
Chambersburg PA
CBHW051256200926
51612CB00002B/58
9781580465083